Carole Rend...
Haig...

Integrate

CW00607360

Integrated Clinical Science

Other titles:

Cardiovascular Disease
Professor JR Hampton

Musculoskeletal Disease
Professor RA Dickson,
Professor V Wright

Gastroenterology
Professor PF Jones, PW Brunt,
NAG Mowat

**Human Health and the
Environment**
Professor R Weir,
C Smith

Respiratory Disease
GM Sterling

Hematology
JC Cawley

Nephro-urology
Professor AW Asscher,
Professor DB Moffat

Endocrinology
Professor CRW Edwards

Available at your bookstore through Year Book Medical Publishers

Integrated Clinical Science

Neurology

Edited by

R.W. Ross Russell

Consultant Neurologist, The National Hospital for Nervous Diseases, Queen Square, and St. Thomas' Hospital, London

and

C.M. Wiles

Consultant Neurologist, The National Hospital for Nervous Diseases, Queen Square, and St. Thomas' Hospital, London

Series Editor

George P. McNicol, MD, PhD, FRSE, FRCP (Lond, Edin, Glas), FRCPath, Hon FACP

Principal and Vice Chancellor, University of Aberdeen. Lately Professor of Medicine, The University of Leeds, and Head, The University Department of Medicine, The General Infirmary, Leeds

Distributed by
Year Book Medical Publishers, Inc
Chicago, Illinois

William Heinemann Medical Books
22, Bedford Square, London WC1B 3HH

First published 1985
Reprinted 1987

ISBN 0 433 16606 1

Printed and bound in Great Britain by the Alden Press, Oxford

Contents

Preface

It is clearly desirable on educational grounds to adopt and teach a rational approach to the management of patients, whereby the basic scientific knowledge, the applied science and the art of clinical practice are brought together in an integrated way. Progress has been made in this direction, but after twenty-five years of good intentions, teaching in many medical schools is still split up into three large compartments, preclinical, paraclinical and clinical, and further subdivided on a disciplinary basis. Lip-service is paid to integration, but what emerges is often at best a coordinated rather than an integrated curriculum. Publication of the INTEGRATED CLINICAL SCIENCE series reflects the need felt in many quarters for a truly integrated textbook series, and is also intended as a stimulus to further reform of the curriculum.

The complete series will cover the core of clinical teaching, each volume dealing with a particular body system. Revision material in the basic sciences of anatomy, physiology, biochemistry and pharmacology is presented at the level of detail appropriate for Final MB examinations, and subsequently for rational clinical practice. Integration between the volumes ensures complete and consistent coverage of these areas, and similar principles govern the treatment of the clinical disciplines of medicine, surgery, pathology, microbiology, immunology and epidemiology.

The series is planned to give a reasoned rather than a purely descriptive account of clinical practice and its scientific basis. Clinical manifestations are described in relation to the disorders of structure and function which occur in a disease process. Illustrations are used extensively, and are an integral part of the text.

The editors for each volume, well-known as authorities and teachers in their fields, have been recruited from medical schools throughout the UK. Chapter contributors are even more widely distributed, and coordination between the volumes has been supervised by a distinguished team of specialists.

Each volume in the series represents a component in an overall plan of approach to clinical teaching. It is intended, nevertheless, that every volume should be self-sufficient as an account of its own subject area, and all the basic and clinical science with which an undergraduate could reasonably be expected to be familiar is presented in the appropriate volume. It is expected that, whether studied individually or as a series, the volumes of INTEGRATED CLINICAL SCIENCE will meet a major need, assisting teachers and students to adopt a more rational and holistic approach in learning to care for the sick.

George P McNicol
Series Editor

Contributors

CR Clarke
Consultant Neurologist
St. Bartholomew's Hospital,
and Whipps Cross Hospital
London

DAS Compston
Consultant Neurologist
University Hospital of Wales
Cardiff

RE Cull
Consultant Neurologist
Royal Infirmary
Edinburgh, and
Senior Lecturer in Neurology
University of Edinburgh

AE Harding
Lecturer in Clinical Neurology
Institute of Neurology, and
Royal Postgraduate Medical School
London

PRD Humphrey
Consultant Neurologist
Regional Neurological Centre
Walton Hospital
Liverpool

D Jefferson
Consultant Neurologist
Regional Department of
    Neurosurgery and Neurology
Derbyshire Royal Infirmary
Derby

D Neary
Consultant Neurologist
Manchester Royal Infirmary
Manchester

JD Parkes
Consultant Neurologist and Senior Lecturer
King's College Hospital
London

JP Patten
Consultant Neurologist
Royal Surrey County Hospital
Guildford

DGT Thomas
Senior Lecturer in Neurological Surgery
Institute of Neurology, and
Consultant Neurosurgeon
National Hospitals for Nervous Diseases
London

RG Twycross
Consultant Physician
Sir Michael Sobell House, and
The Churchill Hospital
Oxford

RW Ross Russell
Consultant Neurologist
National Hospital for Nervous
    Diseases, Queen Square, and
St. Thomas' Hospital
London

AM Whiteley
Consultant Neurologist
Derbyshire Royal Infirmary
Derby

CM Wiles
Consultant Neurologist
National Hospital for Nervous
    Diseases, Queen Square, and
St. Thomas' Hospital
London

Advisory Editors

Professor AS Douglas
Department of Medicine, University of Aberdeen

Pathology:
Professor CC Bird
Institute of Pathology
University of Leeds

Anatomy:
Professor RL Holmes
Department of Anatomy
University of Leeds

Physiology:
Professor PH Fentem
Department of Physiology and Pharmacology
Nottingham University

Pharmacology:
Professor AM Breckenridge
Department of Clinical Pharmacology
Liverpool University

Biochemistry:
Dr RM Denton
Reader in Biochemistry
University of Bristol

Approach to the Patient

As in other branches of medicine, the management of a patient with a neurological illness involves giving information and explanation to the patient and his family, making decisions about treatment either curative or palliative, and offering advice to help the patient surmount or accept his condition most effectively by changing the environment. In order best to advise the patient, the doctor requires an accurate diagnosis and appropriate background information. The history is the essential first step to both diagnosis and overall management (Fig. 1.1).

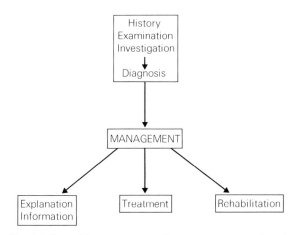

Fig. 1.1 *Essential steps surrounding management of each individual patient.*

HISTORY OF PRESENT ILLNESS

Many patients find it difficult to describe their neurological symptoms clearly, (either because of unfamiliarity or because of educational or cultural background).

The doctor needs to appreciate the extraordinary nature to most people of, for example, a temporal lobe seizure, the sudden loss of use of a limb, or a homonymous visual field loss, and to try and grasp the essential point which each patient is trying to express. Further clarification of symptoms may be obtained through direct questions. Certain symptoms, such as those involving behaviour or memory disturbance, blackouts and giddy spells, as well as disorders in children, require a description from an independent witness since the patient's account alone may be unreliable.

The symptoms usually suggest the anatomical site of disease and are therefore a guide as to where attention should be focused during the physical examination. Occasionally the history may allow quite a precise anatomical diagnosis to be made even in the absence of physical signs (see Fig. 1.2).

Precise details are required about the circumstances of onset of symptoms and how quickly they progressed, whether there were fluctuations or periods of remission, and whether there were generalised symptoms suggestive of systemic illness such as malignancy or infection. It is the tempo, progression and periodicity of symptoms, together with the presence or absence of general features, which give a clue to the underlying pathology (Fig. 1.3).

Some Common Neurological Symptoms

Headache (see also pp 96 and 179)

The site of the headache, the quality of the pain and its pattern of spread, the time of onset in relation to other daily activities, and its duration and periodicity should each be detailed. Associated symptoms suggestive of

Principal symptom	Other symptoms elicited in the history		Possible anatomical sites to explain symptoms
Weakness of right arm -sudden onset	–	?	muscle, peripheral nerve, spinal cord, brainstem, hemisphere
	Mild weakness of right leg	?	Spinal cord, brainstem, hemisphere
	Difficulty finding words	=	Left hemisphere
	Previous episodes of visual loss in left eye	=	Left internal carotid artery lesion causing emboli to left eye and hemisphere

Fig. 1.2 *Indications of anatomical site from clinical features.*

Principal symptom	Evolution of symptoms	Likely pathology
	1. Onset in sleep. No progression.	Vascular occlusion (thrombotic)
	2. Sudden onset remitting after 30 seconds.	Transient ischaemic attack (embolic)
Weak right arm and leg; difficulty in finding words.	3. Gradual onset worsening over weeks.	Tumour or other space-occupying lesion
	4. Gradual spread of symptoms arm→ speech/face→ leg over minutes followed by remission over minutes.	Migraine
	5. Progression of symptoms over a few days followed by resolution.	Demyelination

Fig. 1.3 *Progression of symptoms as an indication of possible pathologies.*

constitutional disturbance such as mood change, nausea, abdominal upset or photophobia are particularly helpful in distinguishing migraine from other forms of headache. Information about exacerbating and precipitating factors is valuable; headache worsened by cough, bending or straining may be due to raised intracranial pressure, and a large number of specific precipitants are recognised for migrainous headache, including items of diet, exercise, and menstruation. Any history of eye, ear, tooth, sinus or neck disease may be valuable in analysing the symptoms. Establishing the relationship of headache to sleep may be helpful, since it is rare for migraine or muscle contraction headache actually to cause waking from normal sleep although both may recur soon after waking. On the other hand, the headache of raised intracranial pressure may be exacerbated at night and, in a depressed patient, all symptoms may be more apparent at this time.

Other pains (see also p. 124)

As with headache, a description is gathered about the site of pain, its radiation, quality, exacerbating and relieving features. Sharp stabbing pains (neuralgia) occurring spontaneously or in relation to movement or sensory stimuli suggest irritation of peripheral nerves or nerve roots. This sort of pain may be typified by trigeminal neuralgia, where the sharp lancinating pains last only a few seconds and are triggered by touch, draughts, chewing or shaving; lumbar root irritation, e.g. due to a prolapsed disc, may give rise to severe sharp pains in the appropriate distribution, precipitated by movement, coughing or straining. Frequently, the original neuralgic pain is altered by protective muscle spasm which may itself be painful. Superficial soreness or burning sensations on the skin may follow partial nerve damage due to infection (e.g. herpes zoster) or injury, and the patient may be reluctant to allow contact with the skin even by his clothes. Such pains are often protracted and last for hours at a time.

Giddiness and blackouts (see also p. 107)

It is essential to establish the precise circumstances of the episodes which the patient is describing. For instance, it is valuable to know the time of day, the relationship to the last meal, what the patient was actually doing when the attack started, his posture, and how he felt. When a 'turn' is associated with loss of consciousness or awareness, it is necessary to ascertain whether this is more likely to be due to an impairment of blood flow to the brain (syncope), to an ictal event, or to some metabolic cause such as hypoglycaemia. A variety of features help to clarify this issue and may also throw light on the type of vascular or ictal event.

If consciousness is not lost the patient usually reports giddiness or unsteadiness. If there is a sensation of movement of the environment in relation to the patient, a disorder of the vestibular system is likely, although vertigo may occasionally be part of an ictal event in the temporal lobe. Associated symptoms may provide clues to the site of the lesion; concomitant tinnitus and deafness suggests peripheral end organ disease, while diplopia, paraesthesia over the face, and slurred speech suggest a brainstem disturbance. A relationship to specific head positions characterises benign positional vertigo; a relationship to standing suggests postural hypotension.

Detailed enquiry is made about previous cardiac disease, including valvular lesions (a possible cause of emboli), palpitations, and the relationship of cardiac symptoms to the dizzy turn. Rarely, a history of sudden loss of consciousness with profound pallor followed by rapid recovery with flushing is obtained, suggesting a transient reduction in cardiac output due to heart block, dysrhythmia or obstruction to flow (atrial myxoma, aortic stenosis). It is also recognised that what appear to be primarily ictal events may be precipitated by cardiac dysrhythmia. Giddy attacks or faintness may accompany migraine, anxiety or hyperventilation. The latter diagnosis is suggested by a subjective feeling of breathlessness, sighing, chest discomfort, sensations of panic, paraesthesiae in the hands and around the mouth, and a variety of other somatic complaints.

Visual disturbance

Alteration of vision is a frequent presentation of neurological illness. It is necessary to deduce whether the disturbance is monocular, or a field disturbance affecting both eyes, or a disorder of eye movement. A patient who complains of visual disturbance on the right may mean that the vision in the right eye is abnormal and may have checked that he sees normally through the left eye alone. If he finds difficulty in seeing the right side of objects, bumps into things on the right, or cannot follow a line of print, he is more likely to have a right homonymous field loss. Peripheral disturbances of the ocular motor system usually cause diplopia, which patients may be able to analyse (see p 33). Central defects of ocular movement may result merely in an uncomfortable unsteady feeling when looking in one particular direction, difficulty in 'focussing', or oscillopsia (apparent rhythmic movement of the environment).

Loss of use of a limb (Fig. 1.4)

The concept implied in 'loss of use of a limb' is wide, and involves a number of possible types of disorder. The patient may fail to distinguish between motor and sensory symptoms and describe a purely weak limb as 'numb' or 'dead'. There is considerable overlap in the types of symptom described by patients with disorders

Physical signs	Type of symptom
Spasticity	Stiffness, tightness, poor control, feels useless.
Rigidity, akinesia	Slow, stiff, painful, useless, poor fine movements.
Weak	Weak, numb, inability to perform specific tasks–getting up from chair, climbing stairs.
Ataxic	Clumsy, weak, tires quickly, always dropping things, unsteady, drunken.
Posterior column dysfunction	Feels numb, useless, weak, difficulty with fine movements: positive sensations– tight feelings around limbs, discomfort, tingling, misshapen feeling, paraesthesiae
Loss of superficial sensation	Feels numb, useless. Can't tell temperature of water.

Fig. 1.4 *'Loss of use' of a limb.*

of the various systems concerned with movement and sensation. After establishing the pattern of symptoms in the affected limb, specific enquiries should be made about the relationship of symptoms to daily activity and, in particular, to exercise. A variety of spinal cord lesions, such as those due to demyelination, spinal cord compression, or angioma, may cause prominent symptoms on exercise with rather minimal symptoms in the resting state; radicular pain, numbness and weakness in the legs may be prominent on exercise in cauda equina claudication (see p. 169).

Higher function, language and memory

After asking the patient what seems to be wrong, a relative or friend should be asked to describe how the patient's personality and behaviour appears to have changed. Examples in everyday life should be obtained to provide a firm basis for the type of disturbance being considered. For example, the patient may forget familiar or new names and telephone numbers, may always require a written list before he can shop satisfactorily, or may tend to forget to turn off lights or fires at the appropriate time. Expressive disorders of language are likely to be evident to relatives and friends as halting or incorrect speech, but the existence of a

receptive (comprehension) language disturbance may not be noticed. Descriptions of the patient's reaction to other members of the family and well-known friends, and ascertaining whether his behaviour and speech are appropriate to the situation, are helpful. In obtaining any history concerning higher cerebral functions, the premorbid level of intelligence is established by questions concerning education and work record, some details about personality, motivation and mood, and the typical pattern of activities indulged in at work and leisure prior to the illness. The patient's current behaviour needs to be compared with this norm rather than any general 'average' view of normality.

Categories of Disease

In considering the pattern of symptoms it is useful to think of five major categories of neurological disease: inflammatory, neoplastic, vascular, demyelinating, and degenerative.

Inflammatory disease, e.g. meningitis, cerebral abscess

The onset of symptoms may be over hours, days or weeks depending on the type of infection. The symptoms can be progressive until treated. Since neurological infections are often acquired by spread from other organs such as the nasal sinuses, ears, chest or skin, there may be a history of preceding nonspecific malaise, fever, ear discharge, respiratory or cardiac problem or skin infection. Generalised neurological symptoms, such as headache, photophobia, vomiting or clouding of consciousness, are often more prominent than focal symptoms.

Neoplastic disease

The symptoms are usually of gradual onset over weeks or months. Their rate of progression depends on the site of the tumour and its rate of growth; a critically-placed tumour in the brainstem may produce early symptoms but a tumour in the non-dominant hemisphere may grow to a large size and cause no complaints. The more slowly symptoms progress, the less likely they are to be noticed. Typically, tumours cause progressive local dysfunction at a single site (e.g. focal epilepsy, hemiparesis or hemianopia), later accompanied by general symptoms of raised intracranial pressure (headache, vomiting, clouding of consciousness) due to their volume effects or to the obstruction of flow of cerebrospinal fluid.

Vascular disease

Symptoms of cerebral infarction are usually of rapid onset, with the disability being at its worst within a few minutes and sometimes tending to fluctuate over the first few hours. They then stabilise and begin slowly to improve. The distribution of the symptoms suggests brain dysfunction at a single site, but signs of inflammation or raised intracranial pressure are usually absent. In the case of cerebral haemorrhage the symptoms tend to progress over hours and there is less tendency to fluctuate. Because there is space occupation by blood clot there are general symptoms of raised intracranial pressure.

General symptoms of vascular disease, e.g. angina, intermittent claudication, are often present in other sites and there may be a past history of hypertension, diabetes or cardiac disease.

Demyelinating disease, e.g. multiple sclerosis

Symptoms of multiple sclerosis appear abruptly over hours or days and show remarkable fluctuations, often in response to fatigue or temperature change. The patient may set out for a walk normally and be unable to return because of progressive weakness of the legs. Periods of complete remission are characteristic. The symptoms usually indicate involvement of multiple discrete sites within the central nervous system, e.g. visual blurring and weakness of the legs, and they tend to involve sensory as well as motor function. Systemic symptoms are usually absent.

Degenerative disease, e.g. Alzheimer's disease, motor neurone disease, Parkinsonism, muscular dystrophy

The features, which are of insidious onset and often go unnoticed by the patient, progress slowly but steadily. The type of symptom indicates advancing dysfunction of one system, e.g. extrapyramidal, spinal motor neurones. Generalised symptoms are usually absent.

The history taking, apart from its purely informational content, reveals much of relevance to the neurological examination. By the end of the history the doctor should have a good idea of the patient's orientation, mood, intellectual background, language and memory functions, and will have gained some insight into his personality. An impression may be formed as to whether the patient tends to elaborate symptoms or gloss over them. All these aspects will be relevant in deciding how to handle the overall clinical problem. In addition, because taking a history is a two-way communication, it gives the doctor an opportunity to establish a sympathetic rapport with the patient and gain his trust and understanding – an essential first step in the dual exercise of treating illness and advising ill people.

PAST HISTORY

Relevant details of past medical history are often omitted by patients, who may be quite unaware of their significance in neurological disorders. For example, a patient who complains of loss of sensation and tingling in the feet may not appreciate that the episode of loss of vision and pain in one eye which he experienced eight years previously could be relevant to the diagnosis of multiple sclerosis. Similarly, a history of birth trauma or childhood head injury may be significant as a cause of epilepsy, or a past history of rheumatic heart disease may indicate the cause of a hemiparesis many years later. Many neurological disorders have their roots in childhood and it may be relevant to obtain details from the parents about the patient's birth, early development and milestones, illnesses in early life and later educational, social and physical progress. This is particularly the case where genetically-determined disorders affecting intellectual or motor development are being considered. Finally, specific enquiry should always be made about past and present medication, since many drugs have both short- and long-term neurological complications. The immunisation history of the patient may also be helpful because, occasionally, late side-effects affect the nervous system.

FAMILY HISTORY

In many varieties of neurological disease the existence of a similarly-affected relative may be a strong indicator of a genetic disorder. It should be appreciated, however, that overt disease in relatives may be unnoticed, ignored, denied or actively concealed by the family and it may therefore be necessary to examine other family members, both to reach an accurate diagnosis and to ascertain the mode of inheritance. Detailed knowledge of genetic conditions and of the various modes of inheritance are required by the doctor in interpreting muscle weakness – for example, in the case of a patient presenting with progressive muscle weakness, the discovery that his mother had several miscarriages and that her brother, who died suddenly at the age of 40, had cataracts and went bald in his twenties, would be strongly suggestive of myotonic dystrophy; in an adult man aged 40 years with choreiform movements, the fact that an aunt committed suicide may be a pointer to the diagnosis of Huntington's chorea. In any genetic condition the relationship of the parents should be defined since consanguinity increases the chances of a recessive disorder in the offspring.

Many familial neurological diseases are system degenerations (i.e. they selectively involve specific cell groups or tracts) but these are fairly rare. Common system degenerations such as Parkinson's disease or motor neurone disease show a familial incidence only slightly above the chance level.

SOCIAL AND ECONOMIC FACTORS

Enquiry into the socio-economic and cultural background of the patient, as well as into the record of employment, may yield information of diagnostic value. Poor housing and malnutrition may contribute to the spread of infections of the nervous system, such as tuberculous or meningococcal meningitis. A diet deficient in vitamins may result in polyneuritis (e.g. thiamine deficiency), myopathy (e.g. nutritional vitamin D deficiency in Indian Asian immigrants), or spinal cord disease (e.g. B_{12} deficiency in strict vegetarians). Chronic alcohol abuse may damage a variety of neural tissues, including peripheral nerves, cerebellum and cerebral cortex.

Industrial exposure to heavy metals is now infrequent, but lead neuropathy still occurs from inhalation of fumes in poorly-ventilated workshops, and outbreaks of organophosphorus poisoning occur from time to time due to contaminated cooking oils. Certain occupations may predispose to damage of the peripheral nerves or central nervous system: examples include cervical spondylosis in house painters, lumbar disc disease in nurses, and occupational cramps in musicians.

Geographical factors have a strong influence on the incidence of infectious and parasitic diseases which may involve the nervous system. Knowledge about the epidemiology of major neurological diseases is of direct value in diagnosis; e.g., a twenty-six-year-old African negro who has lived in the UK for only three years is extremely *unlikely* to be suffering from multiple sclerosis as cause for his spinal cord lesions, whilst tuberculous spinal disease might be quite likely. Although most tropical diseases are contracted only after chronic exposure, there are some (e.g. cerebral malaria) which are not. Tropical infections are appearing with increasing frequency in temperate countries as a result of air travel, and details of recent trips should be recorded.

MANAGEMENT HISTORY

The above points about history taking have mainly been directed towards making an accurate diagnosis. The management of two patients of the same age with the same diagnosis may vary greatly, however, depending on several factors (see Fig. 1.5). For the purposes of management it is important to approach symptoms in terms of functional disability related to the environment in which the patient lives. Weakness of the legs may have quite different management implications when: a) the patient cannot stand at all; b) the patient can walk with a frame around his own home; c) the patient can walk outside with assistance. Enquiry should always be made, therefore, about how a disability affects everyday life.

The family circumstances of the patient, his type of accommodation, his type of work (if any), and his financial and social situation will all profoundly influence the impact of a developing neurological disorder. Furthermore, these factors may make certain types of therapy and management beneficial for one patient but entirely inappropriate for another.

At the end of the history it is helpful to summarise the major points. These should always include the age of the patient, relevant features in the past, family and social history, major symptoms, type of onset and the tempo of the illness.

1. Diagnostic history (both a and b)

    Awoke with weak right arm and leg. Non-progressive over last 3 days. Speech impaired.

    Previous history of angina, hypertension and smoking.

    Rt. handed.

    Father had stroke aged 40 yrs.

2. Management history

a) Single man without relatives, lives alone in 3rd floor flat (no lifts)

    Works as musician (violinist).

    Previous history of depression.

b) Married man-wife at home, lives in large house, wife and patient run own shop assisted by son aged 25.

Fig. 1.5 *Relevant history in two 56-year-old men (a, b), each of whom has sustained a right hemiparesis.*

2

Functional Anatomy and Examination

THE MOTOR SYSTEM

The purpose of the motor system is to coordinate movement of body parts and at the same time to maintain posture and balance. The final common pathway involves the α motor neurones and associated segmental reflex connections. The formulation of a willed movement (praxis) and its execution and coordination are functions of the cerebral cortex, basal ganglia, and cerebellum.

Final Common Pathway

Movement is brought about by application of force generated by muscle to the skeletal system of bones and joints. Each α motor neurone innervates between 10 and 2000 muscle fibres (the motor unit) and force is adjusted by recruitment of motor units and variation of their discharge frequency. α motor neurones are arranged in the anterior horn grey matter of the spinal cord and form longitudinal cell columns principally in lamina IX (Fig. 2.1). Those innervating trunk and neck

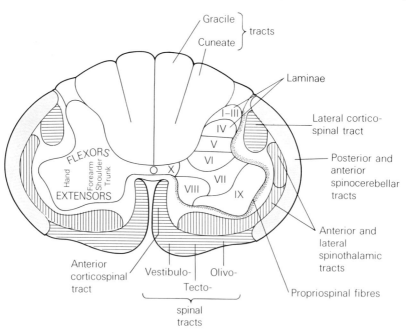

Fig. 2.1 *Diagram of a transverse section of lower cervical spinal cord to show the principal white-matter tracts and structural lamination of the grey matter (RHS), and the general location of anterior horn cells sending axons to specific muscle groups (LHS).*

muscles lie medially whilst the lateral cell columns innervate the limbs.

The spinal cord shortens in relationship to the spinal canal during growth and eventually terminates, in the adult, at the lower border of the first lumbar vertebra. The spinal cord segments, with their associated ventral (motor) and dorsal (sensory) roots, become progressively higher in relationship to the bony canal from the cervical to sacral regions, so that lumbar and sacral roots have a long intraspinal course (cauda equina) (Fig. 2.2). The ventral and dorsal roots unite to form the spinal nerves in the region of the intervertebral foramen through which they exit; because of convergence and branching within the cervical, brachial and lumbosacral plexuses, most peripheral nerves to the limbs contain motor and sensory fibres from several spinal segments. The most prominent feature of injury to the final common motor pathway is muscle weakness.

Clinical examination of muscle strength

The strength of individual muscle groups is estimated by testing manually the force which the patient can produce. The commonest and most satisfactory way of quantifying strength for diagnostic purposes is by applying the Medical Research Council scale:

Grade 0 – no movement

Grade 1 – flicker only

Grade 2 – full range of movement with gravity eliminated

Grade 3 – full range of movement against gravity

Grade 4 – full range of movement against gravity and resistance

Grade 5 – normal power

Techniques for examining specific muscle groups are illustrated in Fig. 2.3, but it is frequently easier to diagnose weakness of the truncal and pelvic girdle muscles by seeing the patient walk, climb stairs, rise from a low chair (see also p. 254). The assessment of strength may be made more difficult if there is pain on movement, sensory loss, or inattention, or if the patient's cooperation is not optimal.

The distribution of muscle weakness may assist in diagnosing its cause. In a root or peripheral nerve lesion, weakness will be confined to those muscles which are deprived of their innervation (Tables 2.1 and 2.2). In muscle disease, weakness tends to be symmetrical, proximal and generalised. Weakness associated

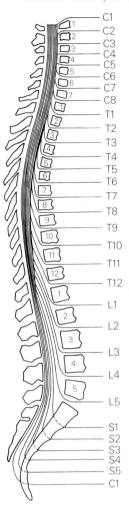

Fig. 2.2 *Diagram to show the relationships to vertebrae of spinal cord segments.*

with lesions of the corticospinal pathways (see p. 11) tends to affect the extensor groups in the upper limbs and the flexor groups in the lower limbs.

When weakness is due to damage to motor units there is usually marked wasting of the muscles at an early stage. However, any reduction in the normal use of muscle may initiate slight wasting. A lesion affecting the corticospinal pathway may therefore eventually cause some loss of bulk but the loss of function is always proportionately greater than would be expected from the degree of wasting. Lesions of the lower motor

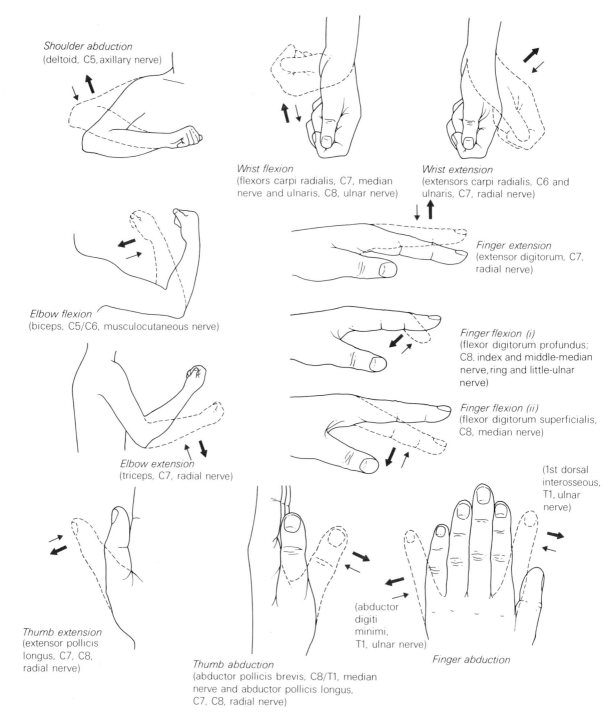

Shoulder abduction
(deltoid, C5, axillary nerve)

Wrist flexion
(flexors carpi radialis, C7, median
nerve and ulnaris, C8, ulnar nerve)

Wrist extension
(extensors carpi radialis, C6 and
ulnaris, C7, radial nerve)

Finger extension
(extensor digitorum, C7,
radial nerve)

Elbow flexion
(biceps, C5/C6, musculocutaneous nerve)

Finger flexion (i)
(flexor digitorum profundus;
C8, index and middle-median
nerve, ring and little-ulnar
nerve)

Finger flexion (ii)
(flexor digitorum superficialis,
C8, median nerve)

Elbow extension
(triceps, C7, radial nerve)

(1st dorsal
interosseous,
T1, ulnar
nerve)

Thumb extension
(extensor pollicis
longus, C7, C8,
radial nerve)

(abductor
digiti
minimi,
T1, ulnar nerve)

Thumb abduction
(abductor pollicis brevis, C8/T1, median
nerve and abductor pollicis longus,
C7, C8, radial nerve)

Finger abduction

Fig. 2.3 *Principal movements tested in upper and lower limbs.*
➤ = *direction of patient's attempted movement,* ➤ = *point
and direction of opposition by examiner. See also Tables 2.1,
2.2.*

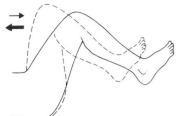

Hip flexion
(iliopsoas, L1/L2, lumbar
plexus and femoral nerve)

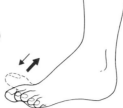

Dorsiflexion of big toe
(extensor hallucis longus,
L5, deep peroneal nerve)

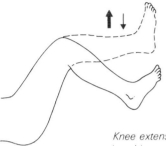

Knee extension
(quadriceps femoris, L3 /L4,
femoral nerve)

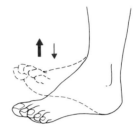

Dorsiflexion of ankle
(tibialis anterior, L4,
deep peroneal nerve)

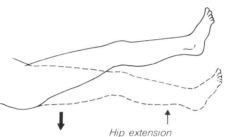

Hip extension
(gluteus maximus, L5/S1/S2
inferior gluteal nerve)

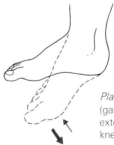

Plantar flexion of ankle
(gastrocnemius – when knee
extended, S1/S2, soleus – when
knee flexed, S1/S2, sciatic nerve)

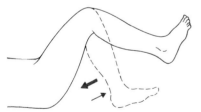

Knee flexion
(hamstrings, L5/S1/S2,
sciatic nerve)

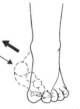

Inversion of ankle
(tibialis anterior and
posterior, L4/L5,
deep peroneal nerve
and posterior tibial
nerve)

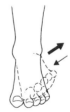

Eversion of ankle
(peroneus longus and
brevis, L5/S1,
superficial peroneal nerve)

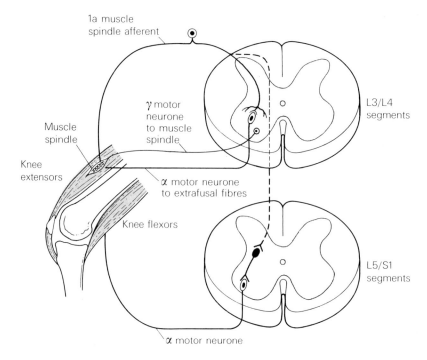

1a muscle
spindle afferent

γ motor
neurone
to muscle
spindle

Muscle
spindle

Knee
extensors

α motor neurone
to extrafusal fibres

Knee flexors

L3/L4
segments

L5/S1
segments

α motor neurone

Fig. 2.4 *Figure to show monosynaptic reflex arc mechanism for the patellar tendon reflex ('knee jerk') with an inhibitory effect on knee flexors via intersegmental collaterals and an inhibitory interneurone.*

neurone (particularly damage to the cell body or the motor root) may be associated with irritability of the motor unit, shown as fasciculations of the affected muscles at rest. In addition, if sufficient α motor neurones or axons are damaged, the tendon reflex is diminished or absent.

Tendon Reflexes

The lowest level of motor control is through the segmental reflex mechanism (Fig. 2.4). Muscle spindles detect length and velocity changes in extrafusal fibres and this information is relayed to the spinal cord in large myelinated afferent (1a) fibres. The gain of the muscle spindle is adjusted through contraction and relaxation of intrafusal muscle fibres innervated by γ motor neurones, whose cell bodies lie mainly in lamina IX (Fig. 2.1). Information about muscle tension is

detected by Golgi tendon organs in series with extrafusal muscle fibres. Sudden passive lengthening of the knee extensors, (Fig. 2.4) – as in testing a tendon jerk – elicits impulses in 1a afferents which monosynaptically excite α motor neurones in the same spinal segment, resulting in an almost synchronous efferent volley and characteristic brief muscle contraction. Concomitantly the antagonist muscles are inhibited (Fig. 2.4). The amplitude of the tendon jerk depends on the stimulus amplitude, the excitability of the motor neurone pool, and the muscle spindle sensitivity – which is determined by the γ efferent discharge. The state of excitability of these cell groups will determine the sensitivity of the reflex arc to passive movement (notably stretch): excessive or reduced excitability depends on the type of lesion (see below). Since the tendon reflexes are only a measure of excitability of the monosynaptic reflex arc in response to a single brief stimulus, their briskness does not always parallel 'tone', which is clinically assessed as the resistance of a limb to passive movement.

Examination

The tendon reflexes conveniently permit the excitability of motor neurones to be examined at a series of levels in the nervous system (Table 2.3). During testing the patient must be relaxed and comfortable. The reflexes on the two sides are compared. When reflexes are very brisk, reducing the stimulus may allow asymmetries to be observed between the two sides. When the reflex is sluggish or absent, a voluntary contraction of some other muscle group may reinforce the response (Jendrassik's manoeuvre). The relaxation phase of the reflex muscle contraction is a reflection of muscle contractility and not of electrical excitability. It is characteristically slowed in hypothyroidism and following cooling.

A tendon reflex will be lost if insufficient muscle fibres can be activated synchronously to produce a visible contraction. This occurs if conduction of impulses in the afferent or efferent pathway is delayed or dispersed due to demyelination of peripheral nerves or if large numbers of 1a afferent or α motor neurones have degenerated (axonal loss) so that the afferent or efferent responses are severely reduced in amplitude. Occasionally, so many muscle fibres have been lost that the reflex muscle contraction is not detectable but this is usually a late development in primary muscle disease.

Tone

'Tone' represents the reflex excitation of muscles in response to passive or active movements. In the clinical examination tone is assessed from passive movements of the relaxed limb, but this only represents a limited sample of ongoing efferent activity in one particular circumstance. During activity, tone is continuously adjusted by a variety of segmental and 'long loop' reflexes.

Clinical examination

The patient should be relaxed, warm and comfortable when tone is examined. In the upper limb, the examiner gently flexes and extends the fingers, wrists and elbow in succession and supinates/pronates the forearm. In the lower limb, the extended limb is gently rolled from side to side to test tone in the hip muscles and flexion/extension movements carried out at the knee and ankle joints.

Two principal patterns of increased tone are easily recognised and usually have quite different clinical significance. Spasticity results from lesions which usually involve the corticospinal tracts and rigidity from lesions which involve the basal ganglia and their connections. The characteristics of spasticity and rigidity are summarised in Table 2.4.

Hypotonia may be caused by a lesion interrupting the spinal reflex arcs or by cerebellar lesions, which probably reduce α and γ motor neurone excitability via

---

TABLE 2.1

Principal Root Values for Main Muscle Groups (see Fig 2.12) for Sensory Distribution

Muscle group	Root values
Sternomastoids	
Trapezius	Spinal accessory: C3, 4
Diaphragm	C3, 4, 5
Deltoid, supra-, infraspinatus,	C5, 6
Rhomboids	C4, 5
Pectoralis major	C5, 6, 7, 8
Serratus anterior	C5, 6, 7
Elbow flexion	C5, 6
Elbow extension	C6, 7, 8
Wrist extension	C6, 7
Wrist flexion	C7, 8
Finger/thumb extension	C7, 8
Finger/thumb flexion	C8
Small muscles of hand	C8/T1
Hip flexion (iliopsoas)	L1, 2, 3
(rectus femoris)	L3, 4
Hip extension	L5, S1, 2
Hip adduction	L2, 3
Hip abduction	L4, 5, S1
Knee extension	L3, 4
Knee flexion	L5, S1, 2
Ankle dorsiflexion	L4, 5
Ankle plantar flexion	S1, 2
Toe dorsiflexion	L5
Ankle eversion	L5/S1
Ankle inversion	L4, 5
Toe flexion	S1, 2
Small muscles of foot	S1, 2

Table 2.2

Muscular Innervation of the Major Peripheral Nerves (See Fig. 2.11 for Sensory Distribution)

Nerve		Muscle
Axillary nerve (C5)		deltoid
Musculocutaneous nerve	(C5, 6)	biceps, brachialis
suprascapular nerve	(C5, 6)	supra-, infraspinatus
Long thoracic nerve	(C5, 6, 7)	serratus anterior
Radial nerve (C6–8)	– branches above elbow	triceps
		extensor carpi radialis
		brachioradialis
	– posterior interosseus nerve	supinator
		extensors carpi ulnaris, digitorum
		indices and pollicis
		abductor pollicis longus
Median nerve (C6–F1)	– in forearm	flexor digitorum profundus I, II
		flexor digitorum superficialis
		flexor pollicis longus
		pronator teres
	– in hand	thenar eminence (except adductor pollicis)
		1st and 2nd lumbrical
Ulnar nerve (C7–T1)	– in forearm	flexor digitorum profundus III, IV
		flexor carpi ulnaris
		all muscles of hand not median supplied
Femoral nerve (L2, 3, 4,)		sartorius, quadriceps
Obturator nerve (L2, 3, 4)		adductors of hip, gracilis
Superior gluteal nerve (L4, 5, S1)		adduction, internal rotation of thigh
Inferior gluteal nerve (L5, S1, 2)		extension of thigh
Sciatic nerve	– L5, S1, 2	knee flexors
	– Common peroneal nerve (L4 – S1)	eversion of ankle
		dorsiflexion of ankle and toes
	– Tibial nerve (L5–S2)	plantar flexion of foot and toes, inversion of foot, intrinsic muscles of feet
Pudendal nerve (S2–4)		perineal muscles

rubrospinal or vestibulospinal pathways. Pure lesions of the corticospinal pathway may cause hypotonia, which is also seen in the early stages of an acute lesion affecting the motor cortex or after spinal cord transection. Hypotonia is not always easy to detect clinically, but may be suggested by hypermobility of joints and

the adoption of certain postures, such as hyperexten sion of the metacarpophalangeal and interphalangea joints with excessive flexion of the wrist on maintainin the arms outstretched, or eversion of the palms of the hands with the arms held above the head. The tendor reflexes (in particular the knee jerk when tested with the

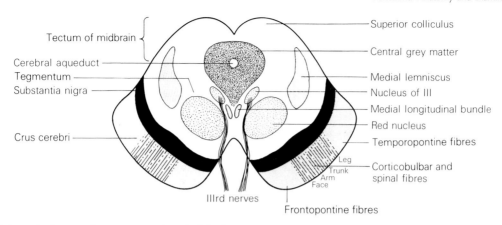

Fig. 2.5 *Schematic diagram of transverse section of midbrain at the level of the superior colliculus.*

Table 2.3

Segmental Innervation of Reflexes

A) Tendon reflexes

Biceps	C5/6
Brachioradialis	C5/6
Triceps	C7
Finger flexion	C7/8
Knee jerk	L3/4
Ankle jerk	S1

B) Superficial reflexes

Abdominal reflexes	
Epigastric	T7–9
Lower abdominal	T11–12
Cremasteric reflex	L1/2
Anal reflex	S4/5

patient's lower leg hanging free) may be pendular, i.e. they are poorly damped and the dependent part of the limb swings to and fro after a single stimulus tap.

Supranuclear and Supraspinal Motor Pathways

Corticobulbar and corticospinal tracts originate in the motor cortex (area 4 of precentral gyrus), sensory cortex (areas 3, 1, 2 of postcentral gyrus) and supple-

mentary motor area (area 6 on the medial aspect of the frontal lobe). Only a small proportion of axons in the medullary pyramids are in fact from the large Betz cells in area 4. After passing in the posterior limb of the internal capsule (closely associated with corticopontine, corticorubral and corticostriatal fibres) they enter the central part of the cerebral peduncles (Fig. 2.5) and are then split up by the pontine nuclei in the ventral pons (Fig. 2.6). 85% of the fibres decussate in the medullary pyramids (Fig. 2.7) and pass down the spinal cord as the lateral corticospinal tract (Fig. 2.1). Most of these fibres synapse on interneurones in laminae IV–VII, but large axons from Betz cells may have monosynaptic connections with α motor neurones in laminae VII–IX. The uncrossed anterior corticospinal pathway is mainly evident in the cervical region. Cranial nerve nuclei receive bilateral supranuclear innervation – with the exception of the lower part of the face (VII), spinal accessory and hypoglossal nuclei, which receive crossed unilateral innervation.

The red nucleus (Fig. 2.5), receiving afferents from cortex, cerebellum and basal ganglia, makes an important contribution to descending motor control via the rubrospinal tract; this pathway shows similar somatotopic arrangement and a similar distribution of synaptic connections in the spinal cord as does the corticospinal tract. Other descending pathways (vestibulo-, reticulo-, and tectospinal tracts) pass ventrally in the spinal cord and terminate more medially in the grey matter (Fig. 2.1).

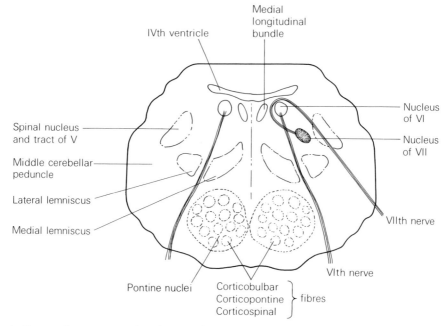

Fig. 2.6 *Schematic diagram of transverse section of pons at the level of the nucleus of VIth nerve.*

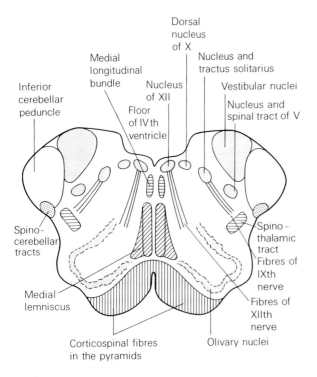

Fig. 2.7 *Schematic diagram of transverse section of the medulla at the level of the inferior olivary nuclei.*

Clinical examination

Loss of fine, rapid and discrete movements is an important effect of damage to the corticospinal pathway, and this may occur independently of spasticity or weakness. It is tested by asking the patient to make rapid repetitive movements of the fingers or toes and to perform fine manipulative tasks. A lesion of the corticospinal pathway frequently leads to spasticity; in the upper limbs this is prominent in the shoulder adductors, elbow, wrist and finger flexors, and in the lower limbs it affects the hip adductors, knee extensors, and plantarflexors of the ankle. Loss of the normal pattern of facilitation leads to weakness in the antagonist muscles, i.e. shoulder abductors, elbow, wrist and finger extensors of the upper limbs and hip, knee flexors and ankle dorsiflexors in the lower limbs. Efforts at voluntary movements in the affected limbs may give rise to complex synergistic reflex responses involving several muscle groups.

The effect of a lesion will clearly depend on its site and extent. A small lesion in the internal capsule may cause a hemiplegia because of close grouping of the corticospinal pathways for arm and leg, whilst a similar lesion in the motor cortex may cause only minor

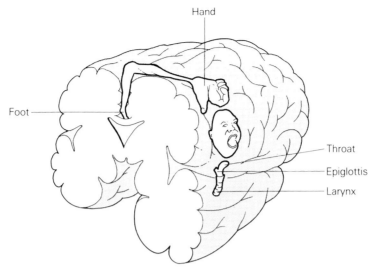

Fig. 2.8 *Somatotopic representation of body in motor cortex (similar pattern in sensory cortex).*

Table 2.4

Clinical Differences Between Spasticity and Rigidity

		Spasticity	Rigidity
1.	Distribution of tone increase	Mainly flexors in upper limbs and extensors in lower limbs	Frequently affects axial musculature: agonists and antagonists at the same time (leadpipe effect) or alternating (cogwheel)
2.	Effect of speed of passive movement	Increases with velocity of muscle stretch	Independent
3.	Variation through movement	Increased at start of movement – clasp knife effect or Repetitive rhythmic contractions after short stretch (clonus)	Unchanged throughout range
4.	Tendon reflexes	Exaggerated	Usually normal
5.	Plantar response	Extensor	Flexor

localised weakness because of the more extensive spatial representation of different parts of the body (Fig. 2.8). In the latter case the lower limb will be involved in a cortical lesion affecting the superior and medial aspect of the motor area, and the face and hand will be involved if the lesion is more lateral. Rarely, weakness of

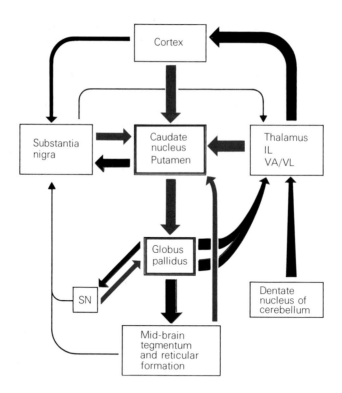

Fig. 2.9 *Block diagram showing some of the main afferent (red) and efferent (black) connections of the basal ganglia ( ), with other structures important in motor control. SN = subthalamic nucleus, IL = intralaminar nuclei of thalamus, VA/VL = ventral anterior and lateral group nuclei of thalamus (see also Fig. 2.14).*

one limb may occur in small selective vascular lesions of the internal capsule or pons.

If the supplementary motor areas of the frontal lobes are damaged, a grasp reflex may be present. This reflex, which is present in the first few months of life but subsequently disappears, is elicited by stroking the palm of the patient's hand towards the finger tips. A positive response is recorded if the patient involuntarily grasps the examiner's fingers.

The plantar response

A characteristic feature of a corticospinal tract lesion is an extensor plantar response (sign of Babinski). A firm sharp stimulus is stroked along the outer aspect of the sole of the foot, curving inwards towards the middle metatarsophalangeal joint. Normally, plantarflexion of the great toe, due to contraction of the flexor hallucis

brevis, is the first movement to be observed. An initial extensor response, with or without fanning of the other toes, is part of the generalised flexion withdrawal reflex and is caused by early contraction of extensor hallucis longus at a latency suggesting a spinal reflex. The extensor response is present in children of less than six months old and in about 75% at twelve months. Extensor responses do not necessarily imply a structural lesion of the corticospinal tracts; they may occur, for instance, in coma from any cause (e.g. hypoglycaemia). The reflex cannot be elicited if the big toe joints are grossly deformed or if the extensor muscle is completely paralysed.

Abdominal reflexes (Table 2.3)

Light stimulation of the skin of the anterior abdominal wall usually results in contraction of muscles in the same quadrant and reciprocal relaxation of posterior trunk muscles. Absence of cutaneous reflexes is associated with a corticospinal lesion, particularly in the spinal cord. Interference with the reflex arc by peripheral nerve or root lesions is sometimes of value in localising lesions of the thoracic spinal cord. However, poor relaxation, obesity, previous pregnancy or abdominal surgery often make these reflexes difficult to elicit. Similar considerations pertain to the cremasteric reflex (segmental innervation L1–2) in which stroking the inside of the thigh results in contraction of the cremasteric muscle with pulling up of the testis and scrotum.

Basal Ganglia

This group of subcortical structures (Fig. 2.9) is closely linked with the cortex and thalamus and its principal efferent pathways are to these sites although there are contributions to descending spinal pathways by vestibulo-, rubro- and reticulospinal tracts. The anato-

mical interrelationship between motor cortex and basal ganglia suggests close cooperation between the two systems in the control of movement. Disorders of the basal ganglia result in slowness of voluntary and postural reflex movements (bradykinesia), muscular rigidity (Table 2.4) and abnormal involuntary movements (dyskinesia) or postures (dystonia). Since the basal ganglia exert an influence on α and γ motor neurones, disease may impair several aspects of motor function, notably the postural reflexes which maintain truncal equilibrium, the reflex adjustment of synergists and antagonists in response to action by a prime mover, and various aspects of speech articulation, breathing and swallowing.

Cerebellum (Figure 2.10)

The smooth coordination of learned and reflex movements is the principal function of the cerebellum. The archicerebellum comprising the flocculonodular lobe (Fig. 2.10) coordinates vestibular function with eye

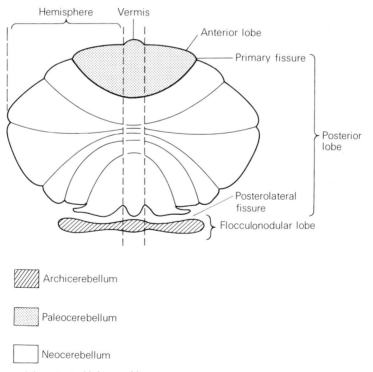

Fig. 2.10 *Schematic diagram of the principal lobes and fissures of the cerebellum.*

movements and other postural mechanisms. The anterior lobe of the cerebellum (paleocerebellum) projects to the fastigial, vestibular and red nuclei and, via descending pathways, influences muscle tone and the control of posture and equilibrium. The most recent part of the cerebellum in evolutionary terms – neo-cerebellum – receives numerous afferents from the cerebral cortex via the pontine nuclei and is primarily concerned with the control of learned movements of the limbs. Afferent fibres to the cerebellum travel mainly in the inferior and middle cerebellar peduncles. Fibres from the limbs pass in the spinocerebellar tracts (Fig. 2.1) to the anterior lobe, from the olivary complex principally to the vermis, from the cortex and pontine nuclei to the neo- and paleocerebellum. The principal efferent pathways pass, via deep cerebellar nuclei, to the thalamus, cerebral cortex, brainstem nuclei and spinal cord.

Clinical examination

Neocerebellar lesions result in decomposition of the normal sequence of a movement, i.e. dyssynergia. The movement may be imprecise in direction (past point-ing), distance (dysmetria) or force. Rapid alternating movements are performed clumsily (dysdiadocho-kinesis) and force of contraction can only be adjusted slowly and inaccurately. Irregular and inappropriate contractions of muscles around the shoulder and pelvic girdle give rise to clumsy movements of the limbs (ataxia) which are typically tested by the finger/nose test, by the heel/shin test, and by watching the patient walk. Irregular tremor on action is a notable feature of cerebellar disorders, especially when deep cerebellar nuclei are involved. The tremor is principally the result of involvement of the proximal musculature but is transmitted distally mechanically. Hypotonia probably results from reduced cerebellar inhibition of the red nucleus and descending rubrospinal pathways. The muscles of articulation may be involved, resulting in a characteristic 'scanning' speech. Typically lesions of one cerebellar hemisphere cause ipsilateral limb signs. Nystagmus is often present more on deviation of the eyes towards the side of the lesion.

Lesions of the anterior lobe and flocculonodular lobe, particularly if affecting the vermis, have a profound effect on truncal equilibrium and may result in a rolling drunken gait with an inability to stand. This may occur despite normal power, coordination and sensation of the limbs when the patient is tested on the bed.

THE SENSORY SYSTEM

Whilst the sensory system includes the special senses and visceral sensation, this section is concerned with general somatic sensation which may either be extero-ceptive or proprioceptive. Exteroceptive sensation gives information about the external environment and thus includes sensory modalities such as tactile sensa-tion, pressure, temperature and pain. Proprioceptive sensation gives information about body position and movement (kinesthesia) obtained from receptors in joints, ligaments, tendons and muscles. Although sensory nerve endings and receptors are not now regarded as being strictly modality specific, some specialised receptors transduce certain forms of energy particularly efficiently and hence are more sensitive to certain types of stimuli (see p. 239).

Peripheral Sensory Fibres

Free nerve endings associated with unmyelinated or thinly myelinated afferents are widely distributed over the whole body and appear to have a particular role in the detection of noxious, painful and thermal stimuli. One type of specialised free nerve endings (Merkel discs) have a particularly low threshold to light touch. Some nerve endings are encapsulated. Meissner's corpuscles are prominent in the papillae of the dermal ridges in the fingers and toes, hands and feet, and are concerned with 'discriminative' sensory function. So-called Ruffini and Pacinian corpuscles also appear to respond to tactile stimuli. Vibration is mainly detected by Pacinian corpuscles which excite large myelinated afferents, and joint position/kinesthetic sensation depends both on receptors in muscle (muscle spindles and tendon organs) and receptors around joints which include Ruffini and Pacinian corpuscles as well as free nerve endings.

Sensory nerve fibres enter the spinal cord principally through the dorsal root, and the cell bodies lie in the dorsal root ganglia. The sensory distributions of the

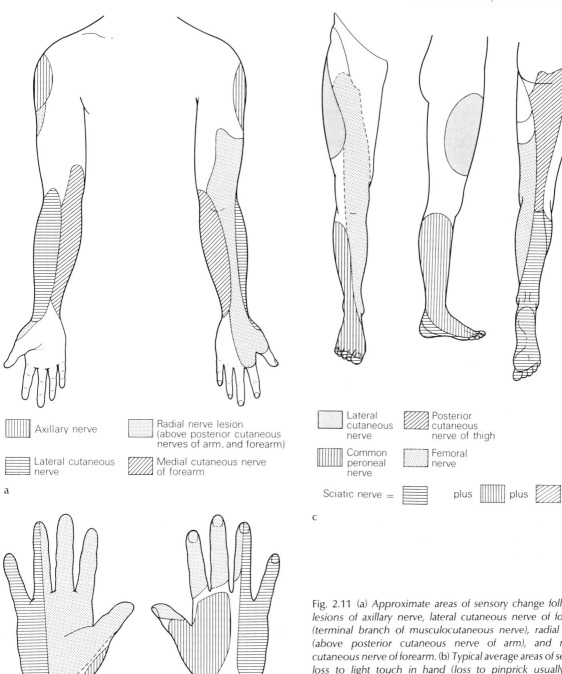

Axillary nerve

Lateral cutaneous nerve

Radial nerve lesion (above posterior cutaneous nerves of arm, and forearm)

Medial cutaneous nerve of forearm

a

Median nerve Ulnar nerve Radial nerve

b

Lateral cutaneous nerve

Common peroneal nerve

Posterior cutaneous nerve of thigh

Femoral nerve

Sciatic nerve = plus plus

c

Fig. 2.11 (a) *Approximate areas of sensory change following lesions of axillary nerve, lateral cutaneous nerve of forearm (terminal branch of musculocutaneous nerve), radial nerve (above posterior cutaneous nerve of arm), and medial cutaneous nerve of forearm. (b) Typical average areas of sensory loss to light touch in hand (loss to pinprick usually less) following individual division of the median, ulnar or radial nerves. (c) Approximate areas of sensory change following lesions of lateral cutaneous nerve of thigh, femoral nerve, superficial branch of common peroneal nerve (unshaded area between hallux and second toe supplied by deep peroneal nerve), sciatic nerve, (peroneal branch shown separately), and posterior cutaneous nerve of thigh.*

principal peripheral nerves and of the dermatomes corresponding to the sensory root are shown in Figures 2.11 and 2.12. The dermatomes supplied by adjacent dorsal roots and the area of supply of peripheral nerve overlap considerably and vary in size depending on sensory modality, so that after an acute nerve section the loss of light touch sensation is more extensive than pin prick or temperature loss. Lesions of dorsal root or peripheral sensory nerve fibres may give rise to irritative symptoms such as sharp pains in their peripheral distribution, burning pain, tingling paraesthesiae and oversensitivity as well as negative symptoms such as numbness, loss of pain and temperature sense. See below for technique of examination.

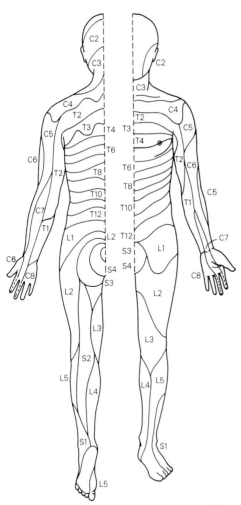

Fig. 2.12 *Cutaneous areas (dermatomes) supplied by each spinal root.*

Spinal Cord (Fig. 2.1): **Dorsal Columns**

In the spinal cord, sensory fibres enter either the dorsal columns or the posterior horns of grey matter. The predominantly myelinated fibres in the posterior columns (the central processes of cells in the dorsal root ganglia) are principally concerned with position sense, detection of movement and discriminative cutaneous sensation. Vibration sense is probably conveyed both by spinothalamic pathways in the anterolateral columns and by the posterior columns. Fibres in the posterior columns are somatotopically arranged, with those from the lower limb being medially placed while fibres from higher segments are fed in laterally. After synapsing in the gracile and cuneate nuclei second-order neurones decussate and ascend in the medial lemniscus to the ventral posterolateral nucleus of the thalamus in close relation to similar fibres from the face (Figs. 2.13, 2.14). Third-order neurones project to the sensori-motor cortex (see below).

Symptoms due to posterior column lesions include irritative phenomena such as paraesthesiae, electric shock-like sensations projected to the limbs, tight band-like sensations around the limbs, or odd feelings like water running over the surface of the limb. Deficiency symptoms include a feeling of uselessness, weakness or clumsiness of the limb. On examination, the sense of passive movement (joint position sense) may be impaired resulting in clumsy or tremulous ataxic movements (sensory ataxia). Tactile stimuli are poorly localised and the sense of direction of movement over the body surface is impaired. There is difficulty in discriminating between two or more stimuli placed close together and in comparing different weights held in the hands.

Clinical examination

In examining the patient, his ability to stand erect and maintain balance with and without the eyes closed should be tested (Romberg's sign). The sign is positive if eye closure results in increased body sway. Position sense is tested by asking the patient to perform movements with the eyes closed, e.g. placing the forefinger of the outstretched hand on the tip of the nose. Sense of passive movement is tested initially in the joints of the fingers and toes. It is essential to explain to the patient what movements are to be performed

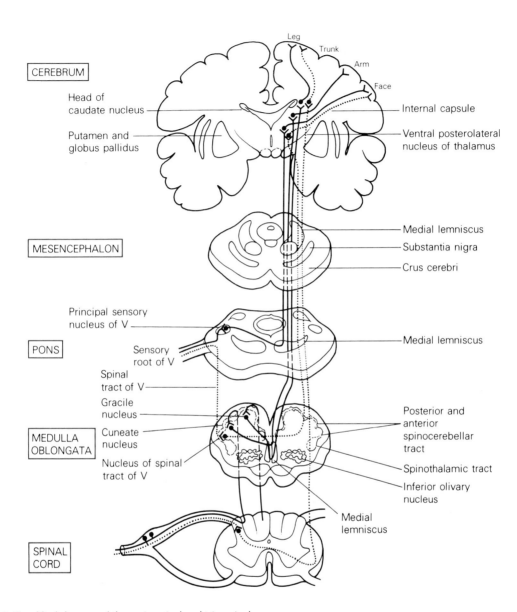

Fig. 2.13 *Simplified diagram of the main spinal and trigeminal sensory pathways.* · · · · = *first, second and third order neurones on 'spinothalamic' pathway and in pathway from spinal tract of V.* ———— = *posterior spinal afferents and their second and third order neurones, and connections from principal sensory nucleus of V (those from mesencephalic nucleus not shown).*

and what response is required, allowing plenty of time for the response to each movement. If joint position sense is judged to be abnormal peripherally, it should then be tested more proximally. Two-point discrimination is tested with blunted points applied separately or simultaneously to the skin. Two-point discrimination is very variable over the body surface, e.g. 2–3 mm on the fingertips, but 2–5 cm in the lower limb. Vibration sense is tested with a 128 c.p.s. tuning fork applied initially to the fingers and toes. The threshold for detection of all the above modalities tends to increase with age, thus in a man aged 70 vibration sense may only be clinically detectable above the knees.

Spinal Cord: Spinothalamic Pathways

Sensory fibres entering the posterior horn grey matter have complex synaptic arrangements, with collaterals often extending over several spinal segments. Fibres carrying impulses destined for the spinothalamic tracts synapse predominantly in laminae VI and VII (Fig. 2.1), second-order neurones decussate over 2 or 3 spinal segments and are then arranged somatotopically in the anterolateral columns (Fig. 2.1). Fibres carrying impulses from the lower limbs are thus progressively displaced laterally (i.e. on the outside) of those from higher segments (Fig. 2.1). Although some fibres of the 'spinothalamic' tract eventually reach the ventral posterolateral nucleus of the thalamus (Figs 2.13, 2.14), many project to the posterior and intralaminar group of thalamic nuclei (Fig. 2.14), to reticular formations and other brainstem structures.

Lesions in the grey matter of the posterior horn or central grey matter of the spinal cord may give rise to loss of pain and temperature sensation associated with preservation of position sense and discriminative function (a dissociated sensory loss). Such lesions may be associated either with spontaneous painful sensations or with numbness which may result in accidental injury such as burns. Impaired temperature sense may be reported as difficulty in detecting how hot the bath water is. A central lesion of spinal grey matter involves first those fibres which have just entered the spinal cord and are decussating: fibres from lower and/or higher segments become involved as the lesion extends longitudinally. The sensory loss thus spreads downwards or upwards from the dermatomes originally

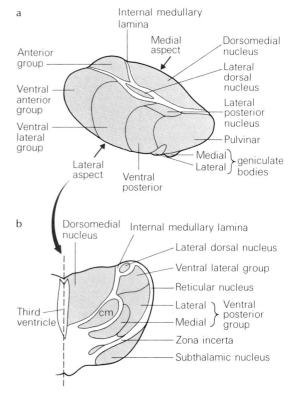

Fig. 2.14 (a) *Dorsolateral view of left thalamus to show major groups of nuclei.* (b) *Transverse section through* (a) *at level of arrows, seen from anterior aspect. C.M. = centromedian nucleus of intraluminar group.*

involved. A lesion which compresses the spinothalamic tract from outside the spinal cord will cause a contralateral disturbance of pain and temperature sense. Because fibres from the lower limb are most superficially placed and fibres at the segmental level of the lesion lie deepest, the sensory level may appear to ascend as the spinothalamic tract is progressively compressed. The upper level of the sensory disturbance is therefore often below the level of the lesion.

Clinical examination

Pain sensation is routinely tested with a sharp pin. The subjective sensation from the test pin should be established on a normal area of skin and, on moving to the abnormal area, the patient should be asked whether he detects anything at all and, if so, how the quality of the sensation differs from normality. It is loss of the sharp 'pricking' quality which is most significant in testing pain sense. The distribution of reduced pain sense should be established by moving from the abnormal area towards the normal area. Many patients are naturally more acutely sensitive to pin-prick in the inguinal region, the nipple area, and the root of the neck. Temperature sensation is assessed by comparing the quality of sensation from objects of different temperatures (e.g. tubes of hot and cold water) or thermal conductivity (e.g. plastic or steel). Light touch sensation, which is probably transmitted in both dorsal and anterolateral columns, is tested with cotton wool. The patient should be familiarised with the sensation and then asked whether sensation is subjectively altered. With his eyes closed he is then asked to respond each time stimulus is felt.

The areas of sensory loss to the above modalities should be carefully mapped out if they are thought to be of clinical relevance. In routine clinical work it is time-consuming to perform an elaborate sensory examination in every case and, on the whole, abnormalities of light touch, pain and temperature are unlikely to be found in the absence of relevant symptoms. However, abnormalities of dorsal column function are frequently either ignored or misinterpreted by patients, and these modalities should always be tested.

Brainstem and Thalamus

The proximity of the principal sensory pathways to various cranial nerve nuclei and their connections makes localisation of a sensory disturbance from a lesion in this region reasonably simple (Figs 2.5–2.7).

Above the pons the medial lemniscus, spinothalamic pathways and trigeminal lemniscus are in close apposition (Fig. 2.14) so that lesions of the upper brainstem, thalamus and internal capsule may cause a complete hemisensory disturbance affecting discriminative sensation, postural and kinesthetic sense, and causing loss of light touch, temperature and, to a lesser extent, pain sensation. Occasionally an isolated thrombotic vascular lesion in this region may cause a pure 'sensory stroke' without cranial nerve or motor pathway involvement. A feature of sensory loss associated with thalamic lesions may be unpleasant spontaneous pain.

The skin on the affected side may be hyperpathic – i.e. following a stimulus the sensation may be delayed, unpleasantly painful, and seeming to spread and radiate from the site of stimulation. The response is particularly marked after repetitive stimulation.

Cerebral Cortex (Figs 2.8, 2.13)

The distribution of sensory fibres in the cortex is extensive, including not only the primary somatosensory area in the postcentral gyrus and paracentral lobule but also the motor cortex and other related regions. There is at least one, and there are probably several, somatotopic representations of the body in the main sensory cortex, with the area of cortex associated with each part of the body being related to its importance in somatic sensation rather than physical size: thus, the hand, face and mouth are extensively represented. The lower leg, bladder, rectum and genitalia are represented medially on the hemisphere and certain areas, e.g. the face, mouth, pharynx and larynx, probably have bilateral representation. The primary somatosensory area receives a major projection from the thalamus, relaying impulses from the medial lemniscus, trigeminal lemniscus and spinothalamic tract.

Clinical examination

Disturbances of cortical sensory function can cause irritative symptoms such as tingling and paraesthesiae which may spread from one part of the body to the next when anatomically adjacent areas of cortex are involved, as in focal epilepsy or migraine. More commonly an acute cortical sensory lesion results in disturbed appreciation of all the main sensory modalities. Discriminative ability is, however, most severely and permanently affected. Typically, position sense, two-point discrimination and spatial localisation are most impaired. The ability to distinguish textures, to appreciate intensity of stimulation whether painful or thermal, to match weights and to identify objects by touch (stereognosis) is also lost. The threshold to peripheral stimuli is characteristically variable, unlike a peripheral sensory disturbance. If two stimuli are presented simultaneously to the right and left side of the body, that from the side contralateral to a lesion of the sensory cortex may not be consciously detected (sensory inattention or extinction), although the same stimulus applied alone is detected. A more elaborate disturbance of sensory function may result in a failure to recognize objects by tactile and proprioceptive pathways although these are demonstrably intact (tactile agnosia).

CRANIAL NERVES AND CONNECTIONS

Olfactory System and Cranial Nerve I
(Fig. 2.15)

The olfactory epithelium is situated in a small area in the upper part of the nasal septum. The sensory hairs are carried on olfactory rods which extend into the

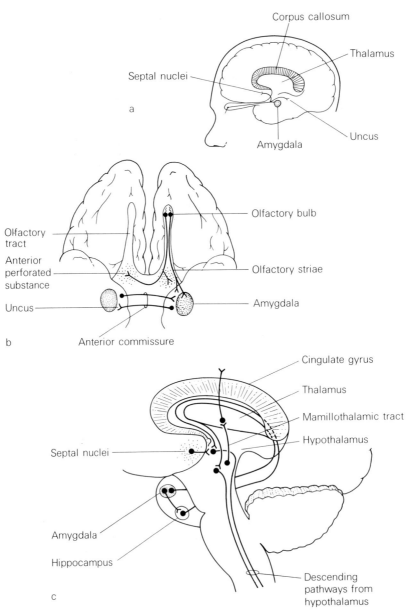

Fig. 2.15 *Olfactory pathways and the limbic system.*

overlying mucus. The geometrical molecular configuration of dissolved substances is thought to determine the olfactory response by fitting into slots or hollows in the surface of the receptors. From the olfactory cells, fibres form a plexiform network in the mucous membrane and 20 or so unmyelinated branches travel through the cribriform plate to end in the olfactory bulb. Each branch has a tubular sheath of dura and pia arachnoid, with an extension of the subarachnoid space along each bundle of nerve fibres. The olfactory nerve fibres converge onto a number of cell types (mitral cells, tufted cells) arranged in layers in the olfactory bulb. From the olfactory bulb, the olfactory tract travels on the under-surface of the frontal lobe. It mainly contains centrally-directed axons, together with a few centrifugal fibres. As it extends caudally, the olfactory tract flattens to become the smooth olfactory trigone and divides into the medial and lateral olfactory striae. The lateral stria carries axons which end in the pyriform cortex and amygdala: most of the medial stria fibres end in the anterior part of the 3rd ventricle. From these areas are numerous secondary connections with the cingulate gyrus, the hippocampus and the hypothalamus.

Clinical examination

Olfaction is tested by asking the patient to sniff a number of test odours (peppermint, camphor, etc.). The eyes should be closed and one nostril is tested at a time. Pungent odours should be avoided since these may stimulate somatic afferents of the Vth nerve.

Lesions of the olfactory system are relatively unimportant compared with the visual or auditory systems. The cribriform plate is an important route of infection into the central nervous system. Olfactory fibres may be sheared off during head injury, sometimes by a surprisingly slight injury. Resultant distortion or loss of smell may be temporary but is more often permanent. The olfactory tract may be compressed by tumour or damaged during surgery, giving rise to unilateral or bilateral anosmia. An hallucination of smell or taste (uncinate aura) is a frequent complaint of patients with temporal lobe epilepsy (see p. 109).

Vision and Cranial Nerve II: Retina (Fig. 2.16)

Derived from an evagination of a central neural tube from the forebrain, the retina consists of an outer layer

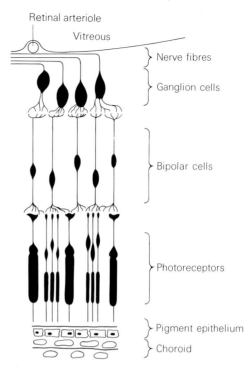

Fig. 2.16 *Diagram of the neural elements of the retina. Note that a large number of rods converge onto a single ganglion cell.*

of rods and cones, an intermediate layer of bipolar cells and Mueller cells (supporting glia), and an inner layer of ganglion cells and nerve fibres. The rods and cones are the photoreceptors and contain in their outer segments a series of laminated discs containing photosensitive pigment, retinene, an oxidative derivative of vitamin A; the inner segments are filled with dense concentrations of mitochondria.

The retina has a steady resting potential generated by the pigment epithelium adjacent to the photoreceptors. When light falls on the eye this potential changes; in the outer retinal layer this is a graded response, but in the retinal ganglion cells it is converted to a series of nerve impulses, with the discharge rate related to the strength of the stimulus. Retinal ganglion cells discharge in a variety of ways: some fire briefly and others continuously, some fire when the retina is illuminated, others in the dark.

The macular region is situated at the point of focus of light entering the eye and consists of cones only. These mediate vision in bright light. Colour discrimination is achieved by three varieties of photoreceptive pigment contained in three different groups of cones. To achieve maximum spatial resolution, cones and small ganglion cells are concentrated at the macula, where the ratio of ganglion cells to cones is 1:1. Scotopic (dark) vision is mediated by rods situated mainly in the periphery of the retina. At the periphery, the ratio of large ganglion cells to rods may be as much as 1:80 – an arrangement giving good contrast resolution.

In the clinic, retinal lesions are usually visible ophthalmoscopically and, if the choroid and pigment epithelium is involved, patches of dark pigment may be visible. Local retinal and choroidal lesions, e.g. toxoplasmosis, cause a scotoma in the visual field of one eye; localised lesions of the inner retinal layers (e.g. due to glaucoma, branch retinal artery occlusions) interrupt conduction in bundles of nerve fibres and produce an arcuate scotoma or sectorial defect. The apex of the defect is at the blind spot. Macular lesions have a marked effect on visual acuity and tend to produce visual distortion and micropsia. Positive unformed visual symptoms, e.g. dazzling, bright spots (photopsia), are a feature of retinal disease. Degeneration of the external layers of the retina results in a loss of photoreceptors; selective loss of rods produces night blindness, whereas selective loss of cones affects mainly visual acuity and loss of colour discrimination.

The blood vessels of the eye derive from two sources; the ciliary arteries supply the choroid, ciliary body, iris and the outer layers of the retina, and the central retinal artery supplies only the inner layers of the retina. The main retinal arteries at the disc have a diameter of approximately 100 microns. In vascular disease (e.g. hypertension, diabetes) the arteries may show irregularity, tortuosity or arteriovenous nipping (caused by thickening of the artery wall). Flame-shaped haemorrhages in the retina lie in the superficial layer and round haemorrhages in the deeper layers. Soft exudates are superficial and consist of swollen axons. Hard exudates are collections of fat-laden macrophages deep in the retina. Microaneuryms and regions of non-perfused capillaries are particularly associated with diabetes.

Cranial Nerve II (Optic) and Chiasm
(Fig. 2.17)

Embryologically, the IInd nerve is also derived from the brain. It consists of myelinated nerve fibres arranged in bundles with prominent fibrous septa. The cell bodies are in the ganglion cells of the retina, but the axons are unmyelinated until they reach the optic disc. At the optic discs the prominent papillomacular bundle which subserves the central part of the visual field enters the temporal side of the disc. This side is normally paler than the nasal side. In the IInd nerve the macular fibres, which make up the majority, travel in the central part. They are smaller and have a slower conduction velocity than those from the outer retina. Immediately anterior to the chiasm all axons from the nasal retina (i.e. those medial to the fovea) separate from those from the temporal retina and cross the mid-line in the optic chiasm (Fig. 2.17). The blood supply to the IInd nerve is derived mainly from the posterior ciliary (not retinal) arteries, with multiple small arteries arising from the ophthalmic artery within the orbit.

Lesions of the nerve fibres in the retina or optic disc, most often produced by vascular occlusion, tend to produce multiple arcuate field defects corresponding to loss of bundles of nerve fibres. In many cases, lesions of the nerve head lead eventually to optic atrophy. If this occurs without previous swelling of the disc it is termed primary. The disc is pale, the edge is clear-cut, and the vessels are normal. The pallor is due to gliosis and loss of capillaries. Optic atrophy which follows disc swelling is termed secondary. In this case the margin of the disc is hazy and the vessels are sheathed.

Lesions of the IInd nerve (Table 2.5) tend to produce central defects in the visual field, with early impairment of visual acuity and colour vision. In these cases, conduction in the optic nerve fibres may be completely abolished; lesser degrees of damage may block rapid trains of impulses or may slow conduction over a damaged segment (continuous rather than saltatory conduction). Acute lesions near the disc may cause transient swelling of the nerve head, whereas more chronic lesions cause optic atrophy. Interruption of fibres subserving the pupillary light reflex causes a reduction in amplitude and speed of the direct pupillary reaction (afferent pupillary defect), although the pupils are equal in size (see p. 36).

As in the optic nerve, the majority of chiasmal fibres subserve the central 20° of the visual field. Those subserving the field immediately lateral to the point of fixation cross in the posterior part of the chiasm. The chiasm is well protected from trauma and seldom involved in vascular occlusion since it is supplied by a

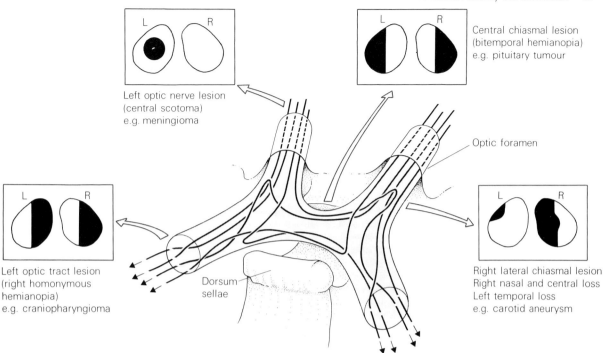

Central chiasmal lesion
(bitemporal hemianopia)
e.g. pituitary tumour

Left optic nerve lesion
(central scotoma)
e.g. meningioma

Optic foramen

Left optic tract lesion
(right homonymous
hemianopia)
e.g. craniopharyngioma

Dorsum
sellae

Right lateral chiasmal lesion
Right nasal and central loss
Left temporal loss
e.g. carotid aneurysm

Fig. 2.17 *To show the arrangement of the retinal projection at the optic chiasm; the fibres from the nasal half of the retina decussate. Note that the fibres from the lower nasal retina cross in the anterior part of the chiasm and sweep towards the contralateral optic nerve.*

number of small blood vessels. It is, however, vulnerable to compression from pituitary tumours, and other suprasellar masses, e.g. craniopharyngioma and meningioma. The mark of the chiasmal lesion is a break at the vertical meridian in the centre of the visual field, with preferential loss of the temporal field. This is due to involvement of crossing fibres. Optic atrophy of the whole disc is usually present and visual acuity is often reduced.

Optic Tracts and Radiation (Figs 2.18, 2.19)

Fibres subserving either the right or left half of the field pass to the opposite optic tract and, mainly, to the lateral geniculate body. Lesions of the optic tract produce homonymous hemianopia which is usually incongruous (i.e. affecting one eye more than the other). Optic atrophy is usually present. Optic tract lesions are rare. About 60% of the million axons in each

optic nerve terminate at the lateral geniculate nuclei, which are small triangular bodies with six layers of neurones. The crossed and uncrossed fibres end in adjacent layers of the nuclei in such a way that fibres from corresponding parts of the two retinas terminate close to each other (Fig. 2.18). The main function of the nucleus is to make possible the fusion of the visual images of corresponding parts of the two eyes. After synapsing, a second axon travels in the optic radiation (Fig. 2.19) to terminate in the primary visual cortex (striate cortex).

The optic radiation is spread over a wide area: its lower fibres pass through the temporal lobe, and the upper fibres pass through the parietal lobe on their way to the occipital cortex. The radiation has a dual blood supply from the middle and posterior cerebral arteries.

The remaining 40% of optic nerve axons bypass the lateral geniculate body to terminate in the superior colliculus and in the tectum of the midbrain (Fig. 2.5).

Table 2.5

IInd (Optic) Nerve Lesions

Type	Clinical feature	Diagnosis
Demyelinating (retrobulbar neuritis)	Papillitis Optic atrophy Central scotoma	Look for other signs of MS. Do VEP. Examine CSF
Compressive e.g. meningioma, pituitary adenoma, aneurysm, glioma of nerve	Optic atrophy Central scotoma Chiasmal signs	Always x-ray skull. Check field in other eye. Enhanced CT scan
Vascular e.g. occlusion of ciliary arteries, temporal arteritis	Ischaemic papillitis Arcuate defects	Look for small vessel disease. Check BP. Exclude diabetes Check ESR
Infective e.g. spread from sinus infection or orbital cellulitis	Papillitis Artery occlusion Optic atrophy Orbital signs	Nasal discharge. X-ray changes
Toxic e.g. tobacco, alcohol, ethambutol	Centrocaecal scotoma (bilateral) Disc normal	Radiology negative. Reversible visual loss
Raised intracranial pressure e.g. cerebral tumour, benign intracranial hypertension	Papilloedema – secondary atrophy Peripheral field contraction esp. lower nasal Enlarged blind spot	CT scan may show cerebral tumour or hydrocephalus Lumbar puncture to confirm raised pressure only *after* exclusion of space-occupying lesion

These fibres are concerned with unconscious visual fixation reflexes (superior colliculus) and with the pupillary light reflex (midbrain tectum, Edinger–Westphal nucleus of IIIrd nerve).

Visual Cortex (Figs 2.19 2.20)

The visual cortex on each side is situated almost entirely on the medial surface of the hemisphere. It includes the region around and buried within the calcarine sulcus. There is point-to-point representation of the half retina on each side and the lower retina projects to the lower part of the visual cortex. Fibres subserving central vision project to the more posterior part, and peripheral fibres more anteriorly (Fig. 2.20). Individual cells and columns of cells respond to stripes or edges of light at a specific orientation falling on one or both eyes. Simple cells respond to such stimuli only at a fixed point in the retina, but more complex cells respond to appropriately orientated stimuli regardless of their position in the field.

Surrounding the primary visual cortex, which is concerned with conscious detection and elementary discrimination of shapes, are a number of secondary regions concerned with the analysis of visual information. These regions receive projections from the visual

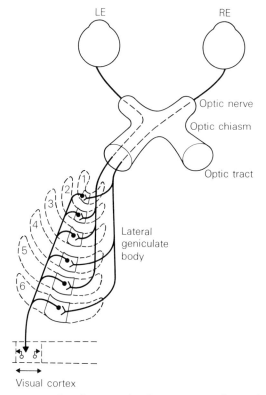

Fig. 2.18 *To show how impulses from corresponding regions of the two retinas project to vertical columns in the lateral geniculate body and thence to the visual cortex.*

cortex but probably not directly from the retina or lateral geniculate body. The functions of these regions have been deduced by mapping the type of visual stimulus required to excite the individual cells. The prestriate cortex immediately adjacent to the calcarine area is concerned with the analysis of visual form and the discrimination of such qualities as contour, brightness and size. Cells in the occipitotemporal region are coded for colour perception, and in the parietal regions they are concerned with the localisation of visual stimuli and the orientation of gaze.

More complex functions involve some degree of hemisphere specialisation. The left hemisphere plays the dominant part in visuoverbal tasks such as reading and verbal memory, and also in object recognition, whereas the right hemisphere is dominant for tasks involving visuospatial judgement, the recognition of faces and scenes, and the memory of nonverbal material.

Lesions in the visual cortex and occipital lobe produce loss of the opposite half of vision (homonymous hemianopia), but central visual acuity remains intact. In many types of lesion there is sparing of a small region of the central field around the fixation point (macular sparing). This is usually a reflection of the large proportion of visual cortex devoted to central vision and does not indicate bilateral macular representation

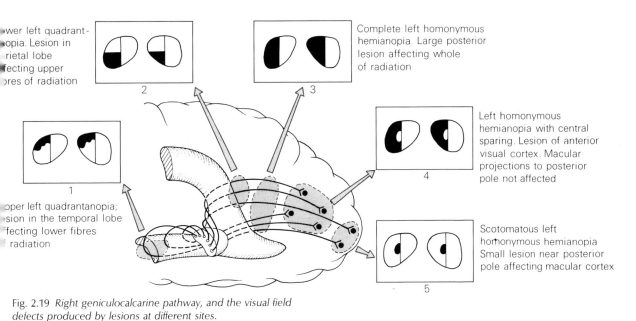

Fig. 2.19 *Right geniculocalcarine pathway, and the visual field defects produced by lesions at different sites.*

(Fig. 2.20): a further factor is the alternative blood supply to the posterior pole, where central vision is represented. Smaller lesions of the occipital cortex may produce quadrantic or scotomatous hemianopias and the defect is usually identical in each eye (congruous). Loss of vision within the field defect may be absolute or relative and some patients may retain some visual functions while losing others, e.g. they may be able to see moving but not stationary objects, or they may be able to detect a stimulus but be unable to locate it (visual disorientation).

Bilateral lesions (usually vascular) cause loss of vision in both halves of the visual field. Complete blindness may result but more often a small island of vision is retained. The pupillary reaction to light is unaffected.

Clinical examination

Visual acuity is measured in each eye by a standard test card at a distance of six metres (Snellen) or at reading distance (Jaeger) under standard lighting conditions. The patient's eyes are corrected for any refractive error.

A normal visual acuity is 6/5 (Snellen), N2 (Jaeger). Acuity measured in this way is a relatively crude test of visual function. Methods which test the patient's contrast sensitivity, such as the ability to see a faint pattern or grating, are more sensitive to minor degrees of damage. Visual fields are tested by confrontation, when the examiner compares the patient's field with his own by holding a small object equidistant between them. More accurate methods employ a perimeter (Bjerrom screen, Goldman) with standard objects and illumination. Isopters for standard objects of different size are recorded on a chart (quantitative perimetry).

The visual field is roughly circular around the fixation spot, with the temporal field being a little more extensive, and the field shows generalised contraction when illumination is reduced or when a smaller object is used. The blind spot corresponding to the optic disc is situated on the temporal side of fixation.

Defects in the visual field are of two types, depressive or scotomatous. In depressional defects there is constriction of the field or part of the field. In the scotomatous type there is a circumscribed 'hole' where

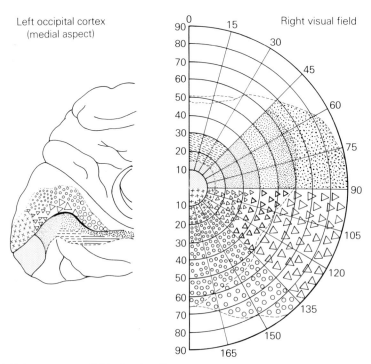

Fig. 2.20 *Diagram of right homonymous field, showing the projection of the various parts of the visual field in the left occipital cortex.*

an object cannot be seen. The defect can be absolute (no object, however bright or large, can be seen) or relative (only small or dark objects are lost).

Colour vision is tested by the ability to read the Ishihara or other pseudoisochromatic plates.

Ocular Movements and Cranial Nerves III, IV, and VI (Figs 2.21 and 2.22)

The eyes are moved by the extraocular muscles, innervated by the IIIrd (oculomotor), IVth (trochlear) and VIth (abducens) nerves. The actions of these nerves in ocular movements are shown in Table 2.6. The actions of the superior and inferior recti and oblique muscles depend on the position of the globe. Thus the superior rectus primarily elevates the abducted globe but internally rotates the adducted globe: the superior oblique primarily depresses the adducted globe but internally rotates (intorts) the abducted globe. Most ocular movements depend on activity in at least two muscles. For example, elevation of the eye in mid position is the result of contraction of the inferior oblique and the superior rectus, and depression of the eye is due to superior oblique and inferior rectus.

Normally the visual axes of the two eyes remain parallel and their movements are yoked together (conjugate gaze). The movements of the two eyes are integrated together within the IIIrd nerve nuclei and through the medial longitudinal fasciculus (MLF) (Fig. 2.21). Lateral movements of the eyes are coordinated in the pontine paramedian reticular formation (PPRF: Fig. 2.21) and vertical eye movements are coordinated in the midbrain.

The IIIrd nerve passes ventrally from the midbrain to the interpeduncular fossa, below the origin of the posterior cerebral artery and parallel and lateral to the posterior communicating artery. It then runs between the posterior clinoid process and the free edge of the tentorium (where it is closely related to the medial temporal lobe), and enters the cavernous sinus. The nerve enters the orbit through the superior orbital fissure and supplies the extraocular muscles (Table 2.6), levator palpebrae superioris, and preganglionic para-sympathetic fibres to the ciliary ganglion. The IVth nerve passes dorsally from the midbrain, decussates with that from the other side, passes around the midbrain and then follows a similar course to the IIIrd nerve to supply the superior oblique muscle.

The VIth nerve passes ventrally from the lower border of the pons and penetrates the dura of the clivus below the posterior clinoid processes, passes near the apex of the petrous bone and the inferior petrosal sinus, and then enters the cavernous sinus where it is closely related to the internal carotid artery. It subsequently enters the orbit through the superior orbital fissure.

Supranuclear control of eye movements

Commands for saccadic (fast voluntary or reflex) eye movements in the horizontal plane probably originate in the pre-motor 'frontal eye fields'. Fibres pass in the anterior limb of the internal capsule, decussate in the upper pons and terminate in the PPRF (Fig. 2.21). Pursuit or tracking movements appear to depend on intact connections of the PPRF with the ipsilateral cortical visual association areas. The control of eye position in relation to head position is partly dependent on reflex connections with the vestibular nuclei. Head accelerations detected by the semicircular canals result in reflex changes in eye position (vestibulo-ocular reflexes). In the absence of visual fixation, these reflexes are predominant so that a sudden rotatory movement of the head to the left will, after an initial lag when the eyes look to the right, result in re-centering of the visual

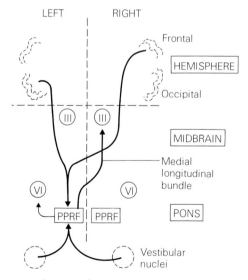

Fig. 2.21 *Schematic diagram of main pathways controlling horizontal ocular movements to the left.*

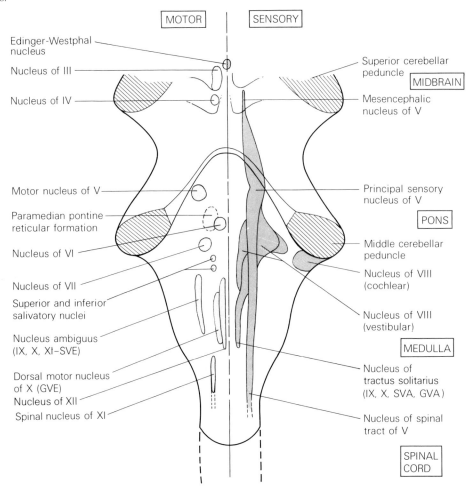

Fig. 2.22 *Schematic dorsal view of infratentorial cranial nerve nuclei seen in longitudinal section. Efferent (motor) cell groups on left, afferent (sensory) cell groups on right. SVE and GVE = special and general visceral afferent components.*

axes (oculo-cephalic – doll's head – eye movements). Similar reflexes occur in the vertical plane.

Pupil light reactions

The afferent pathway for the light reflex passes from retinal ganglion cells to the IInd nerve. Decussation in the optic chiasm results in bilateral transmission of light information to the pretectal area and rostral midbrain. The efferent fibres to the iris sphincter originate in the Edinger–Westphal nucleus (Fig. 2.22: part of IIIrd nerve nucleus) and pass to the IIIrd nerve where they lie

grouped superficially in the early part of its course. These parasympathetic fibres travel in the branch to the inferior oblique muscle and synapse in the ciliary ganglion: postganglionic fibres pass, via short ciliary nerves, to the iris. A light shone into one pupil results in pupillary constriction in the test eye and constriction of similar amplitude and velocity in the other eye (consensual reflex). Parasympathetic fibres to the ciliary muscles (for accommodation) originate in the rostral part of the Edinger–Westphal nucleus and, under normal conditions, accommodation is associated with pupillary constriction. (See also p. 36.)

Table 2.6

Eye Movements

Muscle	Nerve supply	Principal action for clinical testing
Lateral rectus	VI	Abduction
Medial rectus	III	Adduction
Superior rectus	III	Elevation of abducted globe
Inferior rectus	III	Depression of abducted globe
Inferior oblique	III	Elevation of adducted globe
Superior oblique	IV	Depression of adducted globe
		Intorsion of abducted globe

Sympathetic pathways

The sympathetic supply to the eye and face originates in the hypothalamus, passes uncrossed through mid-brain, pons and lateral medulla and exits from the spinal cord at T1. At this site preganglionic fibres are in close relation to the apex of the lung as they ascend in the paravertebral sympathetic chain. Postganglionic fibres originate in the superior cervical ganglion. Those sympathetic fibres destined for the eye form a plexus around the internal carotid artery whilst fibres concerned with facial sweating and pilo-erection follow branches of the external carotid artery. The internal carotid group enter the orbit with the ophthalmic artery and oculomotor nerves and supply the pupil dilator and smooth muscle in the levator of the upper eyelid (Mueller's muscle).

Clinical examination

After inspecting the eyes generally, the position of the eyelids in relation to the iris is noted – if necessary, measuring the width of the palpebral fissure. If a patient is able to make voluntary eye movements, the saccadic and pursuit systems are both tested. The purpose is to see whether eye movements are conjugate, to detect diplopia and analyse it, and to detect nystagmus. Saccadic movements are examined by asking the patient to look left, right, up and down as quickly as possible. In testing pursuit movements, an object is held 40–50 cm from the eyes and the patient asked to follow a slowly moving point throughout the range of

binocular vision in the horizontal and vertical planes. The patient reports whether the object appears double.

Nerve lesions

In a severe nerve lesion affecting one eye the cause of diplopia is usually obvious. Thus, in a complete VIth nerve lesion the eye fails to abduct beyond the midline, while in a complete IIIrd nerve lesion there is ptosis, the globe points downwards and laterally due to the unopposed actions of the lateral rectus and superior oblique, and the pupil is enlarged and unreactive. A IVth nerve lesion is suggested by diplopia on reading or looking down and results in incomplete depression of the globe in adduction (or failure of intortion of the eye when the globe is depressed in abduction).

In less severe or more complex lesions the cause of diplopia can be analysed by following certain rules. The eye position in which the two images are furthest apart is the direction of the main action of the paralysed muscle – thus, if diplopia is maximal on looking upwards and to the right, either the left inferior oblique or the right superior rectus is weak. The peripheral image of the pair arises from the paralysed eye – thus, in the latter example, if the peripheral image disappears when the right eye is covered then the right superior rectus is weak. It is useful to know whether the images are separated from side to side, vertically or obliquely, as clearly a pure lateral or medial rectus lesion is unlikely to be accompanied by major vertical or oblique separation of images. If diplopia persists on covering one eye then the cause is either monocular due to a refractive defect of the lens or cornea or may be hysterical.

The site of a lesion causing an oculomotor nerve palsy may frequently be deduced from signs caused by damage to related anatomical structures. Isolated IIIrd and VIth nerve palsies occur, due to lesions at a variety of sites along their course (see Table 2.7). When ocular movements are bilaterally impaired the lesion may be in the brainstem, or due to bilateral nerve disorders, or due to disorders of the ocular muscles such as dysthyroid eye disease, myasthenia gravis or ocular myopathy.

Internuclear ophthalmoplegia

A lesion of the medial longitudinal fasciculus (MLF) gives rise to an internuclear ophthalmoplegia. For example, on left lateral gaze the MLF allows synchronous abduction of the left eye and adduction of the right eye to maintain conjugate gaze. Thus impulses from the PPRF (Fig. 2.21) go to the left VIth nerve nucleus and to the right IIIrd nerve nucleus via the MLF. A lesion of the MLF results in intact abduction but slowed or absent adduction, which is often most easily seen during fast pursuit or saccadic eye movements. Nystagmus is commonly seen in the abducting eye. The lesion may be unilateral (i.e. occurs in one direction of gaze) or bilateral. The cause is usually a plaque of demyelination (see Chapter 9) or a discrete vascular lesion.

Gaze palsies

A lesion of supranuclear pathways from one frontal lobe results in impaired horizontal conjugate gaze to the contralateral side; a lesion in the brainstem involving the PPRF may cause impaired gaze to the ipsilateral side (Fig. 2.21). Irritative foci of the frontal lobe, as during a focal epileptic fit, may result in forced deviation of the eyes to the contralateral side. Failure of upward gaze is usually the result of an upper midbrain lesion, most frequently due to a supratentorial mass (see Chapter 6), or a more localised compression of the dorsum of the midbrain, e.g. by a pineal tumour. Impaired upward gaze is also a feature of some extrapyramidal disorders (see p. 10).

The eyelid

The upper eyelid is maintained in position and elevated by the levator palpebrae superioris muscle, innervated by the IIIrd nerve, and by a thin sheet of smooth muscle innervated by sympathetic fibres. Overactivity of the latter leads to the lid retraction and lid lag seen in hyperthyroidism and in lesions of the midbrain.

Ptosis (drooping of the lid) may be congenital or acquired. The commonest acquired lesions are those of the sympathetic (as part of Horner's syndrome) or IIIrd nerve (associated with oculomotor paresis). Disorders of muscle notably myasthenia, myotonic dystrophy and progressive external ophthalmoplegia (see Chapter 17) cause ptosis, most often bilaterally. Occasionally, orbital disease or trauma may also cause ptosis. Ptosis should be differentiated from blepharospasm, which is due to contraction of orbicularis oculi (VIIth nerve) resulting from photophobia, local ocular irritation, an extrapyramidal disorder or, occasionally, hysteria.

The pupils

The innervation of the pupil has already been outlined (p. 34). On examining the pupils particular attention should be paid to their shape, to their size under normal ambient lighting conditions, and to the direct and consensual responses to light and the response to visual fixation on a near object.

Afferent pupil defect: A unilateral lesion of the optic nerve results in a reduced or absent direct response when light is shone into the eye and a similarly reduced consensual response in the other eye, the two pupils being equal in size. When light is shone into the normal eye, both pupils constrict normally. Thus when a light is swung from the normal to the abnormal side both pupils may dilate due to the reduced afferent input from the abnormal side (Marcus–Gunn pupil).

Horner's syndrome: The sympathetic innervation to the eye may be damaged at any point over its extensive course (see above); the features of the fully developed Horner's syndrome are a small pupil (miosis), a partial ptosis, with the ipsilateral face being warm, hyperaemic and anhidrotic due to loss of sweating and vasoconstrictor fibres. Horner's syndrome may result from lesions in the brainstem or cervical spinal cord, from

Table 2.7

Causes of Ocular Paresis

1.	Gaze palsies	horizontal	Hemisphere lesion (eyes deviated to side of lesion)
			PPRF brain stem lesion (eyes deviated to contralateral side)
		vertical	Brainstem compression or distortion
			Dorsal lesions in upper midbrain (e.g. pineal tumour)
			Extrapyramidal disease (Parkinson's, progressive supranuclear palsy)
2.	Nuclear and nerve (III, IV, VI) palsies	brainstem	Tumour, vascular lesion, demyelination, encephalitis, Wernicke's encephalopathy, congenital anomaly, brainstem distortion
		peripheral	Medial temporal lobe herniation (III)
			Any cause of raised intracranial pressure (VI)
			Vascular lesions: diabetes mellitus, atheroma, temporal arteritis, syphilis, aneurysm – (infraclinoid (III, IV, VI) – supraclinoid (III) cavernous sinus – fistula – thrombosis
			Meningeal inflammation or infiltration
			Tumour of skull base (pituitary, chordoma, nasopharyngeal carcinoma)
			Cranial polyneuritis (Guillain–Barré, sarcoidosis, neoplasia)
			Orbital tumour, granuloma, sinus disease, orbital fissure meningioma
3.	Muscle diseases		Myasthenia gravis
			Thyroid eye disease
			Progressive myopathic external ophthalmoplegia (e.g. mitochondrial myopathy)

involvement of the sympathetic fibres by pathology in the apex of the lung or the superior mediastinum, or from injury in the neck. The ocular manifestations alone may occur in lesions of the internal carotid artery.

Light/near dissociation: The Argyll Robertson pupil, one of the hallmarks of late syphilis (p. 234), is characterised by small irregular pupils, often with atrophy of the iris, with an absent or reduced response to light, but preserved near response. Tumours impinging on the tectum of the midbrain may also cause a dissociated light/near response. In such cases the pupils are largish, react poorly to light but well to a near target and there may be impairment of upward gaze and lid retraction (Collier's sign).

Holmes Adie pupil, 'tonic' pupil: This is a common cause of marked pupillary inequality. Observed in light, the involved pupil is large and reacts poorly if at all to bright light but shows a slow contraction to prolonged near convergence effort. Subsequent dilatation of the pupil after near effort is also slow. The iris may show small vermiform movements of its borders and the condition is associated with diminished deep tendon reflexes. There is evidence of denervation and supersensitivity of the iris sphincter, which constricts intensely with a weak cholinomimetic such as 2.5% methacholine (normally no miosis is seen even with a 20% solution). The ocular manifestations are thought to be explained by a lesion in the ciliary ganglion. Slight pupillary inequality (anisocoria) occurs in about 20% of the population.

Vth Cranial Nerve (Trigeminal) (Figs 2.13, 2.22, 2.23, Table 2.8)

The sensory fibres of the Vth cranial nerve innervate skin over the face and front part of head (Fig. 2.23), the mucous membranes of nose, nasal sinuses and mouth, teeth, temporomandibular joints, a large part of the supratentorial dura, and the spindles of the muscles of mastication. The fibres are grouped into ophthalmic, maxillary and mandibular divisions, with the latter division also carrying the motor fibres to the muscles of mastication. The cell bodies of the sensory fibres are in the trigeminal ganglion, apart from some of those

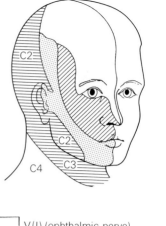

V (I) (ophthalmic nerve)

V (II) (maxillary nerve)

V (III) (mandibular nerve)

C2 and C3 (dorsal rami and ventral rami via cervical plexus)

Fig. 2.23 *Cutaneous areas (dermatomes) of head and neck supplied by the three divisions of the trigeminal nerve, C2 and C3 (C1 has no cutaneous distribution).*

associated with proprioception and muscle spindles which are within the brainstem.

The central processes of these cells enter the lateral pons in close relation to the VIIth and VIIIth nerves in the cerebello-pontine angle. In the pons a substantial proportion of fibres divide into ascending branches (ending in the principal sensory nucleus, Figs 2.13, 2.22 and probably homologous with the posterior column nuclei of the cord) and descending branches which together form the spinal trigeminal tract. In this tract fibres from the ophthalmic division lie ventrally and extend most caudally, while those from the mandibular division lie dorsally, with maxillary fibres occupying an intermediate position. Fibres from the central part of the face terminate more rostrally than those from peripheral parts, which are caudally placed. The fibres synapse in the nucleus of the spinal trigeminal tract (Fig 2.22), which merges caudally with the substantia gelatinosa of the cord.

Second-order sensory neurones, both crossed and

uncrossed, ascend from the main sensory and spinal nuclei in close association with the medial lemniscus and terminate in the ventral posteromedial nucleus of the thalamus (Figs 2.13, 2.14). The principal sensory nucleus probably relays tactile and mechanical stimuli, whilst the spinal nucleus is important in pain and temperature sensation. The mesencephalic nucleus contains the cell bodies of afferent trigeminal fibres, conveying proprioceptive and stretch-receptor impulses concerned with mastication. Collaterals of these fibres also pass to the Vth nerve motor nucleus, establishing a monosynaptic reflex pathway between muscle spindles and motor neurones which is the basis of the jaw-jerk reflex (see p. 11). Trigeminal sensory fibres also project bilaterally and polysynaptically to the VIIth nerve nuclei, providing the basis for the corneal and blink reflexes (see p. 40). The motor nucleus of V (Fig. 2.22) is innervated by corticobulbar fibres both directly and through interneurones in the reticular formations: it usually receives bilateral motor neurone innervation.

Examination of the Vth nerve

Motor function: Wasting of the temporalis muscle is detected by looking for hollowing of the temple and of the masseter by palpation whilst the patient clenches the jaws together. As the mouth is opened, unilateral pterygoid weakness results in deviation of the jaw to the paralysed side. A unilateral upper motor neurone lesion does not cause deviation of jaw opening but occasionally results in contralateral weakness of the masseter, evident on palpation. The jaw jerk is tested routinely: the slack lower jaw is percussed on the chin in a downward direction. An absent jerk has no significance whilst a brisk jerk may suggest a bilateral lesion of corticopontine fibres; it may also be due to nonspecific generalised hyper-reflexia.

Sensation: Light touch, pin-prick and temperature are tested as previously described (p. 23). The distribution of sensory loss (Fig. 2.23) is important in diagnosis. Generalised sensory loss over all divisions suggests a lesion of the sensory root or ganglion whilst a selective generalised loss in one division suggests a more peripheral lesion. The ophthalmic division is particularly prone to involvement by pathology in the orbit or cavernous in the cavernous sinus or the skull base; and

the mandibular division is prone to involvement in the skull base (Table 2.8).

An ipsilateral dissociated sensory loss may result from lesions of the descending tracts/spinal nucleus caused in particular by vascular occlusion (see p. 135) and syringobulbia. An intrinsic ascending cervical lesion (e.g. tumour or syrinx) classically tends to involve the peripheral parts of the face initially, with the nose and mouth becoming involved as the lesion extends rostrally.

The corneal reflex is tested by carefully touching a wisp of cotton wool onto the cornea (not the conjunctiva). Synchronous blinking of both eyes occurs. An afferent defect (Vth nerve lesion) will result in depression or absence of the direct and consensual reflex. An efferent defect (VIIth nerve lesion) will cause an incomplete or absent response on the side of the facial weakness. Contact lenses cause reduced sensitivity. The reflex is depressed at an early stage in tumours expanding in the cerebello-pontine angle; it may also be depressed in contralateral internal capsular lesions, probably because of altered excitability of interneurones in the reflex pathway. Absence of the corneal reflex is potentially hazardous since the cornea may be accidentally damaged and/or infected without the patient being alerted by pain.

VIIth Nerve (Facial) (Figs 2.6, 2.22, Table 2.9)

The VIIth nerve comprises motor fibres supplying the muscles of facial expression and the stapedius muscle, special visceral afferents conveying taste from the anterior two-thirds of the tongue via the chorda tympani (see p. 248), and general somatic afferents from the external auditory meatus and concha of the ear; the sensory fibres have their cell bodies in the geniculate ganglion.

General visceral efferent fibres from the superior salivatory nucleus (Fig. 2.22) pass to the lacrimal gland, to the mucous membrane of the nose and mouth and to the submandibular and sublingual salivary glands. Fibres from the VIIth nerve nucleus (Fig. 2.6) loop around the VIth nerve nucleus before leaving the pons in the cerebello-pontine angle and enter the internal auditory meatus with the VIIIth nerve. The nerve passes in close relation to the middle ear, giving off the chorda tympani branch and the nerve to stapedius, and

Table 2.8

Vth (Trigeminal) Nerve Lesions

1. In brainstem	tumour, vascular lesion, syrinx, demyelination	
2. Roots, ganglion, main divisions	cerebello-pontine angle	Tumour (acoustic neuroma), vascular compression
	petrous ridge	Vth nerve tumour, osteomyelitis of petrous apex
	cavernous sinus (I & II divisions)	Carotid aneurysm, fistula, sinus thrombosis, lateral extension of pituitary tumour
	skull base (II & III divisions)	Tumour (nasopharyngeal carcinoma, metastases, chordoma)
	orbital fissure/orbit (I division)	Sphenoid ridge meningioma, orbital disease
	other	Neoplastic/meningeal infiltration, Guillain–Barré syndrome, other causes of cranial poly-neuritis, idiopathic neuropathy of V, trigeminal neuralgia

leaving the skull via the stylomastoid foramen, after which it is closely related to the parotid gland. The part of the nucleus of VII supplying the upper part of the face receives bilateral (crossed and uncrossed) cortical innervation, whilst that to the lower face receives unilateral crossed fibres. Voluntary and emotional facial expression have, in part, separate supranuclear path-ways.

Examination

The two sides of the face and their movements should be compared whilst observing the patient during conversation. A general lack of facial expression may be caused by severe facial muscle weakness but is also a feature of extrapyramidal disease and depressive illness. The patient is asked to close the eyes tightly and the amount of eyelash still visible is compared on the two sides. Eye closure is also tested against resistance. Movement of the lower face is assessed by asking the patient to show the teeth, blow out the cheeks or whistle.

A lower motor-neurone lesion results in weakness of the whole of the side of the face, giving incomplete eye closure, loss of forehead wrinkling, and impaired movements of the mouth. When acute, the latter may result in slurred speech and drooling of saliva. The palpebral fissure is widened due to sagging of the lower lid and the cornea may be susceptible to damage due to reduced blinking. If all the fibres in the VIIth nerve are damaged there may be hyperacusis due to involve-ment of the nerve to stapedius, loss of normal tear formation, and loss of taste over the anterior part of the tongue.

The commonest cause of a lower motor neurone facial weakness is an idiopathic condition known as Bell's palsy (see p. 248). Other causes of facial weakness are shown in Table 2.9. Intermittent clonic contractions of the muscles of facial expression on one side (hemifacial spasm) are associated with mild facial weakness. The condition is thought to arise from irritation of the facial nerve and requires differentiation from focal motor epilepsy which may also cause twitching of the face. Abnormal irregular facial move-

Table 2.9

VIIth (Facial) Nerve Lesions

1. Brainstem	tumour, vascular lesion syrinx, demyelination	
2. Peripheral	cerebello-pontine angle	Tumour (acoustic neuroma, epidermoid meningioma), vascular compression
	petrous bone	middle ear infection, Bell's palsy, Geniculate herpes zoster
	face	Parotid tumours, trauma
	other	Meningeal infiltration/inflammation (e.g. sarcoid, neoplastic disease) Other causes of cranial polyneuritis (e.g. Guillain–Barré syndrome) Motor neurone disease Muscle disease: myasthenia gravis, polymyositis, myotonic dystrophy, FSH dystrophy

ments may be associated with extrapyramidal disease and neuroleptic medication (orofacial dyskinesias). Facial myokimia – persistent fine rippling spontaneous movements of the facial muscles – is caused by a brainstem lesion, notably demyelination or pontine glioma. Occasional twitches of facial muscles, particularly around the eye, are common in fatigue and have no pathological significance. True fasciculations may occur in motor neurone disease.

Taste

Taste buds, consisting of clumps of ciliated 'taste' cells with supporting cells, are found in the tongue and soft palate in close relation to terminal nerve fibres. Fibres from taste buds in the anterior two-thirds of the tongue travel, via the lingual nerve and chorda tympani, to join the VIIth nerve in the facial canal. The cell bodies are in the geniculate ganglion and gustatory impulses travel to the brainstem in the nervus intermedius. Fibres from the posterior third of the tongue and adjacent soft palate travel in the glossopharyngeal nerve and have their cell bodies in the petrosal ganglion. All taste fibres are distributed to the nucleus of the tractus solitarius in the medulla (Figs 2.7, 2.22). The central connections of the tractus solitarius are uncertain. From the pontine taste area on each side, fibres cross in the upper brainstem, relay in the ventroposterior nucleus of the thalamus, and travel to the cerebral cortex. The cortical taste area is located close to the locus for somatic sensation of the tongue.

Examination of taste

Taste is tested by applying solutions of different types (salt, sweet, bitter) to the tongue and comparing the response of the two sides. The threshold for taste sensation may be objectively measured using a weak electric current. Only peripheral lesions are of any clinical relevance. Lesions of the facial nerve proximal to the middle ear (where the chorda tympani leaves) cause loss of taste (ageusia) over the anterior two-thirds of the tongue. The normal sensation of taste is influenced to some extent by both olfactory and somatic sensation, and lesions of Ist and Vth nerves can sometimes produce dysgeusia or ageusia.

Auditory and Vestibular Systems (Including VIIIth Cranial Nerve Vestibular System) (Figs 2.24, 2.25)

The membranous labyrinth filled with endolymph is enclosed in the compact bony labyrinth of the temporal bone and consists of the semicircular canals, utricle (Fig. 2.24), and saccule. The vestibular receptors are hair cells in the maculae of the utricle and saccule and in the cristae of the semicircular canals. The labyrinthine receptors in the utricle and saccule are sensitive to gravitational and linear forces exerted on small solid crystals (otoliths). The kinetic labyrinthine receptors are sensitive to angular acceleration and deceleration forces produced by movements of the endolymph. The central processes of the bipolar vestibular cells make up the vestibular nerve which passes through the internal auditory meatus in company with the cochlear and facial nerve. It then enters the lower border of the pons and most of the fibres divide into ascending and descending branches to pass to the four main nuclei: superior, lateral, medial and descending. The majority of fibres enter the lateral nucleus (Fig. 2.25).

The vestibular nuclei are connected with the spinal cord, cerebellum, brainstem and reticular formation. There are also many commissural connections between the nuclei on the two sides. The lateral vestibulospinal tract has a facilitatory action on extensor motor neurones in the cord. The medial vestibulospinal tract ends in spinal grey matter over a restricted region of the thoracic cord. Small numbers of vestibular fibres reach the flocculonodular portion of the cerebellum and there is also a larger pathway from the vermis of the cerebellum to the vestibular nuclei. Both afferent and efferent fibres link the vestibular nuclei with the reticular formation. The majority of fibres in the medial longitudinal fasciculus are vestibular in origin and serve to coordinate the oculomotor functions (IIIrd, IVth and VIth cranial nerves) in the brainstem (Fig. 2.25). Vestibular sensations may reach consciousness via a vestibulo-thalamo-cortical pathway. The cortical vestibular region is near the face area in the somatosensory cortex. Alternative pathways to the cortex may exist via the cerebellum and reticular formation.

Clinical vestibular disorders and nystagmus

Vestibular dysfunction produces vertigo – an unpleasant subjective sensation of movement, usually rota-

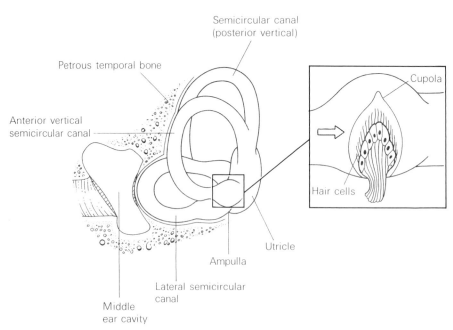

Fig. 2.24 *Structure of the semicircular canals and utricle.*

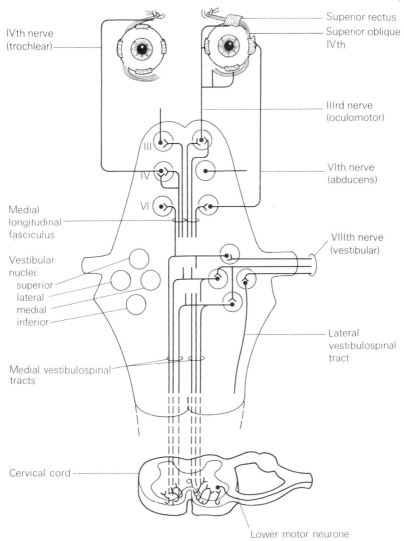

Fig. 2.25 *Central vestibular pathways — with cortical connections omitted. N.B: The levator palpebri superioris and superior rectus muscles are innervated by both IIIrd nerve nuclei.*

ory. Vertigo results from an imbalance in tonic vestibular activity in the brainstem (vestibular tonus). It is often accompanied by nausea, vomiting, oscillopsia, unsteadiness of gait and dysmetria of the arms with past pointing. A characteristic sign is nystagmus, which is a rhythmic oscillation of the eyes.

Activity in opposing pairs of extraocular muscles, and hence eye position, depends on the integration of a variety of reflex mechanisms which involve the visual and vestibular systems and muscle spindle afferents in the extraocular muscles, together with proprioceptive inputs from the muscles and joints of the head and neck. An acquired imbalance in tonic activity results in a slow drift away from the point of gaze which, in the conscious patient, may be corrected by a fast saccadic movement in the opposite direction (the vestibulo-ocular reflex). The direction of nystagmus is named according to the direction of this fast component. Nystagmus occurring only on gaze in the direction of the fast component is called first degree; in the mid position it is called second degree; and on gaze in the opposite direction it is known as third degree.

Nystagmus which is congenital or secondary to poor vision or fixation is often pendular in type, i.e. movement velocities are similar in either direction, of similar amplitude in both eyes, and horizontal in all positions of gaze. It is not associated with a subjective sensation of movement but may be associated with an oscillation of the head (titubation).

During clinical testing nystagmus is looked for in the primary position of gaze and during pursuit movements within the binocular field. If present, the following points are noted:

i. are the movements horizontal, vertical or rotatory?

ii. are the movements equal in both eyes?

iii. what is the direction of the nystagmus?

iv. in which direction of gaze is it most prominent?

v. does the direction of the nystagmus change with the position of gaze?

vi. is the nystagmus dependent on head position? (see below).

The effects of a peripheral vestibular lesion may be mimicked by cold caloric testing. For instance, with the subject supine and head flexed to thirty degrees, cold (30°C) water is flushed through the left external auditory meatus. This produces convection currents in the endolymph of the lateral semicircular canal which lie in the vertical plane. The effect is to cause a tonic deviation of the eyes to the left and accompanying fast corrective saccades to the right (3° nystagmus to the right). If standing, the subject would tend to stagger to the left and the outstretched limbs would drift to the left. In an unconscious patient the corrective saccades are suppressed and a tonic deviation to the left is seen. Warm (44°C) water in the *right* ear produces similar changes (nystagmus to the right). A peripheral vestibular lesion therefore results in horizontal or rotatory nystagmus directed away from the side of the lesion; it is worse in the dark and minimised by optic fixation. The associated symptom of vertigo is often intense but tends gradually to wear off over days or weeks. Such a lesion is often accompanied by deafness and/or tinnitus because the auditory component of the VIIIth nerve or cochlea is likely to be involved.

In benign positional vertigo a temporary disturbance of otolith function results in giddiness with certain postures of the head, typically precipitated by rolling over in bed, sudden standing or head rotation. Static labyrinthine testing may elicit the symptoms and signs. The supine patient's head and neck are extended over the end of the examination couch and the head is rotated. After a brief latent period a rotatory nystagmus beating towards the lower ear is seen, which is accompanied by vertigo. The nystagmus fades over some seconds, and immediate repetition of the test results in a reduced or absent response.

Lesions of central vestibular pathways usually cause less pronounced vertigo but often vague and more protracted giddiness and unsteadiness. The nystagmus is usually evoked by gaze to either side (gaze evoked) and is bidirectional. Nystagmus which is different in the two eyes, or is vertically beating or obliquely beating, is always central in origin. A down-beating vertical nystagmus, more prominent on lateral gaze, is characteristic of a lesion in the region of the foramen magnum (e.g. Chiari malformation). Positional vertigo of central origin usually continues for as long as the abnormal position is held, has no latent period, and does not fatigue.

Caloric testing (see above) may be useful in evaluating different types of vestibular disturbance. Labyrinthine or VIIIth (vestibular) nerve lesions cause a depression of both 'hot' and 'cold' responses from the affected side (canal paresis), whilst a central lesion causes a more complex disturbance usually with depression or enhancement of nystagmus in one or other direction (directional preponderance).

Hearing (Figs 2.26, 2.27)

Vibration of the tympanic membrane by sound waves is transmitted by the ossicles to the foot process of the stapes. At the oval window this causes displacement of endolymph which, in turn, moves the basilar membrane, thus stimulating the auditory receptors – the hair cells of the cochlear duct. The cochlea has a spiral arrangement, with receptors at the basal end being stimulated by high-frequency sound and those at the apex by low frequencies. Nerve fibres radiate through small bony channels towards the spiral ganglia, a continuous row of ganglion cells. The cochlear (auditory) nerve is composed of the axons of the bipolar spiral ganglion cells. It passes through the internal auditory meatus with the VIIth and vestibular nerve and enters the brainstem at the lower border of the pons (Fig. 2.27).

Cochlear fibres are arranged by frequency in the

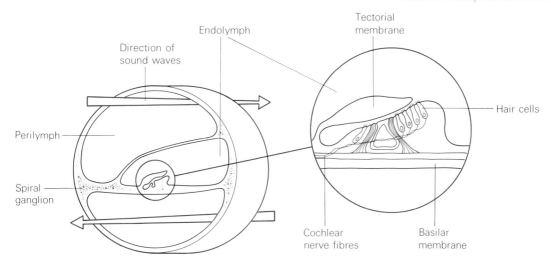

Fig. 2.26 *Structure of the auditory hair cells in the cochlea.*

cochlear ganglion and pass to the cochlear nuclei. Second-order neurones cross the brainstem to form the lateral lemniscus and reach the inferior colliculus. Some synapse en route in the superior olive. From the inferior colliculus the pathway ascends to the medial geniculate body of the thalamus and, via the auditory radiation, the impulses finally reach the auditory cortex at the superior temporal gyrus. The ascending pathways in the brainstem show frequent commissural connections and the synapses above permit interaction with other sensory inputs and in various auditory reflexes.

Clinical disorders of hearing

Unilateral deafness may result from impaired conduction of sounds in the external auditory meatus and the middle ear (conductive deafness) or from dysfunction of the auditory receptors of the cochlear nerve (sensorineural deafness). In conductive deafness, when using the classical tuning fork (256 c.p.s.) test, bone conduction is better than air conduction (−ve Rinne test); and in the Weber test, the sound is heard loudest on the affected side. Pure-tone audiometry is used to measure the degree of impaired hearing at different frequencies but speech audiometry may show impaired function before any defect of pure tones is present. Disease of the temporal bone may affect the cochlea, or the cochlear nerve, or both. Deafness is accompanied by tinnitus and vertigo. Disease affecting the receptor cells, e.g. Menière's syndrome, is characterised by loudness recruitment, i.e. the difference between the affected and unaffected ear is more obvious with soft than with loud noises. Cerebellopontine angle tumour and disease of the temporal bone tend to affect adjacent cranial nerves and the brainstem (see p. 103).

Central lesions do not usually cause deafness unless they involve the ascending pathways on both sides of the brainstem, but minor lesions causing a delay in transmission (e.g. multiple sclerosis) can be detected by recording the auditory brainstem evoked responses (p. 62). Hemisphere lesions do not cause deafness unless there is bilateral damage. There may be some impairment in the ability to localise sounds. Tinnitus and auditory hallucinations are rarely present.

IXth (Glossopharyngeal) and Xth (Vagus) Cranial Nerves (Figs 2.7, 2.22, Table 2.10)

The main components of the IXth and Xth cranial nerves are summarised in Table 2.10. The IXth nerve is predominantly sensory; it mainly supplies the posterior pharynx, the posterior third of the tongue and the carotid sinus. The Xth cranial nerve is more complex. With a minor addition from IX, it supplies the striated muscle of the pharynx, larynx and upper oesophagus.

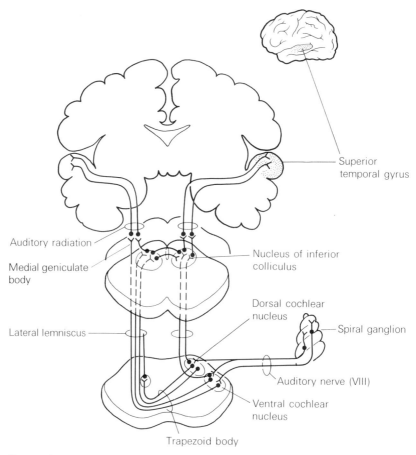

Fig. 2.27 *Central auditory pathways.*

General visceral efferent fibres from the dorsal motor nucleus of the vagus form preganglionic parasympathetic fibres. The special and general visceral afferents of IX and X terminate in the nucleus of the tractus solitarius (Figs 2.7, 2.22) which is extensively connected to the thalamus (conveying taste), to the reticular formations (where it is linked with the regulation of respiration, cardiovascular autonomic function and vomiting), and to the dorsal motor nucleus of X, phrenic nerve nucleus and intercostal muscle motor supply (which are involved in respiration, coughing and vomiting).

Clinical examination

The upper airway, phonation and articulation of speech, swallowing, palatal movement and sensation of the posterior pharynx are examined. If the vocal cords are partially paralysed there may be evidence of upper airway obstruction causing stridor particularly during sleep, speech may be hoarse or altered in volume, and the cough may lose its explosive quality and become 'bovine'. If the patient is unable to swallow adequately, repeated bouts of coughing may interrupt drinking and eating or may occur apparently spontaneously due to aspirated secretions. If there is uncertainty about swallowing the patient should be observed drinking water. Palatal weakness results in nasal regurgitation of fluid as well as giving a 'nasal' quality to the voice due to escape of air during speech. The palate should be observed at rest and during phonation or coughing. Impaired movement is usually obvious and the uvula is pulled to the stronger side if weakness is lateralised. Posterior pharyngeal sensation and the gag reflex are tested with a stimulus (e.g. an orange stick) applied to either side of the posterior

Table 2.10

Functional Subdivisions of IXth and Xth Cranial Nerves

		IX	X
1.	General somatic afferents	Cutaneous sensation on back of ear, posterior wall of external auditory meatus	
2.	General visceral afferents	Tactile, pain and temperature sense on posterior third of tongue, posterior wall of pharynx, tonsils, carotid sinus	Pharynx, larynx, respiratory tract, abdominal viscera
3.	Special visceral afferents	Taste on posterior third of tongue	Taste from region of epiglottis
4.	General visceral efferents	Inferior salivatory nucleus	Dorsal motor nucleus X
		preganglionic parasympathetic outflow (see Table 2.13)	
5.	Special visceral	Nucleus ambiguus (including cranial IX)	
		↓	
		Pharynx, larynx, upper third of oesophagus (striated muscle)	

pharyngeal wall. Both afferent and efferent lesions may occur. The routine examination may need to be supplemented by direct or indirect examination of the vocal cords. The upper motor neurone innervation for palatal and pharyngeal movement is bilateral: there is no significant dysfunction with a unilateral lesion.

XIth Cranial Nerve (Accessory)

The XI nerve (accessory) cranial root comes from the nucleus ambiguus (Fig. 2.22) and supplies the pharynx. The 'spinal root' originates from the upper five cervical segments and lower medulla: rootlets pass up through the foramen magnum, exit through the jugular foramen with the IXth and Xth nerve, and supply the sterno-mastoid and trapezius. The supranuclear innervation for mastoid is mainly from the ipsilateral hemisphere, but for trapezius it is mainly contralateral.

Clinical examination

Wasting of the sternomastoid is frequently obvious from direct observation of the neck. The patient is asked to rotate the head to one side against resistance, when the sternomastoid on the other side will then

stand out and can be palpated. Maintaining a flexed head posture against resistance causes both muscles to stand out. The trapezius is examined by observing the curve of the body between the neck and shoulder and comparing the two sides. Weakness is detected by asking the patient to shrug the shoulders against resistance. Palpation of the contracting trapezius muscle may reveal minor asymmetries of muscle bulk. In an upper motor neurone lesion the ipsilateral sternomastoid is usually weak, impairing head-turning towards the paralysed side. By contrast, the trapezius is weak on the paralysed side.

XIIth Cranial Nerve (Hypoglossal)

This nerve contains general somatic efferent fibres to the tongue and afferent fibres from the muscle spindles in the tongue. The nucleus (Fig. 2.21) is innervated mainly by corticobulbar fibres, reticular formations, the nucleus of the solitary tract, and the spinal nucleus of V.

Clinical examination

The tongue should be observed lying at rest in the floor of the mouth for evidence of wasting, fasciculation or involuntary movement. The tongue is then protruded. In lateralised weakness the tongue curves round to the affected side due to the unopposed action of the normal genioglossus muscle. Rapid movements of the tongue are impaired either because of gross wasting or, more commonly, because of bilateral corticobulbar lesions. In a unilateral upper motor neurone lesion, movements of the tongue are not usually affected. Deviation of the tongue towards the paralysed side, however, occasionally occurs.

Bulbar palsy (Table 2.11)

Damage to the lower (IX–XII) cranial nerve nuclei may occur from lesions in the medulla due to vascular or degenerative disease (e.g. motor neurone disease), tumours, syrinx, and infections such as poliomyelitis. The peripheral course of the nerves may be involved individually by tumours in the neck or skull base or diffusely by meningeal infection and infiltration; certain neuropathies, e.g. Guillain–Barré syndrome or diphtheria, typically result in bulbar dysfunction. The left recurrent laryngeal branch of the vagus may be involved by tumour, lymph nodes or aneurysm in the chest. The pharyngeal or laryngeal muscles themselves are sometimes severely affected in myasthenia gravis, inflammatory myopathy and certain dystrophies. A pseudobulbar palsy is usually caused by bilateral corticobulbar lesions. The palate moves poorly on phonation, the tongue is spastic and slow in movement, speech is dysarthric (see p. 49) and swallowing may be impaired. The jaw jerk and gag reflexes are usually brisk (see p. 38) and there may be emotional lability. This syndrome occurs typically in bilateral vascular disease, motor neurone disease and multiple sclerosis.

Table 2.11

Neurological Causes of Bulbar Palsy (IX–XIIth Nerves)

1. Supranuclear (pseudobulbar palsy)	bilateral (hemisphere) vascular disease, motor neurone disease, demyelination, extrapyramidal disease, tumour
2. Nuclear/brainstem	medullary infarction, tumour, syrinx, encephalitis (rabies, polio, herpes simplex), motor neurone disease
3. Peripheral nerve	cranial polyneuritis: Guillain–Barré diphtheria sarcoidosis meninges: neoplastic infiltration inflammatory disease skull base infiltration: chordoma metastases glomus tumour skull base anomaly: Chiari malformation local infiltrative disease in neck
4. Muscle disease	myasthenia gravis polymyositis dystrophy (myotonic, oculopharyngeal)

ABNORMALITIES OF SPEECH AND SOME HIGHER CEREBRAL FUNCTIONS (Fig. 2.28)

Dysarthria

The normal articulation of speech requires correct coordination of the tongue, lips, pharynx, larynx and respiratory muscles. Cerebellar, extrapyramidal and corticobulbar pathways and bulbar apparatus are involved in articulation so that lesions of any of these, as well as muscular weakness or structural disease of the mouth, pharynx or larynx may result in dysarthria.

Clinical examination

Speech will already have been heard during the history taking, but detection of dysarthric abnormalities may be assisted by asking the patient to repeat certain phrases, e.g. 'British Constitution'; 'Thirty-seven West Register Street'; 'baby hippopotamus'. In extrapyramidal disease the voice is soft and monotonous and there is a tendency to run the syllables together. In cerebellar disease speech is slurred (but irregularly so) and there may be an irregular staccato or scanning quality. In a pseudobulbar palsy the speech is described as 'sticky' and is associated with brisk gag and jaw jerk reflex. Lower motor neurone disorders cause various selective dysarthrias and in myasthenia gravis there may be dysarthria which tends to worsen as speech continues.

Dysphasia

Dysphasia may be defined as a disorder of language which gives rise to impaired formulation or comprehension of speech. Language functions are executed in the left hemisphere of most right-handed people and in about half of left-handers. Disorders of speech formulation (expressive dysphasia) arise from lesions in the frontal lobe, particularly the inferior frontal gyrus

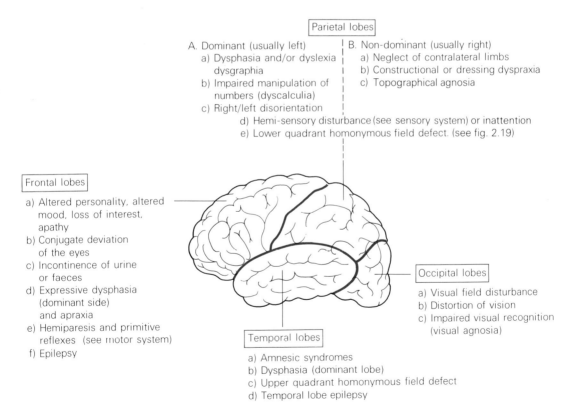

Parietal lobes

A. Dominant (usually left)
  a) Dysphasia and/or dyslexia dysgraphia
  b) Impaired manipulation of numbers (dyscalculia)
  c) Right/left disorientation
    d) Hemi-sensory disturbance (see sensory system) or inattention
    e) Lower quadrant homonymous field defect. (see fig. 2.19)

B. Non-dominant (usually right)
  a) Neglect of contralateral limbs
  b) Constructional or dressing dyspraxia
  c) Topographical agnosia

Frontal lobes

a) Altered personality, altered mood, loss of interest, apathy
b) Conjugate deviation of the eyes
c) Incontinence of urine or faeces
d) Expressive dysphasia (dominant side) and apraxia
e) Hemiparesis and primitive reflexes (see motor system)
f) Epilepsy

Occipital lobes

a) Visual field disturbance
b) Distortion of vision
c) Impaired visual recognition (visual agnosia)

Temporal lobes

a) Amnesic syndromes
b) Dysphasia (dominant lobe)
c) Upper quadrant homonymous field defect
d) Temporal lobe epilepsy

Fig. 2.28 *Diagram to summarise the principal clinical features resulting from damage to the main lobes of the cerebrum.*

(Broca's area), whilst defects of comprehension arise from more posterior lesions – in the superior temporal or parietal lobes (Fig. 2.28).

Clinical examination

Most information is gained by engaging the patient in conversation. In an expressive dysphasia, fluency of speech is lost; both the content and the phrase length are reduced, and such speech as there is tends to be composed of nouns and verbs which may be incorrectly enunciated or incorrectly structured (paraphasias). The speech is usually hesitant, circumlocutious, and accompanied by considerable effort and frustration as the patient struggles to express himself. Occasionally the speech is frankly dysarthric. Speech may be so severely limited that the patient is virtually mute or confined to a few single words. Reading out loud and writing are usually also impaired but comprehension is relatively intact so that the patient will understand questions and attempt to convey meaningful answers.

With a severe defect of comprehension, speech may be fluent and even rapid but lacks meaningful content. The patient fails to engage in appropriate efforts to answer questions and does not understand his own errors of speech. In certain types of dysphasia the structural link between the auditory cortex in the superior temporal gyrus and Broca's area remains relatively intact so that repetition by the patient of words and phrases given by the examiner may be preserved although spontaneous speech may be very poor (transcortical dysphasia). Conversely, this structural link is occasionally the major site of disruption so that the patient has extremely poor repetition despite moderate or good fluency and comprehension (conduction dysphasia).

Apraxia

Apraxia is an inability to formulate and/or execute movements although there is no major corticobulbar/spinal, extrapyramidal, sensory or cerebellar deficit. A willed movement appears to be formulated in the dominant (usually left) frontal lobe but, in order to be executed by the left-sided limbs, must be transferred to the right motor cortex via the corpus callosum. Execution by the right-sided limbs requires transfer

within the left frontal lobe. Apraxia may therefore involve both sides of the body (left frontal lesion) or only the left side (corpus callosum lesion).

Clinical examination

Having established that comprehension, power, tone, coordination and sensation are reasonably intact, the patient is invited to perform or mime various actions such as waving, making a fist, knocking at a door, combing the hair, shaking hands, blowing out a match, pretending to light a match. The patient may be unable to do these on command but may achieve them spontaneously at other times (ideomotor apraxia), or his formulation of complex acts may be impaired at all times (ideational apraxia). Bilateral frontal lesions may give rise to an apraxia of gait.

Lesions of the non-dominant (usually right) parietal lobe result in defective analysis of spatial relationships, so that complex tasks such as dressing and constructional tasks such as drawing a cube or a clock face or copying a geometric design are impaired (dressing and constructional apraxia). In addition, disorders of the non-dominant parietal lobe may result in a disabling neglect or inattention of the left-sided limbs. A summary of the main features of lesions of the cortex is shown in Fig. 2.28.

Memory

Disorders of memory occur as a result of damage in several areas of the brain. The temporal lobes and deep structures, including the fornices, hippocampi, mammillary bodies and their connections, appear to be of particular importance.

Clinical examination

Immediate recall is tested by asking the patient to repeat a series of digits starting with three or four and working up to about seven. Most people will remember six or seven and be able to repeat four or so backwards. Short-term memory (ability to retain new information over a period of minutes) is tested by asking the patient to remember three or four objects or a name and address over 5 minutes, having first ensured that it can be retained for immediate recall. Most amnesic disorders predominantly affect short-term memory whilst leaving long-term memory relatively intact. This is demonstrated by contrasting memory for events within the period of the illness with those in the more distant past, e.g. news events in the last week and the present Head of State compared with items concerning events some years previously such as where the patient was born, and the dates of the Second World War.

CONSCIOUSNESS, COMA, AND BRAIN DEATH

Consciousness depends on integrity of both cerebral and brainstem function. The brainstem has an essential activating effect on the cerebrum via the ascending reticular formations of the medulla, pons and midbrain. This system projects most notably to the nonspecific midline and intralaminar nuclei of the thalamus which, in turn, project to the basal ganglia and cortex via the ventral anterior group of nuclei (Fig. 2.14). A second important pathway appears to ascend to the hypothalamus. The descending reticular pathways influence motor activity and exert control of sensory input via reticulospinal fibres and are closely involved in respiratory function, particularly in the medulla. Impaired consciousness may result from a diffuse insult to the cerebrum or a more localised insult to the brainstem. The cerebrum cannot function without ascending pathways from the brainstem, and recognition of this fact has led to an appreciation that death of the brainstem is functionally equivalent to brain death and death of the patient (see p. 53).

Examination of the Confused or Comatose Patient

In any confused or comatose patient where the diagnosis is uncertain, it is essential to ensure adequacy of ventilation, to check circulatory status and to exclude major pathology or injury in the abdomen, chest, limbs and spine before proceeding to a detailed neurological examination. For practical purposes, hypothermia and hypoglycaemia should also be excluded at an early stage.

Level of consciousness

Many causes of confused behaviour eventually lead to a depressed level of consciousness, and to coma if untreated. The mental state of a patient who is alert and responsive is assessed by his general behaviour and the content of his speech. With such an alert patient it is important at the outset to decide whether he is in fact confused or has a receptive dysphasia (or both).

Asking the patient about his whereabouts, the date and his name will draw an inappropriate response if the patient is grossly dysphasic but, if he is merely confused, the response is likely to be appropriate but incorrect. If the patient cannot be engaged in conversation, his level of arousal may be assessed by the response to simple questions such as asking his name or how he is feeling. If there is no response, brief commands such as asking him to open his eyes or hold up his arms should be tried. Responses may vary from being appropriate with normal speech accompanied by opening of the eyes (if previously closed), through vague vocalisations and mumbling (with or without eye opening), to no significant response. The presence of spontaneous speech and its content should be carefully noted. Occasionally a patient lies apparently awake but mute and immobile with the eyes open and fixating on people or objects around the room. This state, known as akinetic mutism, is usually the chronic sequel to a severe brain injury, anoxic or ischaemic damage to the frontal lobes, or lesions in the region of the 3rd ventricle.

Examination of head, neck and spine

The skull is examined for evidence of local injury and, after known head injury, the ears and nose are specifically checked for leakage of cerebrospinal fluid and the question of injury to the neck is considered. Rigidity of the neck may be due to local injury, meningeal inflammation due to infection or blood, or tonsillar herniation due to raised intracranial pressure. Neck retraction may be due to meningitis, tetanus or hysteria associated with hyperventilation.

The response of the limbs to stimulation

If the patient does not respond (or responds abnormally) to verbal arousal, a painful stimulus is used after having first noted the general posture of the body. Vocalisation, eye opening, grimacing and the movement of the limbs on both sides of the body are noted in response to painful stimulation on face or trunk. The patient may localise the painful stimulus and try to push it away with the arms; a lower-grade response is non-purposive flexion of the limbs. Flexion of the upper limbs with extension of the lower limbs (decorticate posture), and extension of all four limbs (decerebrate posturing) represent successively impaired responses. Having noted the overall pattern of limb response to central stimulation, it can be helpful to examine tone in each limb and the response of the arm and leg on one side may give clear evidence of a focal neurological disturbance in addition to the general depression of consciousness. The best limb response should be carefully noted, as well as any asymmetries (see also Glasgow coma scale, Chapter 5). The plantar responses are frequently extensor whatever the cause of coma.

The cranial nerves

Most of the cranial nerves may be examined to some extent in the non-cooperative or unconscious patient. The visual fields may be crudely assessed by response to a menacing movement of the hand from the right or left side. The optic fundi are examined for papilloedema suggesting raised intracranial pressure, and for haemorrhages occurring in association with severe hypertension and subarachnoid haemorrhage.

The pupils are usually normal in cerebral hemisphere disease (unless brainstem and/or IIIrd nerve compression occurs). Herniation of the medial temporal lobe leads to a wide dilatation of the ipsilateral pupil (6–10 mm) with evidence of developing IIIrd nerve palsy. If there is substantial midbrain distortion, the contralateral pupil also dilates. Apart from midbrain compression, an important cause of widely dilated pupils is the use of drugs with anticholinergic properties (topically or systemically). A lesion in the pons (notably haemorrhage) leads to small reactive pinpoint pupils as a result of bilateral sympathetic pathway damage.

In assessing brainstem function, eye movements have particular importance. The eyes are usually conjugate in position in cerebral lesions which have not influenced the brainstem, with the gaze directed towards the affected hemisphere in destructive frontal

lobe lesions and driven to the contralateral side during the irritative phase of a focal fit. Dysconjugate eye position either suggests brainstem involvement or an ocular palsy.

Whatever the apparent level of consciousness of the patient, pursuit movements in the horizontal and vertical planes should be carefully tested. Occasionally eyelid closure and vertical eye deviations are the only voluntary movements preserved in a patient with a high brainstem lesion. Such a patient can be fully conscious ('locked in' syndrome). Reflex eye movements are tested by passively turning the head from side to side and flexing and extending the neck to note whether oculocephalic reflexes (doll's-head eye movements) are present (see also p. 43).

A vestibulo-ocular reflex can be elicited by syringing the external auditory meatus with 20 ml of ice cold water, having first ascertained that there is no perforation of the tympanic membrane (see also p. 44). If the reflex is present, the eyes tonically deviate to the side of the stimulus.

The Vth and VIIth nerves are assessed by testing the corneal reflexes bilaterally and looking for grimacing following unilateral painful stimulation such as pressure on the superior margin of the orbit. The lower cranial nerves are assessed by noting the ability to clear secretions, and the presence of a cough and gag reflex. Spontaneous swallowing movements are subserved by medullary and lower pontine reflexes and cough and hiccup may only be abolished in advanced medullary failure.

Respiration

The pattern of respiration is sometimes helpful in diagnosis and in anticipating whether artificial support is likely to be required. The question of the adequacy of respiratory muscle strength and hence ventilation when the airway is clear is dealt with in Chapter 17.

Cheyne–Stokes respiration is normally associated, in the neurological context, with supratentorial lesions causing diencephalic and early brainstem compression. Following an apnoeic period, tidal volume gradually increases with successive breaths but then wanes again to be followed by a further apnoeic period. In central neurogenic hyperventilation, tidal volume is usually increased and there is a regular tachypnoea of 40–70 breaths per minute; this condition is associated with pontine lesions. Brainstem disturbances can give rise to a variety of more unusual patterns of breathing including ataxic (irregularly irregular) breathing and apneustic breathing, which consists of prolonged inspiratory gasps, often with a pause at full inspiration. The 'automatic' control of breathing may be impaired in patients with medullary lesions. Once asleep, these patients may fail to breathe adequately due either to upper airways obstruction or central hypoventilation. Conversely, lesions of the cervicomedullary junction have been described, where 'automatic' breathing is intact but patients cannot exert normal voluntary control. For instance they may be unable to voluntarily take a deep breath or to hold their breath.

Type of brain dysfunction

Following neurological and general examination of a patient in coma, it is frequently possible to decide whether the signs are more suggestive of diffuse brain injury or of focal brainstem dysfunction. However, diffuse cerebral injury may give rise to secondary disturbances in the brainstem as a result of mechanical compression and displacement or secondary vascular events, and it may be impossible to distinguish between the two possibilities unless the evolution of the physical signs is known from an early stage. The principal causes of coma are given in Table 2.12 together with relevant initial investigations.

In general with progressive supratentorial lesions, two principal sequences of events are discernible. A unilateral lesion may cause initial focal neurological signs, then gradually expand to displace midline structures with herniation of the temporal lobe into the tentorial hiatus, causing an ipsilateral IIIrd nerve palsy and compression of the upper brainstem. Alternatively a centrally placed lesion, without clear lateralising signs, or diffuse swelling in the supratentorial compartment, may cause direct compression and distortion of the upper brainstem. This results in a deterioration in level of consciousness, impaired upgaze and bilateral extensor plantar responses. Subsequently, brainstem function fails in a rostrocaudal manner, shown by impaired ocular movements and reflexes, pupil response, altered patterns of respiration, flexed and later extensor posturing of the limbs and eventual medullary failure. A primary brainstem disturbance is likely to display localising signs at an early stage in relationship to the level of consciousness.

Brain death

The ability to maintain respiration by mechanical means, and the circulation by pharmacological means, has lead to re-evaluation of traditional notions of death. The brain is considered dead if the brainstem is irreversibly functionless. The diagnosis of this state has become a matter of considerable practical importance because of the advent of transplantation surgery.

In the United Kingdom the diagnosis of brain death, under circumstances where respiration is artificially supported, must be made by two doctors who are experienced in performing the appropriate tests and who are not part of any transplantation team. For practical purposes there must be a clear diagnosis of the structural brain damage which has led to the patient's state; common causes are trauma to the head, intracranial haemorrhage and anoxic brain damage (e.g. following cardiac arrest). Any possibility of drug intoxication or neuromuscular blockade must be carefully excluded. Hypothermia must also be excluded; using a low-reading thermometer, the core temperature should be greater than 35° centigrade. There should be no spontaneous movements, whether epileptic in nature or due to decerebrate or decorticate posturing, and no response to external stimulation including voice, pain, noise or light. Brainstem reflexes – including pupillary responses to a bright light, oculocephalic reflexes and ocular responses to cold caloric stimulation, corneal reflexes, gag and cough reflexes in response to pharyngeal or laryngeal suction – must all be absent. Spinal-tendon reflexes may be preserved. Spontaneous respiration is absent. In testing for apnoea the patient is first preoxygenated with 100% O_2 for about 10 minutes and then given 95% O_2 and 5% CO_2 for 5 minutes, which permits the arterial P_{CO_2} to rise to about 5.3 kPa (40 mmHg). The patient is then disconnected from the ventilator. It is recommended that the arterial P_{CO_2} is allowed to rise to at least 6.65 kPa (50 mmHg) before the patient is said to be apnoeic.

It should be appreciated that severe craniofacial injuries resulting in cranial nerve palsies or a history of severe chronic obstructive airways disease (with a raised arterial P_{CO_2}) may make interpretation of these

Table 2.12

Common Causes of Coma and Relevant Investigations

A. Diffuse brain dysfunction	Diagnosis
1. Drug overdose/side-effects Alcohol	Relevant history; blood/urine samples
2. Hypo-, hyperglycaemia	History of diabetes; blood glucose
3. Hypoxic/ischaemic injury	History of possible cardiac arrest, suffocation, drowning: BP measurement, ECG
4. Respiratory, renal, hepatic failure	History; blood gases, urea/electrolytes, evidence of liver disease
5. Hyponatremia	Recent i/v fluids, oat cell carcinoma of lung, meningitis; plasma/urinary osmolalities
6. Hypothermia	Elderly, hypothyroid; check rectal temperature, thyroid function
7. Head injury	History; plain x-rays, CT scan
8. Epilepsy	History, drugs; later an EEG
9. Subarachnoid haemorrhage	Neck stiffness; CT scan, lumbar puncture
10. Meningitis/encephalitis	History of contact, vaccination, foreign travel; blood cultures, CT scan, examination of csf, blood tests for parasites e.g. malaria
11. Hypertensive encephalopathy	History of hypertension, pregnancy (eclampsia); check blood pressure

B. Focal brain dysfunction			Diagnosis
1. Brainstem disease	vascular	'locked in' syndrome basilar occlusion cerebellar haemorrhage arteritis	Examination Ocular signs CT scan ESR
	tumour demyelination		History
2. Hemisphere disease with secondary brainstem compression	tumour, haematoma, abscess, swelling after trauma, infarction, infection, encephalitis		History, lateralising signs, CT scan, EEG

tests particularly difficult and sometimes impossible. It is advisable to repeat the above tests on two separate occasions some hours apart before drawing any final conclusions. Although not essential in the UK criteria, there are occasional clinical situations where an electroencephalogram confirming the presence of a flat unresponsive recording or cerebral angiography to confirm the absence of cerebral blood-flow may be helpful in overall management.

AUTONOMIC SYSTEM

The sympathetic and parasympathetic systems both contain efferent and afferent neurones. The efferent pathway consists of a thinly-myelinated preganglionic neurone whose cell body is within the central nervous system and an unmyelinated postganglionic neurone whose cell body is peripheral. Preganglionic sympathetic fibres arise in the intermediolateral cell column of the thoracic and upper lumbar cord segments, pass from the spinal cord in the ventral root, and reach the sympathetic chain and related ganglia whence post-ganglionic fibres are distributed to the whole body, where they have particular influence on the control of blood flow to various organs, blood pressure, heart rate, sweating, piloerection and pupillary responses (see p. 34). The parasympathetic outflow is grouped into nuclear complexes in the brainstem and there is a further grouping in the sacral spinal-cord segments S2–S4 (see Table 2.13). Activity of the sympathetic and parasympathetic system is partially reflex in nature at a segmental level, although subject to numerous descending influences which are, at least in part, integrated in the hypothalamus and reticular formations of the brainstem.

The hypothalamus contains a number of nuclei and has extensive afferent connections from the septal region, the amygdala and hippocampus, periaqueductal grey matter, and reticular formations. Its efferent projections reach the reticular formations, other brainstem structures, and the intermediolateral cell column of the spinal cord. The hypothalamus is vital for the normal regulation of many activities concerned with

the maintenance of internal homeostasis (see Table 2.14) such as temperature, water/electrolyte balance, wakefulness and appetite.

The peripheral distribution of autonomic neurones will not be considered in further detail, with the exception of distribution to the bladder and genital organs. The motor supply to the bladder is through parasympathetic fibres from S2–4 supplying the detrusor muscle, and via somatic efferent fibres from the same segments travelling in the pudendal nerves to the external sphincter. The parasympathetic fibres from these segments are also concerned with the mechanism of erection. Sympathetic fibres from T12–L2 segments descend in the hypogastric plexus to supply the trigone and upper urethra and are also concerned with the mechanism of ejaculation.

Afferent fibres from the bladder ascend in the hypogastric plexus to T12–L2 segments and presumably play a role in detecting changes in intravesical pressure and volume. Further afferent fibres return to the S2–4 segments of the spinal cord to complete the reflex pathway responsible for bladder emptying. Sensation from the bladder probably reaches consciousness by the lateral columns of the cord, and awareness of micturition and related events is dependent on

---

Table 2.13

Parasympathetic Outflow

1. Edinger–Westphal nucleus	IIIrd nerve	pupil sphincter, ciliary muscle
2. Superior salivatory nucleus	VIIth nerve	glands of nose and palate, submaxillary/sublingual glands
3. Inferior salivatory nucleus	IXth nerve	parotid gland
4. Dorsal motor nucleus of vagus	Xth nerve	pharynx/oesophagus, trachea/larynx/bronchi, lungs/heart, gut to transverse colon
5. Sacral outflow	S2–S4	gut below transverse colon, external genitalia, bladder, sphincters

Table 2.14

Functions of Hypothalamus

1. Integration of sympathetic and parasympathetic activity
2. Temperature regulation
3. Thirst and water balance, osmoreception
4. Control of pituitary endocrine function
5. Appetite and weight
6. Influence on sleep pattern
7. Influence on emotional expression

intact frontal lobe function. Inhibition of bladder-emptying reflexes appears to depend on intact descending control via corticospinal pathways.

Clinical examination

Several areas of hypothalamic and autonomic function may require special investigation. From a clinical point of view, evidence of bladder and sexual dysfunction will be gained from the history. The eyes are checked for the presence of ptosis and pupil size. Impaired cardiovascular reflexes cause loss of normal sinus arrhythmia, postural hypotension often with a fixed heart rate, and loss of the vagally-mediated reflex bradycardia following a Valsalva manoeuvre. Considerable information can be gained from palpation of the pulse and measurement of blood pressure at the bedside. The skin is examined for evidence of sweating, and regional differences of skin temperature noted. The abdomen is palpated to exclude an enlarged bladder and the anal sphincter checked at rectal examination.

Autonomic dysfunction may arise from interruption of peripheral pathways, most commonly by various drugs which interfere with normal synaptic transmission. Certain neuropathies may selectively involve smaller-diameter fibres and cause marked autonomic symptoms (see p. 246). Focal lesions of the spinal cord and brainstem may interrupt descending pathways and there are a variety of degenerative conditions of the central nervous system which can present with features of autonomic failure (see p. 194).

From the neurologist's point of view, impairment of micturition, defaecation and sexual function are fairly frequent. Damage to the conus medullaris or cauda equina interrupts the normal reflex bladder-emptying mechanism and may thus cause retention of urine leading to a distended bladder. Defaecation and penile erection are also impaired. Selective lesions of the afferent pathways from the bladder cause it to become atonic and enlarged due to loss of the normal reflex emptying mechanism and failure of conscious detection of fullness.

Complete interruption of spinal cord pathways results in loss of conscious awareness of bladder fullness but, after a time, reflex emptying of the bladder may become established – usually at lower bladder volumes than previously. Partial interruption of descending pathways results in urgency and frequency of micturition as a result of reduced inhibition of the reflex emptying mechanism. Finally, lesions of the frontal lobes may result in incontinence with little apparent awareness of the event.

SUMMARY

Inevitably, it is essential during the neurological examination to focus attention on those aspects of the nervous system indicated by the history. It is important, however, to look at the whole patient and, at least briefly, to consider all the seven parts of the neurological examination indicated in Table 2.15.

Table 2.15

Summary of the Neurological Examination

1.	Higher functions	level of consciousness orientation memory and intellect speech and language functions mood
2.	The coverings of the nervous system	skull meninges spine
3.	Gait, balance and posture	
4.	Cranial nerves	
5.	Motor system	tone power coordination reflexes praxis
6.	Sensory system	joint position vibration pain, temperature, light touch discriminative ability
7.	Autonomic system	pulse blood pressure sweating sphincters/bladder

3

Neurological Investigations

A wide range of clinical expertise may be required for the investigation of any neurological problem: detailed examinations of the eyes, ears, vocal cords and nasopharynx, the heart or the bladder frequently entail referral to the appropriate specialist. Selective haematological, metabolic or immunological tests are helpful when directed towards a specific clinical problem but, as in other branches of medicine, they are rarely justified as screening procedures. Syphilis serology, blood glucose, sedimentation rate, thyroid function tests, electrocardiogram and chest x-ray are examples of investigations which do sometimes yield important abnormalities and hence are frequently requested with a low index of clinical suspicion.

The investigation of the cerebrospinal fluid is dealt with in Chapter 4 and electroencephalography in Chapter 7. Some of the other main neurophysiological and neuroradiological investigations used are outlined below.

NEUROPHYSIOLOGICAL INVESTIGATIONS

Nerve Conduction Studies

Motor conduction

The conduction of electrical impulses along distal and proximal segments of peripheral motor and sensory nerves can be studied routinely. Motor conduction is usually investigated by recording the compound muscle action potential evoked by a supramaximal stimulus in the nerve of interest. The latency from a distal stimulus site to the start of the muscle action potential (distal motor latency) depends on the propagation time in the terminal ramifications of the nerve, a delay due to neuromuscular transmission and muscle fibre conduction time (Fig. 3.1). The amplitude of the muscle action potential depends on the number of muscle fibres depolarised, which is in turn a function of the number of motor fibres in the nerve and the number of muscle fibres in each motor unit. The temporal dispersion of the response will be influenced by the spectrum of conduction velocities in component axons and the effect of this on synchronous muscle fibre excitation. Marked temporal dispersion of a response leads to a reduced amplitude.

When the latencies from a proximal and distal stimulation site are measured, the distal component is common to both. The difference between the two latencies is the time for conduction to occur in the fastest fibres between the two stimulus points. The nerve conduction velocity in these fastest fibres can therefore be calculated (Fig. 3.1). More complicated procedures exist for estimating the conduction velocities of the slowest fibres.

Demyelination of nerve fibres (see Chapter 16) leads to slowing of conduction velocity with relative preservation of action potential amplitude, although some increased temporal dispersion may be seen (Fig. 3.2). Sometimes actual conduction block is present in demyelinated fibres, so that stimulation distally gives rise to a muscle action potential whilst proximal stimulation (or voluntary contraction) fails to evoke a response. If damage is primarily to the axons, the amplitude of the response is reduced whilst there is a relative preservation of conduction velocity since a proportion of fast-conducting fibres are still intact.

F and H reflexes

Supramaximal stimulation of many motor nerves also

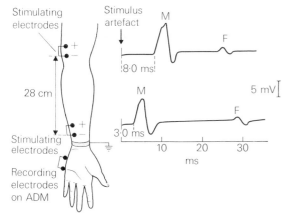

Motor conduction velocity (elbow-wrist)

$$= \frac{0 \cdot 28 \times 1000}{8 \cdot 0 - 3 \cdot 0} = 56 \text{ m/s}$$

Fig. 3.1 *The compound muscle action potential (M wave) from abductor digiti minimi (ADM) following supramaximal ulnar nerve stimulation at the wrist and elbow. The difference in latencies and the known distance allow conduction velocity to be calculated. The F waves (see text) are also shown. Note how the latency to the F wave is shorter following more proximal stimulation.*

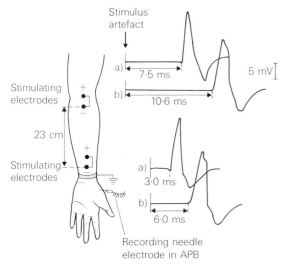

a) Motor conduction velocity: 51 m/s
b) Motor conduction velocity : 50 m/s
  (elbow-wrist)

Fig. 3.2 *The measurement of distal motor latency and forearm conduction velocity in (a) normal subject and (b) patient with median nerve compression at wrist. A concentric needle electrode is inserted into abductor pollicis brevis (APB). Note the prolongation of distal motor latency due to compression in the carpal tunnel (b) with a normal forearm conduction velocity.*

results in a late potential or F wave (Fig. 3.1) due to antidromic invasion of the motor root and subsequent orthodromic excitation of the nerve and muscle. The presence and latency of an F wave is therefore evidence of the integrity of the proximal segment of peripheral motor fibres. Submaximal stimulation of the posterior tibial nerve may be followed by a reflex response recorded from the gastrocnemius at a latency of about 35 ms: this response decreases with increase in the stimulus amplitude and corresponds to a mono-synaptic reflex (H reflex). The H reflex provides an index of excitability of anterior horn cells but can only be elicited routinely in gastrocnemius.

Repetitive nerve stimulation

Routine nerve conduction studies are carried out using single shocks at low frequencies e.g. 0.5–1 cps. In myasthenia gravis, supramaximal repetitive stimulation at faster rates, e.g. 2–3 cps, leads to an abnormal decrement in compound muscle action potential amplitude. The abnormal motor end plates result in a reduced safety margin for neuromuscular transmission and, with repetitive stimulation, a proportion of ter-minal axons fail to activate muscle fibres, resulting in a reduced amplitude of the compound potential (Fig. 3.3). A brief voluntary contraction causes an enhanced response (facilitation) caused by a transient increase in acetylcholine release and hence an increased safety margin for transmission. In presynaptic disorders (Eaton–Lambert syndrome, botulism – see Chapter 17) there is impaired transmitter release at low stimulation rates, resulting in only a few muscle fibres depolarising and hence a small compound action potential: during high frequency stimulation there is very marked facilitation (Fig. 3.4).

Nerve action potentials

A compound muscle action potential is some millivolts in amplitude, but nerve action potentials are in the microvolt range. The advent of signal averaging tech-niques, however, has made it possible to record nerve action potentials routinely. Sensory nerves, for instance the digital nerves (Fig. 3.5), may be supramaximally stimulated and the volley in the median or ulnar nerves recorded at the wrist and elbow. The amplitude of the response gives some indication of the number of intact axons, whilst the latency of response, the conduction velocity in the forearm (if measured), and the dispersion of the recorded potential give information about the speed of conduction. Similarly, mixed (motor and sensory) nerve action potentials can be recorded following stimulation of nerve trunks, e.g. ulnar nerve at the wrist or the deep peroneal nerve at the ankle.

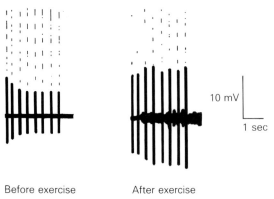

Before exercise   After exercise

Fig. 3.3 *Myasthenia gravis: supramaximal ulnar nerve stimulation at the wrist at 2cps: surface electrodes on ADM. The initial action potential is of normal amplitude and decreases on repetitive stimulation. After a 20-second maximum voluntary contraction there is facilitation of the response. (Courtesy Dr NMF Murray, The National Hospital for Nervous Diseases.)*

Electromyography (EMG)

The primary purpose of a routine EMG is to determine whether muscle symptoms (usually weakness) are due to neurogenic or myopathic disease (see p. 256). In neurogenic lesions, the technique may be of value in determining the distribution (segmental or peripheral nerve) and extent of the abnormality; in myopathy, specific abnormalities may be observed which aid diagnosis.

When a recording needle electrode is inserted into relaxed muscle there is a brief burst of 'insertional' activity followed by electrical silence. During a weak voluntary contraction, motor units are recruited, some fibres of which will be more or less close to the electrode. A number of different and discrete motor unit potentials may be seen on the oscilloscope and also heard over the loudspeaker, and the frequency content of such potentials have a characteristic sound. These units typically have fewer than four phases (potential changes), and a normal range of amplitudes is established. As the force of contraction increases, further motor units are recruited and the discharge rates of others increase so that individual units can no longer be clearly defined and an interference pattern occurs.

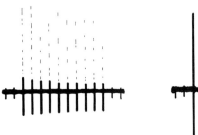
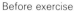
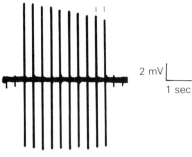

Before exercise   After exercise

Fig. 3.4. *Myasthenic syndrome: supramaximal ulnar nerve stimulation at the wrist at 2cps: surface electrodes on ADM. The initial action potential is small (note different scale from Fig. 3.3) and there is slight decrement. After a 20-second maximum voluntary contraction there is very marked facilitation which rapidly starts to decline. (Courtesy Dr NMF Murray, The National Hospital for Nervous Diseases.)*

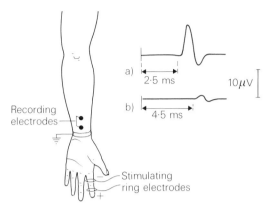

Fig. 3.5 *Measurement of sensory nerve action potential in* (a) *normal subject and* (b) *patient with median nerve compression at wrist. Supramaximal stimuli are given through ring electrodes to the digital nerves of the index finger. Surface recordings are made over the median nerve at the wrist and the signal is averaged over a number of responses. Note how the latency is increased and the amplitude reduced due to median nerve compression in the carpal tunnel. The response is usually compared with that from the little finger (ulnar-supplied), which should be normal.*

Denervation

In denervation, spontaneous muscle fibre depolarisations occur and are best recorded in the relaxed muscle (fibrillations, +ve sharp waves). Occasionally whole motor units discharge at rest (fasciculations) and this can often be seen clinically as well as recorded electrically. Although the extent of fasciculations can be determined from needle sampling, they are of such an amplitude that they may be recorded at the skin using surface plate electrodes. This has the advantage that large areas may be sampled at once and, using a multichannel recorder, recordings may be made from all four limbs simultaneously. This type of recording is of particular use in suspected anterior horn cell disorders (e.g. motor neurone disease) where fasciculations can be infrequent; it cannot be used for detecting individual muscle fibre potentials.

The number of motor units is reduced in denervation and hence the interference pattern is incomplete, often comprising a few discrete units firing at high (30 cps) rates during a full effort. If terminal sprouting and collateral reinnervation (see p. 240) has taken place, the remaining motor units are larger than normal and have an increased number of components, resulting in polyphasia and increased duration. An upper motor neurone (corticospinal tract) lesion will cause reduced recruitment and firing rate of motor units, resulting in a reduced interference pattern but not showing specific features of denervation of muscle fibres (fibrillations) or reinnervation (large polyphasic units).

Myopathy

In myopathy, individual muscle fibres from each motor unit are damaged so that the motor unit potentials are reduced in amplitude. In addition, this loss of components leads to reduced duration and increased polyphasia, which results in an increased high-frequency content heard over the loudspeaker as a high-pitched crackle. The reduction in motor unit size (but not number, initally) means that more units need to be recruited to produce a given force and hence the interference pattern is complete at a lower than expected force and remains complete until a very extensive loss of muscle fibres has occurred.

In primarily myopathic disorders, spontaneous electrical discharges at rest are sometimes seen. Fibrillations may be prominent in inflammatory myopathy and occasionally give a clue to rare metabolic conditions such as acid maltase deficiency (see p. 261), where they may represent denervation of individual muscle fibres. Characteristic waxing and waning high-frequency discharges following needle movement, muscle percussion or contraction are seen in myotonic disorders (see p. 259) and are of help in diagnosis: a different pattern of high-frequency discharge is sometimes seen in neurogenic disorders.

Quantitation

The degree of polyphasia, and duration and amplitude of discrete motor unit potentials can be measured during low force contractions and compared with normal values. Alternatively the interference pattern at a standard absolute or relative force may be analysed for the number of potential changes per unit time and the mean amplitude of each potential change; characteristic values occur in myopathic and neurogenic disorders. In addition, signal analysis techniques may be applied to determine the frequency distribution and power to yield a 'power spectrum'. This has been of particular use in the study of muscle fatigue.

Single fibre EMG

Single-fibre EMG techniques allow the relationship between the discharges of individual muscle fibres within the same motor unit to be studied using a very fine electrode which records from a very limited volume of muscle. The normal variation in time (jitter) between muscle-fibre discharges in the same unit is small (20 μs) but increases when the terminal ramifications of a motor axon, or the neuromuscular junction, are affected by disease. Thus, in myasthenia gravis, increased jitter is a frequent finding and direct evidence of blocking of conduction to some fibres is also seen (see above). A single-fibre electrode at any one site records from, on average, one to three muscle fibres belonging to the same motor unit and this is therefore an estimate of the 'fibre density' of the motor units. The 'fibre density' increases if significant collateral reinnervation has occurred (see Fig. 3.5), but tends to remain the same if demyelination is prominent without loss of axons.

Evoked Potentials

Reference has been made to the detection of peripheral nerve action potentials by averaging the electrical response following successive stimuli. Similar techniques allow the central nervous system response to be detected using surface electrodes following a range of sensory stimuli. Since the on-going EEG signal is 50–100 μv in amplitude, the signal-to-noise ratio is unfavourable for recording potentials of a few microvolts only, and a computer is used to detect the evoked response, which is time-locked to the stimulus. The responses commonly measured are potentials evoked by visual, auditory and somatosensory stimuli (VEP; AEP; SEP). Electrodes are attached to the skin over the brain or spinal cord and the responses to 250–2000 stimuli (depending on the signal-to-noise ratio) are averaged. The major positive and negative waves (P or N waves) correspond to activation of certain CNS structures and, in a normal population, occur at standard latencies with bilateral symmetry and, given the same stimulus parameters and recording techniques, have a defined range of amplitudes.

Visual evoked potentials (VEP)

The stimulus usually consists of an alternating (usually 2 cps) black and white chequerboard pattern but, if visual acuity or patient cooperation is poor, a simple on/off flash response is used. Recording electrodes are placed on the scalp in the midline occipital region and on either side (Fig. 3.6a). The patient fixates on the centre of the chequerboard with each eye (whole field stimulation) and, subsequently, the right or left halves of the screen are covered up to the fixation point to obtain stimulation of the temporal or nasal half-fields (Fig. 3.6b).

The most valuable response parameter at present is an occipital cortical potential, positive in polarity and with a mean latency at about 100 ms ($\overline{P100}$). A lesion anterior to the chiasm will cause a difference in the whole field responses between the two eyes, whereas these are usually of similar latency and amplitude. An increased latency of P100 from one eye is characteristic of demyelinating disease of the optic nerve (see p. 144) but compressive or ischaemic lesions can also cause delay, hence the interpretation of the result is determined by the clinical context. A reduction in amplitude of $\overline{P100}$ is seen in many ocular conditions which reduce acuity (e.g. cataract, retinal disease) as well as optic nerve compression, infiltration or toxic damage. Chiasmatic or more posteriorly placed lesions produce bitemporal or homonymous asymmetries in amplitude or latency corresponding to the half-fields involved.

The clinical value of VEPs is most apparent in the diagnosis of optic nerve demyelination, and a clear prolongation of latency in one eye (in the absence of ocular disease) is strong evidence of a previous episode of optic neuritis even in the absence of neurological or ocular signs: the test therefore helps to establish the presence of multiple lesions in a patient who clinically may only have a single lesion such as a paraparesis (see also p. 153). In addition, subclinical abnormalities can be found in toxic or genetically-determined conditions (e.g. vitamin B_{12} deficiency, Friedreich's ataxia), optic pathway compression or infiltration (e.g. optic nerve glioma).

Auditory evoked potentials (AEP)

The stimulus consists of a series of electrically-generated square wave 'clicks' applied at standard amplitude

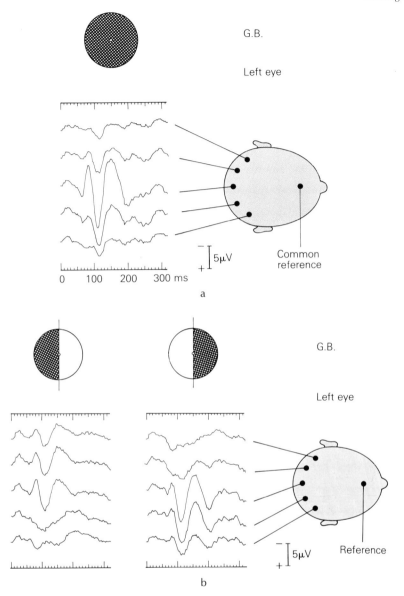

Fig. 3.6 (a) *Pattern reversal visual evoked potential to a 0–16°
checkerboard recording from the left eye of a healthy person.
(Courtesy Dr AM Halliday, Institute of Neurology, London.)*

(b) *Pattern reversal visual evoked potentials to left and right
half-field stimulation from the left eye of the same person
whose left full field response is shown in (a) (Courtesy of Dr AM
Halliday, Institute of Neurology, London.)*

and at 10 c.p.s. monaurally or binaurally through
headphones. Responses are recorded from scalp electrodes at the vertex and the mastoid processes (or ear
lobes).

The brainstem auditory evoked responses (BSAEPs)
comprise a series of potentials (I–V) and are currently of

most clinical value, although a variety of later subcortical and cortical responses may be recorded. Wave I
corresponds to activation of the VIIIth nerve and acts as
evidence of effective stimulation. Waves II/III correspond to activation of the cochlear and olivary nuclei,
wave IV corresponds to the nuclei of the lateral

lemniscus, wave V to the inferior colliculus, and waves VI and VII to subcortical structures. Latencies are often measured from wave I (Fig. 3.7).

AEPs have a wide application but are of particular value in the diagnosis of acoustic neuroma in a patient with sensorineural hearing loss and prolongation of interwave intervals (e.g. I–V, III–V) and can be useful in confirming a brainstem disturbance which is either only suspected clinically on the basis of the history or is entirely subclinical.

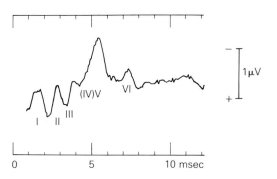

Left ear-lobe referred to vertex
Binaural clicks 70 dB HL 20/sec
4000 responses

Fig. 3.7 *Auditory evoked potentials (averaged response) to 4000 binaural click stimuli at 70dB above hearing threshold recorded with surface electrodes on the ear lobe and the vertex. Generators of the main potentials are situated as per text. (Courtesy of Dr AM Halliday, Institute of Neurology, London.)*

Somatosensory evoked responses (SEPs)

The stimulus is electrical stimulation of peripheral sensory fibres, usually in the fingers. Surface electrodes are applied to the skin of the neck and over the scalp. The evoked responses of greatest clinical interest are N9, which corresponds to activation of the brachial plexus, N13 corresponding to the cervical spinal cord, and N19 – a cortical response. The time between N13 and N19 is a measure of central conduction time. Recordings can also be made following stimulation of the lower limbs (Fig. 3.8).

These potentials may be particularly useful in confirming the presence of a plexus or spinal cord lesion or in determining the site of an unknown lesion causing a sensory disturbance. Central conduction time has also

been used for monitoring cortical and subcortical function in vascular lesions, e.g. ischaemia following stroke or subarachnoid haemorrhage.

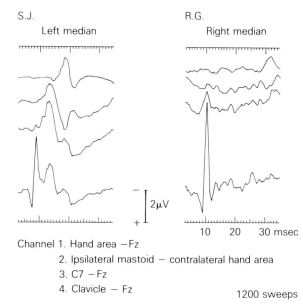

Channel 1. Hand area −Fz
2. Ipsilateral mastoid − contralateral hand area
3. C7 − Fz
4. Clavicle − Fz

1200 sweeps

Fig. 3.8 *Somatosensory evoked potentials in response to electrical stimulation of the median nerve at the wrist recorded over the contralateral sensory cortex (Channel 1), a cervical electrode (Channel 3) and a supraclavicular electrode (Channel 4). Channel 2 is from the contralateral sensory cortex referred to ipsilateral mastoid reference. The large $\overline{N9}$ wave (Ch.4) corresponds to brachial plexus activation, the $\overline{N13}$ wave (Ch.3) a cervical cord response, the $\overline{N19}$ wave (Ch.1) the cortical response. (Courtesy of Dr AM Halliday, Institute of Neurology, London.)*

RADIOLOGICAL INVESTIGATIONS

Plain X-ray

X-ray of the skull is a routine investigation in any patient with an undiagnosed brain lesion. Plain x-rays, which may include lateral, anteroposterior, Townes and basal views, may give valuable information in the following conditions.

Trauma: fractures of the vault or base of the skull may be seen (undisplaced or depressed), and mid-line shift from intracranial haematoma may be indicated by displacement of a calcified pineal gland.

Tumour: osteolytic bone metastases may be seen as defects in the skull, and nerve exit foramina may be expanded by local tumour erosion (e.g. acoustic neuroma). Raised intracranial pressure may be indicated by separation of sutures (children only), erosion of the skull base, and pituitary fossa (Fig. 3.9). Pituitary tumours usually cause distension and enlargement of the sella (Fig. 3.10). Meningiomas may cause local bone overgrowth (hyperostosis) either on the inner or outer table of the skull. Some low-grade glial tumours and craniopharyngiomas may be calcified.

Vascular: a large aneurysm may cause local bone erosion similar to tumour. It may also show calcification deposited in the wall. A localised haematoma, whether intra- or extracerebral, may cause pineal shift.

Congenital: developmental defects may result in premature fusion of the skull bones (craniostenosis) as well as a variety of dysraphic defects. In various developmental abnormalities in the foramen magnum region, the upper cervical vertebrae are displaced upward indenting the posterior fossa (basilar impres-sion). Some vascular malformations (Sturge–Weber syndrome) show cerebral calcification (Fig. 3.11).

Inflammatory: abnormal opacification or local bone erosion in the region of the paranasal sinuses may indicate chronic infection which has spread to involve the brain or orbit.

Angiography

In cerebral arteriography, serial x-rays are taken following the injection of an iodine-containing dye into an artery (aorta, carotid or vertebral). The injection may be made directly into the carotid artery or via a catheter introduced at another site such as the femoral artery. Angiograms show occlusion or irregularity of the lumen of large arteries, either extracranial or intracranial, and later films show details of the capillary circulation and venous circulation. Cerebral angiography is widely used to detect small aneurysms in relation to the circle of Willis in patients with subarachnoid haemorrhage (Fig. 3.12). This normally requires angiography of all four

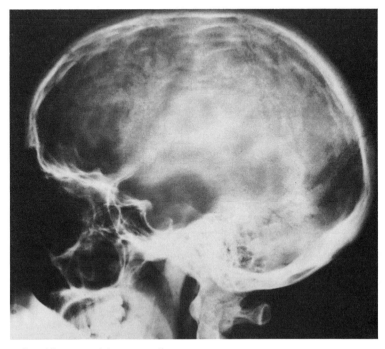

Fig. 3.9 *Thinning of the vault and flattening of the pituitary fossa in a patient with raised intracranial pressure.*

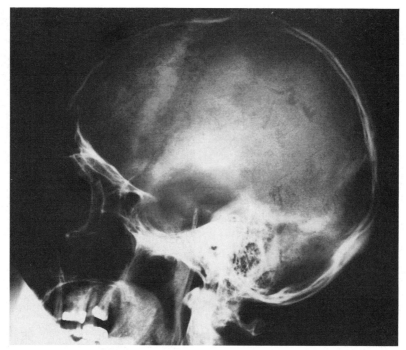

Fig. 3.10 *Expansion and destruction of the pituitary fossa by a pituitary adenoma.*

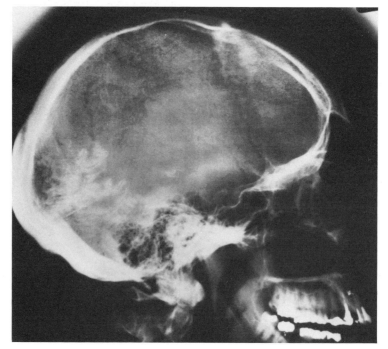

Fig. 3.11 *Calcification in occipital cortex in a patient with Sturge–Weber syndrome (trigemino-cerebral angiomatosis).*

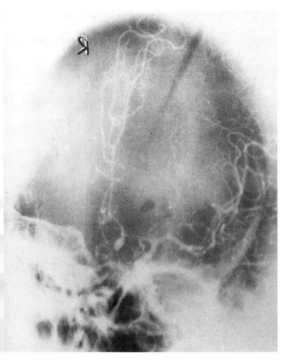

Fig. 3.12 *Berry aneurysm of anterior communicating artery with vascular spasm, from a patient with subarachnoid haemorrhage.*

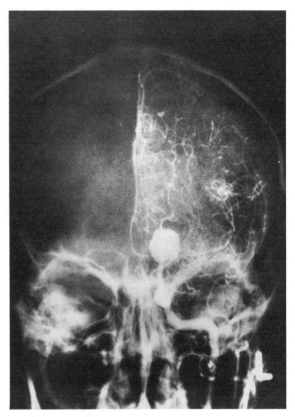

Fig. 3.13 *Giant terminal carotid aneurysm which compresses the optic chiasm.*

main arteries. Larger aneurysms which act as space-occupying lesions (and arteriovenous malformations) are more easily shown (Fig. 3.13). Angiography is now giving way to CT scanning in the detection of cerebral tumours, but may still be valuable in indicating the type of tumour (malignant glioma or meningioma). In addition, displacement of vessels caused by the tumour or by a haematoma and details of the vascular supply of the tumour are important to the neurosurgeon (Figs 3.14 and 3.15).

Recent advances in angiography include digital subtraction angiography, a computer-assisted enhancement technique giving greatly improved contrast sensitivity. This enables adequate visualisation of the major neck vessels and large cerebral vessels after an intravenous injection of contrast medium (Fig. 3.16). The introduction of flexible catheters into extracranial and intracranial arteries under fluoroscopic control has enabled the radiologist to introduce artificial emboli with the objective of reducing the growth of tumours or blocking arteriovenous fistulae.

Dangers of arteriography

Accidental damage to the artery at the site of injection may cause a local haematoma, occlusion of the artery, dissection of the artery or dislodgement of emboli. Complications from the injected solution include allergic reactions to iodine and cerebral vascular damage from excessive concentrations of contrast. These are usually temporary and occur most often in patients with severe atherosclerosis and hypertension after vertebral arteriography.

Air Encephalography

Air, introduced into the subarachnoid space at lumbar puncture with the patient upright, rapidly enters the ventricular system as well as entering the basal cisterns.

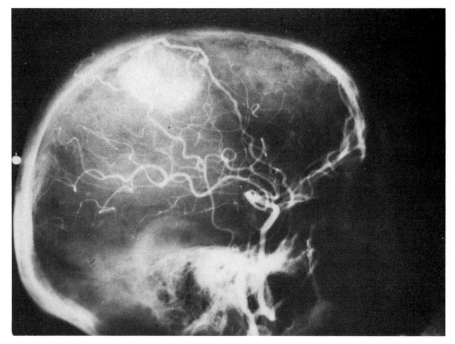

Fig. 3.14 *Meningioma supplied by branches of external carotid artery. Vascular blush shows position of tumour.*

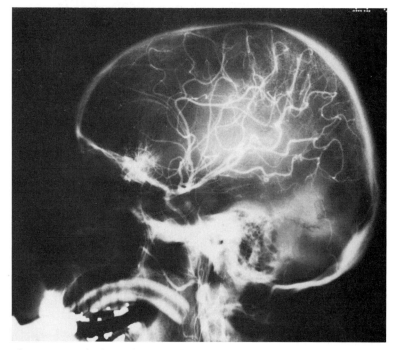

Fig. 3.15 *Large subfrontal meningioma displacing the terminal carotid and anterior cerebral arteries.*

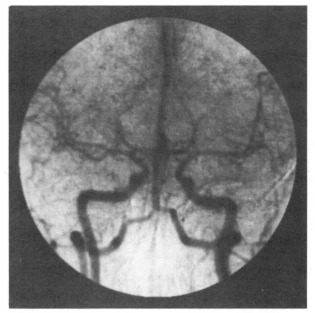

a

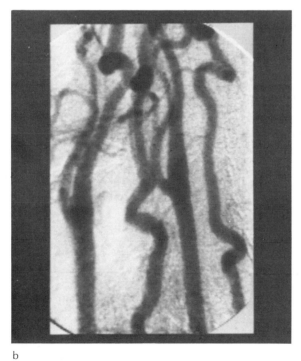

b

Fig. 3.16 (a) *Digital subtraction angiogram showing carotid and vertebral arteries in the neck.*
(b) *View of intracerebral arteries and circle of Willis.*

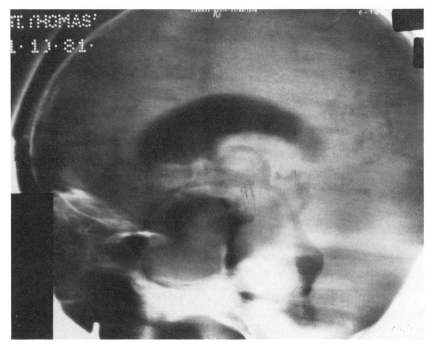

Fig. 3.17   *Air encephalogram showing upward displacement of the 3rd ventricle by a tumour arising in the pituitary fossa.*

X-ray tomography of the brain following such an injection may show displacement of structures caused by tumour or other space-occupying lesions. The technique has largely been replaced by CT scanning but it is still sometimes used for small lesions, especially those in the region of the pituitary fossa (Fig. 3.17). Lumbar air encephalography is dangerous in patients with raised intracranial pressure or large cerebral tumours as it may cause further displacement and brainstem compression.

CT Scanning

This technique, the major recent advance in diagnostic radiology, produces a series of two-dimensional brain maps showing the x-ray density of a series of horizontal brain sections (Fig. 3.18). Computer reconstructions in sagittal and coronal planes are also possible. The ventricles and sulci of the brain are visible as radiolucent areas. Certain other material, such as fresh blood, calcium deposits and some types of tumour, may show increased density. The diagnostic potential of the method is increased by carrying out a second scan after an injection of iodine-containing contrast, which is taken up selectively by some tissues (enhancement). The main uses of CT scanning may be summarised as follows:

Trauma: extra- or intracerebral haematomas, oedema or brain contusion or displacement are well seen (Fig. 3.19).

Vascular lesions: infarction appears after 36–72 hours as a wedge-shaped low-density region showing some enhancement but usually little displacement (Fig. 3.20). Intracerebral haemorrhage is well shown as a radiodense lesion, with or without brain displacement. Subarachnoid haemorrhage is visible in the ventricles, basal cisterns and sulci. Angiomas show as irregular serpiginous lesions, sometimes only seen on enhancement. Large aneurysms may also be shown.

Tumours: many tumours have similar radiodensity to brain but may show irregular regions of increased density (Fig. 3.21). Surrounding the tumour there is often low-density oedema and evidence of displacement of normal structures. Cysts or cystic tumours appear as well-defined low-density areas. After contrast injection most tumours enhance strongly, especially meningiomas and pituitary tumours (Fig. 3.22).

Degenerative lesions: brain atrophy is shown by enlargement of the ventricles as well as the sulci on the surface (Fig. 3.23). Correlation between the amount of brain atrophy and the intellectual performance of the patient is not close. A degree of brain atrophy occurs in most elderly people.

Hydrocephalus: obstruction of the circulation of CSF either within the brain or in the basal cisterns may also cause ventricular enlargement. In this case, however, there is no evidence of cortical atrophy and the sulci are not widened.

Demyelinating disease: large plaques of multiple sclerosis situated in cerebral white matter may be visible on CT scanning and may show contrast enhancement. However, they are likely to be better shown by the new techniques of magnetic resonance imaging.

Inflammatory lesions: a chronic bacterial abscess appears as a rounded encapsulated lesion which enhances with contrast. There is usually marked surrounding oedema (low density). Focal encephalitis, e.g. in the temporal lobe, resembles oedema in scan appearance.

Spinal Radiology

The principal object of spinal radiology is to distinguish patients with diseases causing external compression of the spinal cord and roots from those with intrinsic disease. Some information may be gained from plain film, but compressive lesions are usually confirmed by contrast myelography: a water-soluble or lipid-soluble contrast material is introduced into the subarachnoid space and is screened throughout the length of the spinal theca by tilting the patient.

Trauma: plain films of the spine may indicate fracture or fracture–dislocation, and separate views in flexion and extension may indicate subluxation of one vertebra on the next, a potential cause of damage to the cord.

Tumour: metastases may cause erosion of the vertebral bodies visible on the plain films. Long-standing benign lesions may expand the spinal canal or foramina and cause erosion of the pedicles. Myelography shows a partial or complete blockage to the passage of contrast and may indicate whether the block is extradural, intradural, or intrinsic in origin. Smaller tumours may show as filling defects.

Inflammation: chronic inflammatory disease of the spine (e.g. tuberculosis) often involves both vertebrae and discs and may be visible on the plain films. An acute epidural abscess will be shown on myelography as a complete block.

Vascular: angiomas of the cord or cauda equina may be shown on myelography by a characteristic coiled outline. The vascular nature of the mass can be confirmed by segmental spinal angiography (of the lumbar arteries).

Degenerative: some degree of osteoarthritis or disc degeneration is visible in spinal x-rays of most normal middle-aged and elderly patients. Myelography is necessary to show the level of the compression and the extent of the narrowing of the canal by disc prolapse (Fig. 3.24). A congenitally narrow spinal canal either in the cervical or lumbar region predisposes to neurological damage. Lumbar disc prolapse causing a root compression can be shown by the more limited technique of radiculography.

Complications

Myelography may sometimes precipitate clinical deterioration with a compressive lesion, and urgent surgery may be necessary. Allergy to iodine is only a relative contra-indication; severe reactions can usually be prevented by prior treatment with corticosteroids. Metrizamide and other water-soluble contrast media may cause a confusional state, and sometimes seizure, if much enters the head. Patients are therefore kept in bed with the head elevated for six hours after the procedure and prophylactic anticonvulsants such as

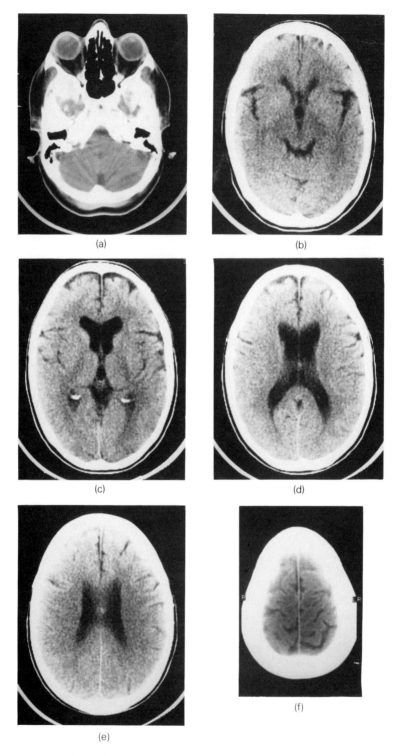

Fig. 3.18 *Normal appearances on CT scanning.*

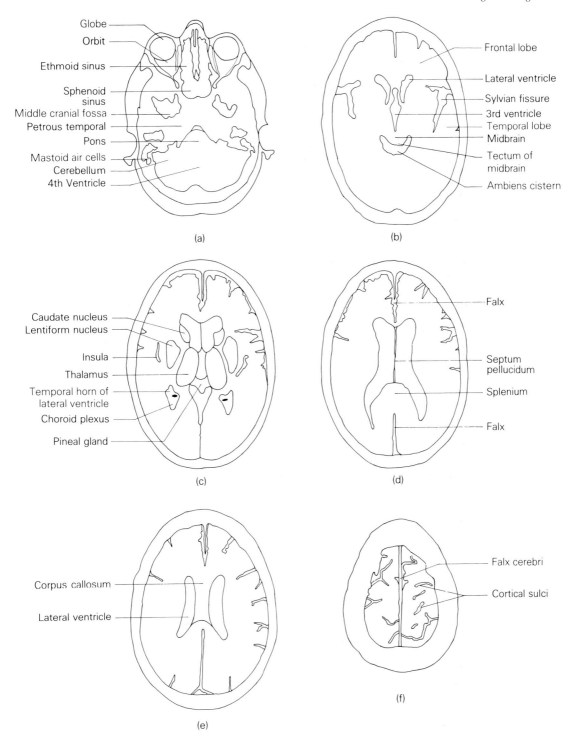

(a)

Globe
Orbit
Ethmoid sinus
Sphenoid sinus
Middle cranial fossa
Petrous temporal
Pons
Mastoid air cells
Cerebellum
4th Ventricle

(b)

Frontal lobe
Lateral ventricle
Sylvian fissure
3rd ventricle
Temporal lobe
Midbrain
Tectum of midbrain
Ambiens cistern

(c)

Caudate nucleus
Lentiform nucleus
Insula
Thalamus
Temporal horn of lateral ventricle
Choroid plexus
Pineal gland

(d)

Falx
Septum pellucidum
Splenium
Falx

(e)

Corpus callosum
Lateral ventricle

(f)

Falx cerebri
Cortical sulci

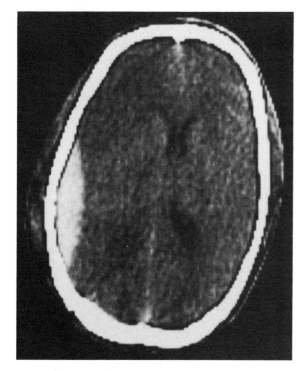

Fig. 3.19 *Extradural haematoma causing displacement and midline shift.*

phenobarbitone are sometimes recommended. Oily contrast materials occasionally cause progressive arachnoiditis and it is probably wise to remove contrast material after myelography.

Body CT Scanning

In spinal disease, this is of most value when combined with subarachnoid contrast injection. Transverse scans give a clear view of the spinal cord within the bony canal and allow the detection of cord expansion more easily. Contrast may be seen within a syrinx. In the lumbar region the technique allows the roots to be seen in the lateral recesses of the canal, which is difficult with radiculography alone. Sagittal, parasagittal and coronal reconstructions are of great value in defining structural defects at the foramen magnum. In addition, CT allows bone erosion to be seen, associated paraspinal masses (e.g. with neurofibromas or tuberculous disease) to be

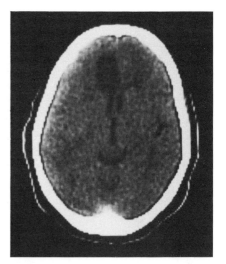

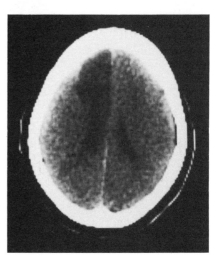

Fig. 3.20 *Infarct in anterior cerebral artery territory (low density).*

detected, and in myasthenia gravis it is helpful in the detection of thymomas.

Other Techniques

Emission computed tomography utilizes the radiation from short-lived isotopes (e.g. oxygen-15, or fluorine-18 labelled deoxyglucose) which are generated by a cyclotron. The sections of brain imaged yield data about local blood flow, oxygen or glucose uptake, and

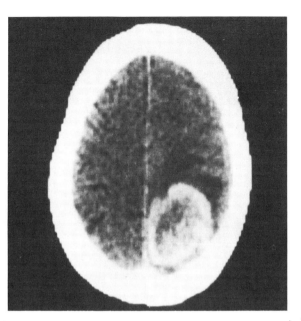

Fig. 3.21 *Malignant glioma right occipital region with surrounding oedema (enhanced CT scan).*

provide a more dynamic view of brain metabolism than is possible with CT scanning.

Magnetic resonance imaging (MRI) utilises the properties of protons aligned in a strong magnetic field and pulsed with radiofrequency waves at right angles to generate images of the brain. Preliminary work suggests that this technique will be of particular value in studying disease of white matter. The posterior fossa and spinal cord can be imaged particularly well.

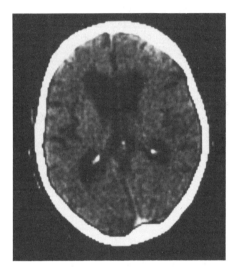

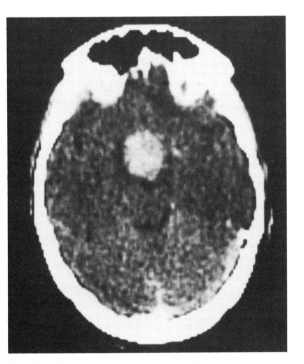

Fig. 3.22 *Pituitary adenoma (enhanced CT scan).*

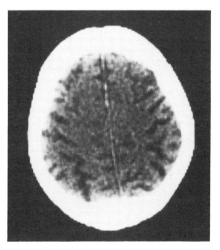

Fig. 3.23 *Cerebral atrophy showing ventricular dilatation and prominent cortical sulci.*

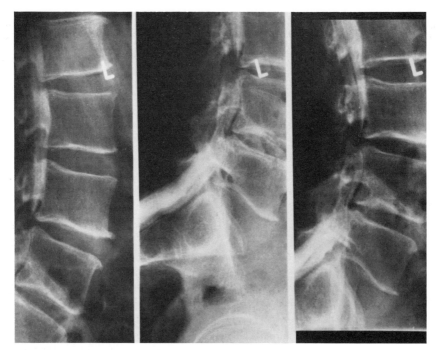

Fig. 3.24 *Lumbar myelogram to show indentation of the myodil column by posterior prolapse of intravertebral discs.*

4

Cerebrospinal fluid, raised intracranial pressure and hydrocephalus

CEREBROSPINAL FLUID (CSF) (Fig. 4.1)

CSF is produced, at the rate of 0.3–0.4 ml/minute, by the choroid plexuses of the lateral, third and fourth ventricles, with a smaller contribution coming from the brain and meningeal capillary bed. Thus the CSF volume of approximately 150 ml is exchanged 3–4 times per day. CSF from the lateral ventricles circulates through the interventricular foramina to the third ventricle, thence to the aqueduct and into the fourth ventricle, from where there is free exchange with fluid in the central canal of the spinal cord. From the fourth ventricle, CSF passes out into the basal cisterns, via the central and the lateral recess exit foramina, and circulates over the surface of the spinal cord and upwards over the hemispheres to be absorbed into venous sinuses by bulk flow through the arachnoid villi. Movement of the CSF is pulsatile, in response to arterial pulsations and venous pressure changes. Normal CSF pressure is between 60–150 mm of CSF when recorded at lumbar puncture in a relaxed adult in the lateral position. It is crystal clear in appearance and contains $0–4 \times 10^6$ lymphocytes/litre, up to 0.4 g/l protein, and 2.8–4.7 mmol/l glucose (usually equal to or greater than 50% blood glucose). Cisternal or ventricular CSF contains even fewer cells and the protein is only 0.1–0.15 g/l, but the glucose is similar to lumbar CSF.

Sampling of CSF

CSF may be sampled by lumbar or cisternal puncture or, as part of a neurosurgical procedure, by tapping the ventricles via a burr hole. The precise indications (Table 4.1) for lumbar puncture and the possible contra-indications (see Table 4.2) should always be carefully considered. A fine (equal to or less than 20 SWG) needle is introduced under sterile conditions below the termination of the spinal cord, usually via the L3/4 interspace, with the patient in the left lateral position and having first infiltrated local anaesthetic. Failure to obtain CSF is usually due to incorrect positioning of the needle, but may occasionally be caused by filling of the lumbar sac by tumour. On entering the subarachnoid space the stilette is withdrawn and, on seeing the flow of CSF, the pressure is measured with a manometer. The patient should be reassured and encouraged to relax while the oscillation of the CSF column with respiration is observed. Ideally CSF is then collected sequentially into three sterile tubes, with a separate 0.5 ml sample taken into a fluoride tube for glucose analysis. A total of 8–10 ml is usually adequate in an adult. A blood sample for glucose or serum protein analysis may be useful for comparison with the CSF.

After lumbar puncture, the patient should be encouraged to relax for an hour or two lying down and to drink plenty of fluids. Headache follows lumbar puncture in up to 50% of cases and is probably due to low pressure resulting from persistent leakage of CSF through the dural puncture site. Protracted bed rest does not seem to prevent post-lumbar puncture headache, but the use of a fine gauge needle does. Once the headache is established, however, it is often only relieved by lying down. Some patients require careful observation afterwards because neurological deterioration may occur some hours after the puncture if there is an undiagnosed spinal cord compression or an intracranial space-occupying lesion.

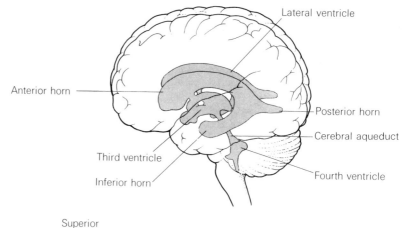

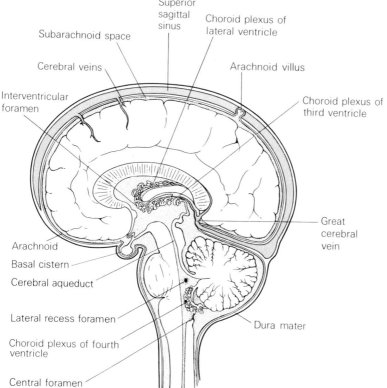

Fig. 4.1 *Circulation of cerebrospinal fluid in relation to brain structure.*

Investigation of CSF

The appearance of the CSF is noted: normally it is perfectly clear. Blood-staining, decreasing in sequential samples, is suggestive of local bleeding caused by the needle. Uniformly blood-stained fluid suggests subarachnoid haemorrhage and this is confirmed by centrifugation of the fresh sample to show a xanthochromic supernatant. This can be detected three hours after subarachnoid bleeding and may persist for up to

Table 4.1

Indications for Lumbar Puncture

1. Diagnostic
   a. Meningitis
      Subarachnoid haemorrhage
      Specific inflammatory disease, e.g. syphilis
      Demyelinating disease (cells, protein analysis)
      Neoplastic disease (malignant cells, tumour specific markers)

   b. Measurement of CSF pressure
         benign intracranial hypertension
         occasionally in communicating hydrocephalus

   c. Access for radiological procedures – introduction of contrast media

2. Therapeutic
   a. Introduction of chemotherapeutic agents
         antimicrobials – in infective disease
         cytotoxic agents – in neoplastic disease

   b. Removal of CSF
         benign intracranial hypertension
         following neurosurgical procedures

   c Anaesthetic purposes

Table 4.2

Contra-indications for Lumbar Puncture

1. Actual or suspected intracranial mass lesion
2. Local sepsis
3. Bleeding disorder (or patient on anticoagulants)
4. Major spinal deformity or anomaly of spinal cord

three weeks. Xanthochromia is also found when the protein concentration is greatly elevated or if the patient is deeply jaundiced.

A cell count is performed on a fresh sample and, if it is elevated, a cytological examination is performed on a centrifuged deposit. Depending on the clinical indication, a raised cell count will also suggest appropriate microbiological studies, including Gram, Ziehl–Nielsen, fungal stains, viral studies and the setting up of appropriate cultures and immunological detection procedures. If a CSF tap is bloody, the white cell/red cell ratio is similar to that in peripheral blood, i.e. approximately 1:1000.

The total CSF protein, which is raised in many neurological conditions, is determined. Occasionally the level is so high that a web or clot is formed in the CSF. The CSF IgG level (normally less than 12% of total protein) is measured by immunodiffusion or immuno-electrophoresis, but any defect in the blood–brain barrier may lead to an excessive level. Protein electrophoresis allows the pattern of CSF proteins to be examined and compared to serum. The technique is most useful in distinguishing leakage of protein across an abnormal blood–brain barrier from local (intrathecal) synthesis. Notably, the presence of restricted bands of immunoglobulins (oligoclonal bands) in the CSF is a feature of several disorders, including multiple sclerosis, syphilis, and sarcoidosis (see Fig. 9.3).

Although syphilis serology is also routinely performed on abnormal CSF, other serological tests for fungal antigens (e.g. cryptococci) and viral antibodies are of value.

RAISED INTRACRANIAL PRESSURE

Intracranial pressure rises if there is expansion of one of the three main components contained within the skull:

the brain/meninges, the cerebrospinal fluid, or the blood volume. The *brain* may expand due to oedema (e.g. following trauma of ischaemia) or in association with a mass lesion (e.g. tumour, abscess or haematoma). The *cerebrospinal fluid* space may enlarge due to overproduction, impaired circulation or absorption of CSF (see below). The volume of *blood* in the head may increase as a result of a rise in arterial PCO_2 (causing dilatation of the vascular bed), or of impaired venous drainage such as following dural sinus thrombosis.

Symptoms and Signs

Headache occurs as a result of stretching of the dura and basal blood vessels. Typically, it is bursting in nature and may waken the patient at night. It is occipital in location or generalised with spread to the neck. It is worsened by manoeuvres which raise intracranial pressure further such as straining, lifting, sneezing, bending or lying down. Vomiting is frequently associated, and may be worse at night. Papilloedema develops and the patient may have brief periods of loss of vision with, ultimately, optic atrophy and blindness if untreated. Rising intracranial pressure eventually leads to impaired mental function and coma. When acute, it may be associated with a reduced cardiac rate and rising blood pressure, IIIrd and VIth nerve palsies, and extensor plantar responses.

Differential diagnosis

The cause of such symptoms and signs may not always be apparent, particularly when there are no focal neurological signs to suggest the diagnosis of a space-occupying lesion. In particular, a number of conditions may present with raised intracranial pressure without focal signs (Table 4.3).

HYDROCEPHALUS: MECHANISM AND PATHOPHYSIOLOGY

The volume of CSF inside the head may be greater than normal if the normal CSF spaces have dilated as a result of loss of cerebral substance following atrophy, infarction or trauma (hydrocephalus *ex vacuo*). The term hydrocephalus usually refers, however, to an excessive accumulation of CSF as a result of impaired production, circulation, or absorption.

Increased production

Choroid plexus papilloma may be associated with excessive CSF production resulting in hydrocephalus, but this is a rare condition.

Impaired ventricular circulation (obstructive hydrocephalus)

Lesions within the third ventricle such as colloid cysts, craniopharyngioma, giant pituitary tumours, or intrinsic tumours of the thalamus or hypothalamus may obstruct CSF flow and cause dilatation of the lateral ventricles. If the obstruction is in the region of the aqueduct, as with congenital narrowing or inflammation causing aqueduct stenosis, or with tumours in the

---

Table 4.3

Causes of Raised Intracranial Pressure Without Focal Neurological Signs

1. Hydrocephalus (see below)
2. Chronic (often bilateral) subdural haematomas (see p. 87), subarachnoid haemorrhage
3. Clinically 'silent' tumours (e.g. non dominant frontal (see p. 97)
4. Venous sinus thrombosis (see p. 141)
5. Benign intracranial hypertension (see p. 82)
6. Meningitis (infective, infiltrative — see p. 224)
7. Diffuse brain swelling due to anoxia, ischaemia, trauma or electrolyte disturbance (e.g. hyponatraemia), severe hypertension

pineal region, the third ventricle is dilated also and may impinge on the hypothalamus, sella turcica, pituitary gland and optic pathways. Fourth-ventricular obstruction can result from congenital anomalies such as a Chiari malformation (see p. 180), the Dandy–Walker syndrome where there is atresia of the fourth ventricle outlet foramina, or any space-occupying lesion in the posterior fossa.

Impaired absorption (communicating hydrocephalus)

In this condition, ventricular circulation of CSF is unobstructed and there is free communication with the basal cisterns. Obstruction to circulation is mainly in the subarachnoid spaces so that the third and lateral ventricles are dilated and the subarachnoid space over the surface of the brain is only poorly seen. When the CSF pressure is monitored, it may be normal or only intermittently raised. Infection, haemorrhage, or neoplastic infiltration in the subarachnoid space may all cause this condition.

When CSF pressure is raised acutely due to hydrocephalus, there is increased absorption across the ependyma lining the ventricles and this gives rise to oedema in the periventricular regions. Nerve fibres may become damaged if the condition is unrelieved.

Clinical Features

Infantile hydrocephalus

In this condition the head characteristically enlarges and, if this occurs in utero, may cause difficulty in delivery. The sutures separate and, as the frontal region bulges forwards, the eyes are depressed forwards and downwards. Signs of raised intracranial pressure may be found but convulsions, optic atrophy, VIth nerve palsies, incoordination and extensor plantar responses, together with a variable delay in mental development, are the main neurological features. Hypopituitarism may result from hypothalamic or pituitary compression by an enlarged 3rd ventricle.

Hydrocephalus in adults

Adults with obstructive hydrocephalus present with typical features of raised intracranial pressure which

quickly brings them to medical attention. Patients with communicating hydrocephalus, however, present with a more protracted history: characteristically there may be dementia, a progressive disturbance of gait and balance and incontinence of urine. They may be found to have apparently normal CSF pressures when an occasional measurement is made. Typically, there is a disturbance of the gait which is broad-based and staggering, with a shortened stride length and a marked tendency to loss of balance; there are also increased tone and tonic grasp reflexes, brisk tendon reflexes particularly in the lower limbs, and extensor plantar responses. Headache and papilloedema do not usually occur.

Investigation

CT scan is the most useful investigation in both confirming the diagnosis of hydrocephalus and in determining its cause. In obstructive hydrocephalus the neurosurgeon may sometimes wish to perform further contrast studies, such as ventriculography, to precisely determine the site and nature of the obstruction. In communicating hydrocephalus, CSF pressure measured at lumbar puncture (after first excluding a space-occupying lesion) may be normal; more prolonged pressure monitoring with, for instance, an intraventricular or subdural catheter, frequently reveals periods of raised pressure ('normal pressure hydrocephalus'), however. Removal of CSF at lumbar puncture may result in a transitory clinical improvement in some patients. The introduction of water-soluble contrast medium into the subarachnoid space and measurement of the time taken for it to pass into the ventricles and over the brain convexities (determined by CT scanning) may help in differentiating cerebral atrophy from communicating hydrocephalus.

Management

The treatment of symptomatic hydrocephalus is either to remove the obstruction or to create a bypass using a shunt. Some of the causes of obstructive hydrocephalus such as colloid cyst or posterior fossa tumours may be amenable to direct surgical removal but, if major surgery is felt to be contra-indicated or inappropriate, useful symptomatic relief of the symptoms of raised intracranial pressure may be obtained by a shunt. Aqueduct stenosis may be treated by a shunt from the lateral ventricle into the cisterna magna (Torkildsen's procedure); most other shunts employ a catheter in the lateral ventricle draining, via a subcutaneous reservoir and one-way valve, into the peritoneal cavity or right atrium. The valve system can be selected to apply to various ranges of intracranial pressure.

Although they are relatively simple to place if the ventricles are enlarged, shunts may cause a significant number of complications, which include blockage, infection, 'low pressure' headache, and subdural haematoma, together with the need for revision in growing children. Ventriculo-peritoneal shunting is probably the commonest method of treating symptomatic communicating hydrocephalus, but the precise indications for when this should be used remain a matter of some controversy.

BENIGN INTRACRANIAL HYPERTENSION

This condition occurs in young females, typically in the third decade, and appears to be due to impaired absorption of CSF from the subarachnoid space across the arachnoid villi into the dural sinuses. There may or may not be associated venous sinus thrombosis (see p. 141). The ventricles, in contrast to hydrocephalus, are usually normal or reduced in size. The patient is often obese and there may be a history of minor trauma, endocrine disturbance, ingestion of certain antibiotics including tetracycline and nalidixic acid, excess vitamin A intake, or treatment with corticosteroids.

Such patients require full investigation to exclude other causes of raised intracranial pressure, including CT scanning and examination of the CSF with concomitant pressure measurements.

The aim of treatment is the relief of symptoms of raised intracranial pressure and the prevention of progressive optic nerve damage – which is shown by a gradual constriction of the visual fields and eventual secondary optic atrophy. Removal of predisposing causes, particularly treatment of obesity, is paramount. Intracranial pressure (and hence symptoms) may be controlled by lumbar puncture and, in a number of patients, raised pressure does not recur. Medical treatments with carbonic anhydrase inhibitors such as acetazolamide or corticosteroids are variably successful. Surgical procedures such as lumbo-peritoneal shunt, optic nerve sheath incision or subtemporal decompression are occasionally performed if vision is deteriorating. The overall prognosis for the condition is usually excellent provided that vision can be preserved.

5

CNS Trauma

INCIDENCE

Approximately 100 000 patients with head injury are admitted to hospitals in England and Wales each year, although the majority of injuries are slight and over 80% are discharged within 48 hours. However, it is a leading cause of death, with peaks of incidence in infancy and in young adults and a further peak in the elderly. In civilian practice the commonest causes of CNS injury are blunt injuries to head and spine from road traffic accidents, falls at home or at work, and assault. Missile injuries, due to bullets or bomb fragments, are other potent causes of CNS trauma. Males considerably outnumber females.

CNS REACTION TO INJURY

Basic Mechanisms of Primary Brain Damage

Impacts on the skull cause direct mechanical deformation of the bone and the underlying brain, as well as imparting translational (linear) and angular (rotational) acceleration to the head. The degree of acceleration depends on the exact mechanical conditions pertaining before, during, and after impact, i.e. site, direction and magnitude of violence. Mechanical deformation (coup at the site of injury) is probably the most important factor. Its consequences may be focal brain contusion and laceration, extra- and intradural haematomas and/or skull fracture. Cavitation produced by sudden deformation of the brain also causes implosion and turbulence locally in cerebral tissue. The resulting stresses and strains tear both axons and small blood vessels.

Translational and angular acceleration are also very important. The brain at body temperature behaves as a viscous fluid and, when subject to such forces, rotates back and forth, impacting on the rigid margins of the anterior, middle and posterior cranial fossae and on the dura of the falx cerebri and tentorium cerebelli. Diffuse white-matter lesions may occur due to shearing of axons throughout the CNS, from the frontal lobes, through the brainstem down to the upper cervical spinal cord, with the magnitude of damage in proportion to the axial and angular acceleration of the brain. Brain surface haemorrhages, and rupture of superficial veins, may also be caused by such forces.

Basic Mechanisms of Primary Brain Damage

The factors causing secondary brain damage are hypoxia, ischaemia and raised intracranial pressure. These important pathophysiological processes are interrelated.

In the unconscious patient, the airway may be compromised by the tongue, by inhaled vomit, or by direct trauma and swelling. Lung function may be impaired by associated chest injury, by aspiration of gastric contents or by pulmonary oedema induced by central neurogenic mechanisms. Such factors reduce arterial PO_2 and may increase PCO_2. The effects of this are cerebral hypoxia, leading directly to cerebral dysfunction, and cerebral vasodilation, leading to increased intracranial pressure.

Low systemic blood pressure may also increase the risk of cerebral ischaemia. Blood pressure may be low when cardiac output is reduced by disturbed neurogenic control from the damaged brain or by hypovolaemic shock in the patient with multiple injuries.

Raised intracranial pressure (ICP) is frequently present after head injury. Several factors contribute, including haematoma formation, cerebral oedema due to contusion or infarction, and vasodilatation due to the raised arterial PCO_2. There may be a constant, persisting, elevation of pressure or, more commonly, intermittent waves rising to a plateau for several minutes and then falling. In damaged brain, normal cerebral blood-flow autoregulation may be impaired so that perfusion becomes critically dependent on the difference between systemic arterial and intracranial pressure. Thus cerebral perfusion may be insufficient if systemic arterial pressure is low, while high systemic blood pressure can increase cerebral flow and blood volume, with a consequent dangerous rise in ICP.

Cellular Response to Injury: Repair and Regeneration

Biochemical changes become detectable within minutes of severe head injury. Cytoplasmic enzymes and membrane antigens are released into the cerebrospinal fluid (CSF) and peripheral blood. Electron microscopic studies of experimental injury in animals have revealed changes in the ultrastructure of neurones and glial cells, as well as in the capillary endothelial cells, within minutes. In patients coming to autopsy 10–14 days after injury, degeneration in myelinated axons may be observed by light microscopy. Marked changes in enzyme biochemistry and shedding of myelin membrane antigen often persists for 2–3 weeks after injury. Natural repair processes operate in the CNS after damage. Lysis and removal of damaged cells occurs with perivascular white-cell infiltration of affected brain, associated with leucocytosis in CSF and peripheral blood. Reactive gliosis takes place in areas of diffuse white-matter damage, areas of frank contusion, and areas of infarction. The volume of brain substance diminishes, with focal or general atrophy.

In adults, regeneration of neurones in the CNS almost certainly does not occur. However, in neonates and infants it is possible that some regeneration of neurones with remyelination of axons takes place. In young children there is also a degree of plasticity in the CNS so that in some cases neurological function may recover when undamaged areas of cortex take over functions which they do not usually subserve.

CLINICAL SEQUELAE OF HEAD INJURY

Skull Fracture

Linear fractures of the skull vault or base are not of themselves dangerous, although they indicate that a significant head injury has occurred. The fracture may rupture a meningeal artery (Fig. 5.1) and so cause extradural haematoma (see below). When a basal skull fracture tears the dura of the floor of the anterior fossa and the nasal mucosa, a CSF fistula is created, allowing *CSF rhinorrhoea*. Sometimes air enters the skull while CSF is escaping and an aerocele is created. The fistula may seal spontaneously in a few days or it may persist. Meningitis can ensue, sometimes within hours, although more commonly it occurs after a delay of days, weeks, or even months if the fistula remains unsealed. *CSF otorrhoea*, due to fracture in the petrous temporal bone, has similar infective risks but in nearly all cases CSF otorrhoea settles spontaneously. *Depressed fractures* in the skull vault also are usually directly *compound* between air and brain. In these cases adequate surgical repair is required to prevent infection, and elevation and debridement lessens the risk of post-traumatic epilepsy due to cortical scarring. Missile injuries produce compound fractures as well as leaving residual foreign bodies (Fig. 5.2).

Primary Brain Damage

Concussion, diffuse white matter injury, contusion, laceration, intracerebral haematoma

In the slightest form of primary brain damage – concussion – no macroscopic changes can be seen in the brain. However, it is assumed that microscopic changes occur which interfere transiently with consciousness. Following return of consciousness there will be a period of post-traumatic amnesia, the length of which is proportional to the severity of brain injury. There may also be a period of retrograde amnesia for

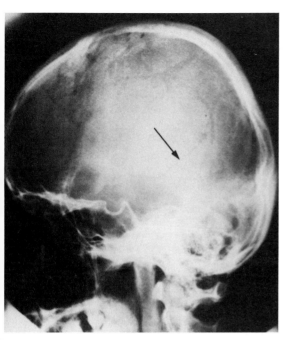

Fig. 5.1 *Lateral skull x-ray. Linear skull fracture in parietal region, crossing vascular marking of posterior branch of middle meningeal artery.*

the period before injury. During a period of post-traumatic amnesia the patient with concussion may be orientated and have no focal neurological deficits. Commonly there will be headache. If shearing occurs in many nerve fibres it may become visible microscopically as axon degeneration in the white matter of the cerebral hemispheres and brainstem. Severe primary diffuse white-matter injury of this kind results immediately in deep and persisting depression of consciousness, often with absence of cranial nerve function and limb responses as well as temporary apnoea (Fig. 5.3).

Macroscopic contusion and laceration are generally most pronounced in the anterior poles of the frontal and temporal lobes, where the rotational impact of brain on skull is greatest (Fig. 5.4). Sometimes these changes may be most evident at a site in the brain directly opposite to where a blow has been delivered (contra coup) (Fig. 5.4). Bleeding due to contusion and laceration may in some cases cause a significant intracerebral haematoma (Fig. 5.5). An intracerebral haematoma may also occur rarely if a deep artery is torn by rotational forces (delayed apoplexy). Evidence of focal neurological injury, e.g. cranial nerve palsy or

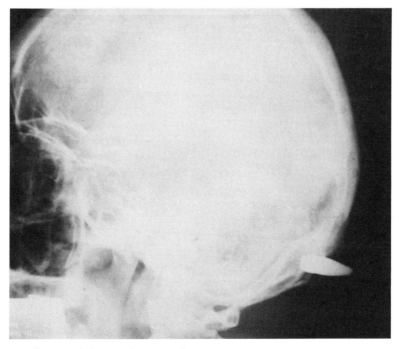

Fig. 5.2 *Lateral skull x-ray. Bullet wound of occipital region, with compound depressed skull fracture.*

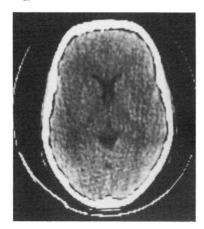

Fig. 5.3 *Diffuse white matter injury. No midline shift, ventricles rather small.*

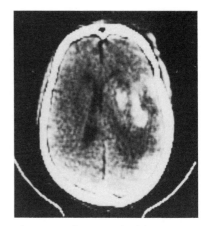

Fig. 5.5 *Right temporal intracerebral haematoma, with surrounding oedema and midline shift to left.*

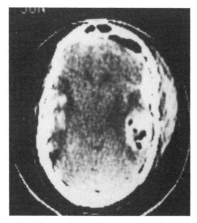

Fig. 5.4 *Bitemporal cerebral contusion with right-sided acute subdural haematoma. Soft-tissue swelling in right temporal region at site of impact with 'contre-coup' injury on left.*

Table 5.1

Factors Predisposing to Late Epilepsy

Post-traumatic amnesia > 24 hours
Dural tear/depressed skull fracture
Persistent neurological defect
Penetrating missile injury
Intracranial haematoma
Early epilepsy
Family history and young age

---

hemiparesis, may be present, as well as signs of raised intracranial pressure and brain herniation (see p. 53).

Epilepsy occurs within the first week in about 2% of head injuries (early epilepsy) and in about 12% of *severe* head injuries within 5 years (late epilepsy). The factors predisposing to late epilepsy are shown in Table 5.1 (see also p. 108).

Extradural Haematoma

The typical cause of extradural haematoma is a blow to the side of the head in the temporal region, associated with linear fracture of the squamous temporal bone in the middle cranial fossa (Fig. 5.1), often with little immediate sign of brain damage. However, at the time of injury the bony fracture has been combined with tearing of the middle meningeal artery, lying in the external surface of the dura.

Subsequently, arterial bleeding occurs and a haematoma forms, compressing the ipsilateral cerebral hemisphere (Fig. 5.6). The brain is shifted so that the midline structures are displaced and the medial part of the temporal lobe (uncus) is herniated down through the tentorial hiatus alongside the midbrain. If not arrested this process of 'coning' progresses rapidly to irreversible haemorrhage and necrosis in vital centres, with fatal apnoea and circulatory collapse (see p. 53).

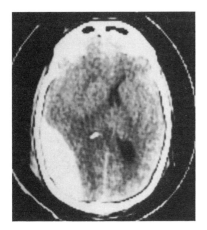

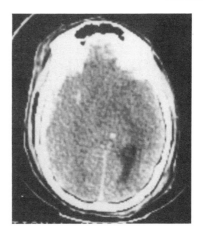

Fig. 5.6 *Left parietal extradural haematoma, with crescentic outline. Midline shift to right (same case as Fig 5.1).*

Fig. 5.7 *Left frontotemporal acute subdural haematoma: 'iso-dense' on CT scan and inferred from compression of the ventricular system and midline shift.*

Subdural Haematoma

Acute/subacute: chronic

Superficial brain contusion and lacerations, as well as torn bridging veins between the brain and the major venous sinuses, may cause haemorrhage in the sub-dural space forming a haematoma of clotted blood, hours or days after injury (Fig. 5.7). An arbitrary distinction may be made between acute (first 48 hours) and subacute (2–14 days) subdural haematomata. Chronic subdural haematoma is a different lesion. It is a watery collection, containing breakdown products of blood and encapsulated in a fibrinous membrane, forming about 6 weeks after slight head injury, usually in the elderly (Fig. 5.8a,b). Such patients may present with no known history of head injury, and with progressive deterioration of intellectual function, leg weakness, and progressive deterioration of conscious-ness.

All these extracerebral haematomas in the subdural plane may cause brain shift and herniation in the same way as extradural haematomas, although generally less rapidly.

Occasionally the mechanisms of CSF absorption will be disturbed, resulting in a delayed onset of hydro-cephalus with symptoms often similar to that caused by chronic subdural haematoma (see p. 80).

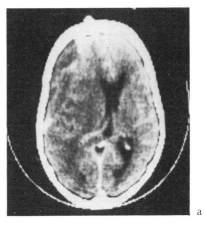

a

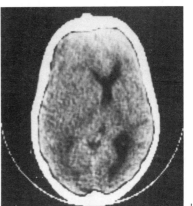

b

Fig. 5.8 *Chronic subdural haematoma in left frontotemporal region before (a) and after (b) intravenous contrast.*

Fat Embolism

A minority of head-injured patients with associated bony fractures of limbs or pelvis develop fat embolism, either shortly after injury or after fracture manipulation. Fat emboli lodge in the cerebral and pulmonary arteries, causing secondary brain damage as well as impaired lung function with hypoxia. These changes are associated with petechial haemorrhages in the face, upper trunk and conjunctivae.

Patterns of Head Injury in childhood

Blunt head injury is common in infancy and childhood, due to accidental falls, road traffic accidents and non-accidental child abuse. Compound depressed fractures of the skull vault as well as penetrating injuries of the orbits by sharp objects are also seen. Early post-traumatic epilepsy frequently occurs and may indicate the formation of a haematoma. Widespread cerebral oedema is also more common in children than in adults. The classical pattern of deterioration, with lateralised signs and depression of conscious level, is often not found in children. Increasing restlessness and rapid changes in the vital signs – blood pressure, pulse and respiration – may be the manifestations of progressive intracranial haematoma requiring urgent investigation. The capacity for recovery from serious head injury is greater in children than in adults.

MANAGEMENT OF HEAD INJURY

Emergency Treatment

In the unconscious patient who has sustained a head injury, attention to the airway must be the most urgent medical priority. Positioning the patient semiprone and the insertion of an oropharyngeal airway are generally sufficient to achieve a safe airway, thus preventing secondary hypoxic damage. In cases where there are facial injuries or where mechanical ventilation is necessary, a cuffed endotracheal tube may be required.

Diagnosis of significant associated injuries, including flail chest and pneumothorax, limb and pelvic fracture, haemorrhage from major vessels, spleen or liver, and perforated abdominal viscus must take next priority. Some of these complications, which may prove even more rapidly fatal than deteriorating head injury, necessitate urgent specific treatment. Thus relief of tension pneumothorax or abdominal laparotomy may occasionally have to take precedence over the careful neurological assessment of the patient. Other complications, such as limb or facial fractures, may await treatment until the patient's neurological state has been assessed and found to be stable.

Drugs and anaesthesia

Sedative drugs or narcotic analgesics are contra-indicated in the head-injured patient because they may depress conscious level directly as well as causing cerebral hypoxia by respiratory depression.

General anaesthesia with volatile anaesthetic agents (e.g. halothane) which increase cerebral blood flow and thus may elevate ICP, is relatively contra-indicated early after head injury. Unfortunately, where general anaesthesia proves essential for treatment of associated injuries it is sometimes found that the patient deteriorates neurologically during anaesthesia and fails to recover.

Initial Neurological Assessment and Continued Observation (see also p. 90)

Assessment of conscious level and specific neurological damage are the next priorities in clinical management. As full a history as possible must be taken from relatives, ambulancemen or, where possible, patients. The conscious patient can himself often estimate the period of unconsciousness he has suffered following injury and may reveal the period of amnesia prior to injury (retrograde amnesia) or post injury (anterograde or post-traumatic amnesia). Others must speak for the unconscious patient. Where possible, it is important to know the cause and circumstances of the head injury, and to know the course of events prior to admission to hospital. Direct questions, e.g. whether the patient has talked after injury, may be necessary to elicit whether there has been a 'lucid' interval. Such a period implies that the primary brain injury was of only mild or moderate severity and raises the important possibility of treatable secondary complications if later deterioration has occurred before admission. Thus, if the patient has recovered consciousness and then lapsed again into unconsciousness, or if the patient has shown signs of responsiveness short of full recovery, and then declined, there is a strong presumption that secondary brain damage has occurred.

Inspection of the skull, sc lp, nose and neck visually and by palpation, as well as of the ears by auroscope, may be required to reveal scalp lacerations, depressed fractures, or CSF otorrhoea and rhinorrhoea. If a neck fracture is suspected because of deformity or localised pain, great care must be taken to avoid further displacement before cervical x-ray has been performed to definitely establish the diagnosis and to allow appropriate stabilisation to be applied.

The neurological examination should be performed as completely as possible to elicit focal deficits, e.g. IIIrd nerve palsy, hemiparesis. For the purposes of monitoring clinical progress, however, a standardised and unambiguous assessment is necessary which can be regularly performed by either medical or nursing staff. The Glasgow Coma Scale is one method which fulfils this need, being based on monitoring of the best verbal response, eye opening and best motor response (Fig. 5.9). Any deterioration is of great importance and must be thoroughly investigated as it may signify a potentially treatable complication.

Radiological Investigation

Plain skull x-ray

The primary purpose of plain skull x-ray, at the time of admission of the head-injured patient to hospital, is to reveal skull fracture – linear or fissured (Fig. 5.1), and possibly depressed (Fig. 5.2). Occasionally, fistula may be evident because of intracranial air, or midline shift, shown by displacement of calcified pineal gland to one side of the midline. In the restless patient it is frequently difficult to obtain satisfactory films and it may be necessary to repeat the examination.

CT scan

Computerised axial tomography of the brain is the most efficient method of investigating a patient who has deteriorated following initial injury. Specifically,

evidence of displacement of midline structures, brain swelling, contusion and intra- or extracerebral haematoma can be seen (Figs 5.3–5.8). If the patient is deeply unconscious, or conscious and cooperative, diagnostic scans are readily obtained. In the uncooperative restless patient, general anaesthesia may be required to permit successful scanning.

Other specialised investigations

Lumbar puncture may be necessary in order to diagnose meningitis complicating CSF fistula. Frequently the organism isolated is *Streptococcus pneumoniae*. Intrathecal injections of radio-isotopes or radiological contrast media may eventually be required to define the site of fistula if it fails to close spontaneously. Angiography may be required to define the site of post-traumatic carotico-cavernous fistula.

Treatment of Head-injured Patients

General

Fluid balance and nutrition must be attended to accurately, which often necessitates intravenous rehydration and feeding, although in other cases nasogastric feeding is sufficient. In the post-injury phase, inappropriate antidiuretic hormone (ADH) secretion is common and, to limit cerebral oedema, it is important to avoid excessive fluid input and to check plasma and urine osmolality.

Nursing care, with attention to pressure areas, mouth and eyes, and regular turning, as well as physiotherapy to chest and limbs, are essential in the unconscious patient. In both the conscious patient with post-traumatic headache and in the restless unconscious patient, the use of non-narcotic analgesics such as codeine phosphate may be indicated.

Specific treatment

Antibiotics: In cases of compound depressed fracture, or of CSF rhinorrhoea and otorrhoea, prophylactic antibiotics are generally used to reduce the risk of meningitis. Penicillin and sulphadimidine are appro-

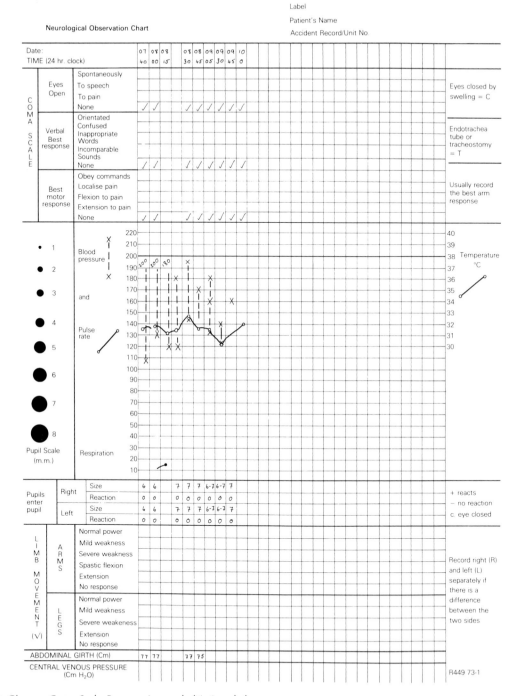

Fig. 5.9 *Glasgow Coma Scale. Eye opening graded 1–4, verbal response 1–5, motor response 1–5. Pupil size and reaction, together with lateralised neurological deficits and vital signs recorded in a case of severe head injury.*

priate unless an organism is cultured and its specific sensitivities determined. If infection is acquired in hospital, local bacteriological advice should be sought.

Anticonvulsants (see pp. 114 and 116) Post-traumatic epilepsy may develop early (in the first week) or later (see above). An initial fit may require control with intravenous diazepam, typically with a bolus injection of 5–10 mg in an adult. Subsequently phenytoin may be used. The use of anticonvulsants routinely after major head injury or following a single early fit is controversial. After more than one fit, however, or in the presence of certain types of head injury often complicated by epilepsy, e.g. gun shot wounds, it is advisable to use an anticonvulsant.

Reduction of ICP: Mannitol: A rapid intravenous bolus of mannitol (40 g in 15 minutes in the adult) temporarily lowers raised ICP. However, if this is repeated at intervals of 4–6 hours over 48–72 hours the beneficial effect is lost. If there is an expanding haematoma inside the skull, the beneficial effect of mannitol is even more temporary. Once mannitol therapy has been started it is important to exclude, usually by CT scan, an operable mass lesion. Corticosteroids, such as dexamethasone, have been widely used in head-injured patients but there is no evidence from clinical trials that they control ICP or improve overall results.

Assisted ventilation

Elective intermittent positive pressure ventilation (IPPV) at a low arterial PCO_2 is an effective way of reducing intracranial pressure, although cerebral blood flow is also reduced. Because the patient may need either sedation or muscle relaxants to achieve this, monitoring of the neurological status is made more difficult or impossible clinically. In these circumstances CT scan is invaluable in excluding a surgically-treatable intracranial mass and intracranial pressure monitoring may be helpful. Similar considerations also apply if a patient requires IPPV for an obstructed upper airway or flail chest. Endotracheal intubation, with or without assisted ventilation, is also frequently necessary in the management of obstructed airway or failure of spontaneous respiration in the unconscious head-injured patient.

Continued observation in the head-injured patient

Some severely head-injured patients are unresponsive and apnoeic from time of injury and die within a short time, before or after admission to hospital. It is presumed that in such cases there has been overwhelming primary brain damage. Many initially unconscious patients, however, gradually improve during a period of general supportive care and regain consciousness within hours or days. In such patients a virtually full recovery may follow.

Treatment of deteriorating head injury

In a general hospital, admitting head-injured patients as emergencies, approximately one patient in 20 will be found to deteriorate rapidly or gradually as he is observed over a period of hours or days. Systemic blood loss, hypoxia or infection may precipitate neurological deterioration. Important intracranial causes are haematoma, meningitis, brain swelling, and epilepsy. The most urgent cause to be considered is an intracranial haematoma. Radiological investigation by CT scan or, in rare emergencies, direct surgical exploration, is essential to confirm or refute the diagnosis and often necessitates the patient's transfer to a neurosurgical unit. Suspected meningitis means that the CSF should be examined either by lumbar puncture, if safe, or by ventricular tap, and appropriate antibiotic treatment started.

Operative Treatment

When a head injured patient is rapidly deteriorating due to suspected intracranial haematoma, exploratory burr holes are cut at the site of any skull fracture and in frontal, temporal and parietal regions, bilaterally, seeking signs of extradural haematoma; if this is not present the dura is opened to look for subdural haematoma. If a haematoma is found, the skull exploration is extended by craniectomy to allow its thorough surgical evacuation. In those cases where preoperative CT scan has shown a haematoma – extradural, subdural, or intracerebral – such exploration is unnecessary and a craniotomy may be performed accurately at the appropriate site. Operative treatment is also required to elevate and debride compound depressed skull fractures, where possible within 12–24 hours of injury. If

CSF rhinorrhoea persists for more than 7 days, surgical repair of the torn dura in the anterior cranial fossa is generally needed. However, such repair is best delayed for 2–3 weeks until the general condition of the patient is improved and cerebral oedema has settled.

Results

Mortality

In spite of modern neurosurgical management, the mortality from intracranial haematomata remains high, about 20% in extradural haematoma and 60–70% in acute subdural haematoma.

Morbidity, late results and rehabilitation

Even following mild injury, minor symptoms such as headache, giddiness, irritability, poor concentration and depression are common. These symptoms probably have an organic basis but other factors such as prolonged litigation about compensation may lead to their exacerbation and cause delay in return to work. A sympathetic attitude to such symptoms is thus warranted even where there has been only very transient loss of consciousness or none at all.

In moderate to severe head injuries there may be specific persisting neurological deficits like dysphasia, hemiparesis or cranial nerve palsies. Of the latter, diplopia, loss of smell, deafness or facial weakness are the commonest manifestations. More global effects of brain damage may become evident as impaired intellectual function, particularly concentration and memory, as well as changes in mood and personality, particularly increased irritability and disinhibited behaviour. A period of time in a rehabilitation unit with facilities for speech therapy, physiotherapy and occupational therapy and close liaison with the disablement resettlement officer (DRO) may be invaluable in assisting return to life outside hospital.

Spontaneous improvement may occur for up to 2 years after injury, but generally it is possible to assess rate of improvement within a matter of weeks and to give a prognosis to the patient and his family. It may become evident that the patient cannot return to his occupation, and in this case early retraining is desirable. In a very small percentage of cases of head injury the patient remains alive but very severely disabled, sometimes with no evidence of contact with the outside world ('vegetative state'). Institutional care over a period of months or years, is required until generally some intercurrent complication supervenes and the patient dies.

SPINAL INJURY

Spinal injury is frequently caused by accidental falls either at work or in the home, by sports injuries or by traffic accidents. Penetrating injuries may also be caused by knife wounds and missiles (bullets or bomb fragments). The spinal cord, anywhere between the upper cervical region, through the thoracic spine to the conus at the first lumbar vertebra may be affected.

In the lower part of the lumbar and sacral spine it is the cauda equina that is injured. Flexion, extension, and compression are the forces that deform the spinal canal, often with bony fracture or acute intervertebral disc prolapse, and sometimes with subluxation or dislocation. Primary damage to the cord, by contusion or laceration, leads to immediate neurological deficit appropriate to the level of injury. In general, after acute complete traumatic spinal cord lesion there is no effective recovery. Partial lesions may gradually improve. Deterioration at some time hours or days after initial injury implies a secondary factor, for example further displacement of the unstable spine or spinal cord compression by disc prolapse or haematoma. Such secondary damage may potentially be prevented or treated. Diagnosis of spinal fracture and assessment of stability depends on radiology – generally plain x-ray, supplemented if necessary by tomography. Spinal compression is diagnosed by myelography, although CT scanning of the spine is being rapidly developed.

Surgical Treatment

Where the spine is unstable, fixation, either externally by traction (weights pulling on calipers applied to skull or halo (metal ring applied to skull and rigidly fixed to pelvis externally), or internally (wires and rods placed at open operation), is often required to stabilise cervical pine fractures. Less commonly, it is required for horacic or lumbar injuries. Spinal decompression, in many cases requiring anterior or lateral approaches to the spine rather then simple posterior laminectomy, may also be indicated in order to remove disc or bone fragments causing deteriorating spinal injury. Open injuries require operative debridement to prevent infection, including meningitis.

Results

Partial cord lesions, spinal root lesions, and cauda equina lesions may all show a degree of functional recovery, spontaneously or after surgical decompression. Complete cord transections do not recover. Early admission to a specialist spinal unit probably reduces urinary tract, pulmonary and skin complications. Active rehabilitation from an early stage is essential to maximise return of useful function or to adapt to complete paraplegia.

6

Intracranial Tumours

INTRODUCTION

Any type of cell within the brain or spinal cord can undergo neoplastic change and give rise to a space-occupying lesion, or tumour. However, the most common primary brain tumours arise from glial cells, particularly astrocytes, whilst tumours arising from neurones are rare. Tumours may also grow from the meningeal coverings of the central nervous system and from bone, in the skull and in the spinal canal. Secondary metastatic tumours may spread to the brain directly by invasion or through the bloodstream. These varied tumours form a heterogeneous pathological spectrum, each with characteristic histology and individual natural history, but with a common pathophysiology as space-occupying lesions. Because the function of normal nervous tissue becomes impaired when it is subjected to erosion or compression, whatever the cause, patients with these lesions generally present with a small variety of syndromes, i.e. those due to general raised intracranial pressure, to focal loss of neurological function, to epilepsy or to spinal-cord compression.

Aetiology and Pathogenesis

The cause of CNS tumours in man is not known. Experimental tumours may be induced in animals by exposure to viruses and to chemicals. Therapeutic radiation to the head in childhood appears to be associated with an increased incidence of meningiomas and of gliomas. Other possible aetiological factors are head injury and occupational exposure in the petrochemical industry.

Metabolism of Brain Tumours

Biochemical studies of human brain tumour tissue removed at operation or autopsy, have shown that its principal energy-producing metabolic pathway is anaerobic glycolysis, in contrast to normal brain tissue where the energy is produced, almost exclusively, by oxidative metabolism of glucose. The enzymes found in brain tumours are those more appropriate to anaerobic metabolism, and increasing malignancy of tumour is paralleled by increasing deviation of enzyme pattern from normal. However, this switch to anaerobic metabolism is not simply related to ischaemia since blood flow and oxygen supply appear ample in many malignant tumours.

Cell Kinetics

In a malignant glioma 15–30% of cells are actively undergoing mitosis at one time (the growth fraction) whilst the equivalent proportion in a benign astrocytoma is about 1%. The time each dividing cell spends in a single cycle is similar, regardless of tumour grade, at about 48–72 hours. The difference in the rate of increase in size of tumours of differing malignancy is therefore dependent mainly on the growth fraction and the rate of cell death and removal.

Microvasculature of Cerebral Tumour: Cerebral Oedema

A prominent feature of many gliomas is surrounding oedema. Electron microscopic studies have shown that the capillaries of cerebral gliomas differ from normal brain capillaries in having fenestrated endothelium, not sealed by tight intercellular junctions. Large hydrophilic molecules, including serum proteins, can readily enter the tumour through such fenestrations, and this ease of penetration by solutes and water is probably a major source for the oedema.

However, disruption of the normal anatomical blood–brain barrier (BBB) is not found throughout the tumour. The penetration of the barrier, particularly at the actively-proliferating marginal zone at the edge of the tumour, is a theoretical difficulty in brain tumour chemotherapy.

PATHOLOGY

The international classification, from the World Health Organisation, offers a logical system for classifying intracranial tumours (Table 6.1). This classification is based on cell type of origin. Thus the most common type of primary brain tumour, the *glioma*, lies within the neuroepithelial cell category. Other relatively frequent tumours like *meningiomas, pituitary adenomas* and *acoustic schwannomas* are each in different categories. The criteria for the diagnosis of 'malignancy' in CNS tumours differ from those applied in other cancers. It is most unusual for primary CNS tumours to metastasise to other parts of the body. However, many have a tendency to invade locally and to recur after excision. Histological grading is based on assessment of cellular differentiation within the tumour as well as the appearance of unfavourable prognostic factors like vascular endothelial hyperplasia, necrosis and haemorrhage. Even histologically benign, slowly-expanding intracranial tumours may ultimately be lethal by virtue of the space which they occupy. In particular sites their local pressure effects on vital functions may be fatal, in

Table 6.1

Classification of Tumours of the CNS

	Cells of Origin	Examples
1.	Neuroepithelial	astrocytoma
		oligodendroglioma
		ependymoma/choroid plexus papilloma
		pineal cell tumours
		neuronal tumours
		poorly-differentiated, e.g. medulloblastoma
2.	Nerve sheath	Schwannoma/neurioma
		neurofibroma
3.	Meninges	meningioma
		xanthoma
		melanoma
4.	Primary lymphoma	
5.	Blood vessels	haemangioblastoma
6.	Germ cell tumours	germinoma, teratoma
7.	Others	craniopharyngioma
		epidermoid or dermoid cyst
		colloid cyst of 3rd ventricle
		lipoma, enterogenous
8.	Vascular malformations	
9.	Anterior pituitary	adenoma
		adenocarcinoma
10.	Local extension to nervous system	glomus jugulare tumour chordoma
11.	Metastatic tumours	
12.	Unclassified	

(Adapted from WHO Classification 1979)

some cases at an early stage. However, taking account both of histological grading, and of typical clinical experience with particular tumour types, numerical grades I (benign), II (semi benign), III (relatively malignant) and IV (highly malignant) can be ascribed to these tumours.

INCIDENCE

Cerebral glioma is the tenth most frequent malignant tumour in males, whilst other tumours are exceedingly rare. There are two age peaks of incidence, in childhood (5–9 years) and middle age (50–55 years). The absolute incidence may be estimated at between 5–15/100 000/year, but many small benign tumours may remain undiagnosed in life.

CLINICAL DIAGNOSIS OF INTRACRANIAL TUMOURS

General Symptoms

Symptoms of raised intracranial pressure (ICP)

Headache, visual failure, vomiting, change in consciousness, 'coning': An intracranial space-occupying lesion within the closed confines of the skull, which is itself rigidly divided into right and left compartments by the dura of the falx cerebri and into supratentorial and infratentorial compartments by the tentorium cerebelli, displaces brain across the midline and upwards or downwards through the tentorial hiatus. An early symptom is headache, due, it is presumed, to stretching of dura and distortion of basal blood vessels. The headache is generally moderately severe, often frontal or temporal and commonly worse on waking in the morning. Raised ICP is transmitted to the optic nerve head causing papilloedema and eventually visual failure. At first intermittent, this may progress to optic atrophy, gradual constriction of the visual field and blindness. Vomiting is the third cardinal feature of raised ICP, and is characteristically unassociated with nausea.

Enlargement of a space-occupying lesion can cause herniation of the brain to such an extent that the brainstem, cranial nerves and arteries may be compressed. A supratentorial tumour will cause the medial temporal lobe to herniate through the space between the midbrain and the tentorium ('tentorial herniation'), the IIIrd and VIth cranial nerves, as well as the posterior cerebral artery, are compressed and displaced. An important early sign is enlargement of the ipsilateral pupil progressing to a fixed and dilated pupil. Finally, it may cause infarction or haemorrhage into the upper brainstem as well as infarction of the posterior part of the cerebral hemisphere, supplied by the posterior cerebral artery. Tumours in the posterior fossa may cause herniation upwards with similar results, but they usually force the cerebellar tonsils downwards through the foramen magnum, causing fatal compression of the medulla. The clinical manifestations of tonsillar herniation are increased headache, neck stiffness, decerebrate posturing and respiratory irregularity, followed by respiratory and cardiac arrest.

Focal Symptoms

Focal neurological dysfunction

Loss of certain neurological functions, such as speech or limb movement, causes a patient to seek medical help quickly. Other symptoms which may be equally serious, such as dementia or deafness, may pass unnoticed for much longer. Both intrinsic tumours (gliomas, metastases) and extrinsic tumours (meningiomas, pituitary adenomas and acoustic schwannomas) can permanently or reversibly damage adjacent normal brain tissue or cranial nerves. Although many tumours may present with both raised intracranial pressure and focal neurological disturbance, some may grow to a very considerable size without focal features. This occurs most often in clinically 'silent' areas such as the nondominant frontal or temporal lobe. In such cases, rather nonspecific mental changes or raised intracranial pressure may be the only clinical features (see also pp. 49).

Epilepsy (see also Chapter 7)

An epileptic seizure is a common symptom of brain tumour and is the first symptom in over one-third of patients with intrinsic tumours of the cerebral hemispheres; tumour at any site may cause epilepsy in children. Extrinsic tumours, e.g. meningiomas in the supratentorial compartment, also cause epilepsy and this symptom can precede the development of other symptoms by many years. Epilepsy of late onset, occurring for the first time after the age of 30 years, should always therefore raise the suspicion of an underlying tumour. Status epilepticus arising in an adult is even more likely to be associated with tumour.

SUPRATENTORIAL TUMOURS

'Gliomas' – neuroepithelial tumours, astrocytomas, oligodendrogliomas, ependymomas

Gliomas are the commonest primary tumours which occur in the cerebral hemisphere of the adult. Most are highly malignant (grade III–IV) and carry a dismal prognosis. Approximately 90% are in either the frontal (Fig. 6.1), parietal or temporal lobes, with other sites such as the corpus callosum (Fig. 6.2), thalamus or occipital lobe being much less common. (See also Fig. 2.28 for focal features).

Frontal Lobe

Personality change, with either irritability or docility, and deterioration of mental function are common. In the dominant left hemisphere, expressive dysphasia develops when the tumour involves the motor speech area, and hemiparesis as the motor cortex is involved.

Generalised seizures and sometimes focal epileptic movements of contralateral face and body, frequently occur (adversive seizures, Jacksonian epilepsy). Physical signs at an early stage include the presence of a grasp reflex (see p. 49), mild facial weakness and an extensor plantar response.

Parietal Lobe

Tumours in the parietal lobe may cause contralateral sensory loss and neglect, often associated with in-attention to objects in the corresponding visual field. In the dominant hemisphere there may be a receptive dysphasia, while similar lesions of the non-dominant hemisphere may cause spatial disorientation and dressing apraxia.

Temporal Lobe

Homonymous hemianopia or quadrantanopia, involving upper quadrants and associated with dysphasia when the dominant side is involved, are the typical features of a space-occupying lesion in the temporal lobe. Epilepsy, either with specific 'temporal lobe' features or with generalised seizures, is common.

i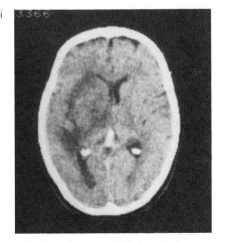

ii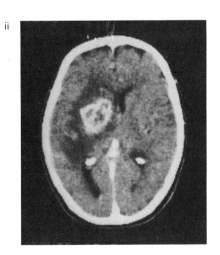

Fig. 6.1 *Cerebral glioma (left frontal) i before, ii after contrast.*

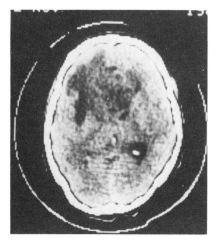 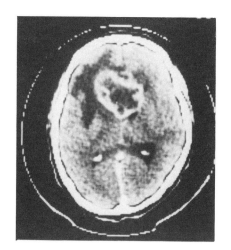

Fig. 6.2 *Corpus callosum glioma, before and after intravenous contrast injection.*

Primary Brain Tumours at Other Supratentorial Sites

Occipital lobe gliomas cause complete homonymous hemianopia and may not be noticed until symptoms of raised ICP supervene. Gliomas in the thalamus tend to cause relatively early hemiparesis and hemisensory loss. Intrinsic tumours of the hypothalamus can lead to disorders of thirst, appetite and temperature control (see p. 56) whilst those in the pineal region (germinomas, teratoma, glioma) cause local dysfunction of the midbrain tectum giving rise to a palsy of upward gaze (see p. 33), loss of pupillary light reaction, and frequently symptoms of raised ICP.

Meningiomas

These space-occupying lesions can arise from any meningeal surface. In the supratentorial compartment of the skull the common sites are: cranial vault (Fig. 6.3), falx, sphenoid wing, olfactory groove and suprasellar region.

Vault (Fig. 6.3): *convexity and parasagittal meningiomas*

Frontally sited meningiomas may cause only subtle personality changes, while those sited posteriorly over the cerebral hemisphere may be clinically silent until the symptoms of raised ICP arise. Those which occur over the middle third of the hemisphere or in the parasagittal region often present earlier with epilepsy or with focal motor or sensory deficits.

Basal: *sphenoid wing* (Fig. 6.4), *olfactory groove, suprasellar*

Meningiomas arising in the outer part of the sphenoid wing grow into the Sylvian fissure and distort the temporal and posterior frontal lobes. Hemiparesis, facial weakness and, on the dominant side, dysphasia may ensue, as may epilepsy. Tumours placed more medially involve the optic nerve and the cranial nerves in the orbital fissure (III, IV, V, VI), resulting in unilateral visual failure, ophthalmoplegia and proptosis. Meningiomas of the olfactory groove initially cause unilateral loss of smell, which is often unnoticed by the patient. Subsequently, symptoms of raised ICP supervene. At this stage optic atrophy may be found on the affected side with papilloedema in the opposite eye (Foster–Kennedy syndrome).

Meningiomas arising on the tuberculum sellae expand in the suprasellar region to compress the optic chiasm. The resulting pattern of visual failure may be very similar to that found in pituitary adenomas or craniopharyngiomas (see pp. 99, 100).

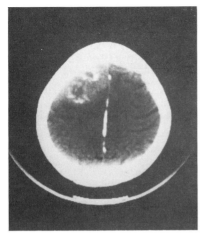 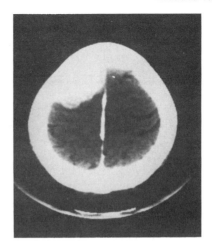

Fig. 6.3 *Vault meningioma, before and after contrast.*

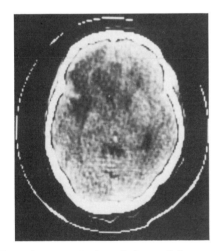 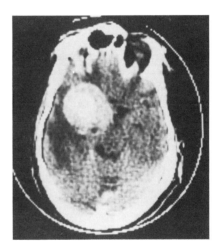

Fig. 6.4 *Sphenoid wing meningioma, before and after contrast.*

Pituitary Adenomas

Chromophobe adenoma, functioning microadenoma

Pituitary tumours present because of their endocrine effects (hypopituitarism, acromegaly, Cushing's syndrome, amenorrhea, galactorrhea) or because of compression of the visual pathways or both. Rarely the presentation is acute due to haemorrhage or infarction causing headache, acute visual failure and hypotension (pituitary apoplexy).

The chromophobe pituitary adenoma (Figs 6.5, 6.6) commonly presents as a space-occupying lesion in the suprasellar region. The tumour extends upwards to stretch and compress the optic chiasm (see p. 29). A bitemporal hemianopia develops, which may progress to complete visual failure if not treated. Asymmetric tumour growth may lead to predominantly uniocular visual loss due to optic nerve involvement, with a minor

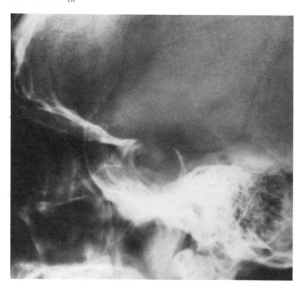

Fig. 6.5 Lateral plain skull x-ray – massive erosion of pituitary fossa by chromophobe pituitary adenoma.

field loss (usually upper temporal) in the other eye. Compression of the remaining pituitary tissue causes hypopituitarism (amenorrhoea, impotence, regression of secondary sexual characteristics, pale smooth skin, cold intolerance).

Pituitary adenomas which secrete abnormal quantities of prolactin, growth hormone or ACTH may present both as space-occupying lesions and with their respective endocrine syndromes. Although microadenomas are small (less than 10 mm) they may be associated with headache and may ultimately expand to cause chiasmal compression (Fig. 6.7).

Craniopharyngioma

Developmental cell rests in Rathke's pouch most commonly present in childhood with obstruction of the 3rd ventricle and hydrocephalus. In adolescence or adult life they form large cystic space-occupying lesions above the pituitary fossa. In childhood, failure of growth and sexual development, together with diabetes insipidus, associated with visual failure due to compression of the visual pathways, are common features. In older patients hydrocephalus, due to

obstruction of the foramina of Munro by expansion of tumour into the 3rd ventricle, may cause mental deterioration or raised ICP.

SECONDARY BRAIN TUMOURS

Metastases (Fig. 6.8)

Almost any malignant tumour in the body can metastasise to the brain, to the subarachnoid space, or to the skull vault or base. Metastases can present like any supratentorial or infratentorial primary tumour and also cause carcinomatous meningeal infiltration with meningism, headache, vomiting, with cranial nerve palsies and hydrocephalus.

INFRATENTORIAL TUMOURS

'Gliomas' – Brainstem, Cerebellar Astrocytoma, Medulloblastoma, Ependymoma, Haemangioblastoma, Cerebellar Metastasis

Most intrinsic brain tumours in the posterior cranial fossa occur in children and young adults. However, haemangioblastoma and cerebellar metastasis occur mainly in adults.

Brainstem glioma

Gliomas which occur within the brainstem cause progressive, but often fluctuating, lower cranial nerve palsies resulting in diplopia, facial weakness, deafness, dysphagia and dysarthria. Long-tract signs tend to occur late.

Cerebellar astrocytoma, medulloblastoma, ependymoma

Tumours in the cerebellar hemispheres (e.g. astrocytoma in children, ependymoma, haemangioblastoma or metastasis) tend to cause lateralised symptoms and signs in the limbs on the same side. Midline tumours of the vermis or the 4th ventricle (e.g. medulloblastoma in

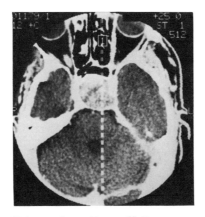

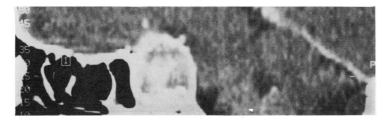

Sagittal

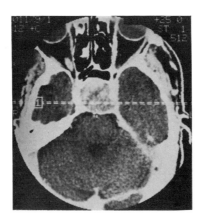

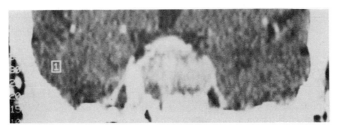

Coronal

Fig. 6.6 *Pituitary adenoma after contrast, coronal and sagittal reconstructions.*

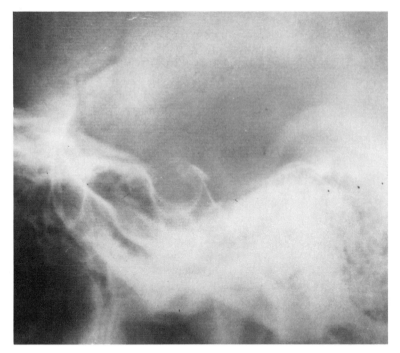

Fig. 6.7 *Erosion of anterior inferior pituitary fossa by micro-adenoma of pituitary.*

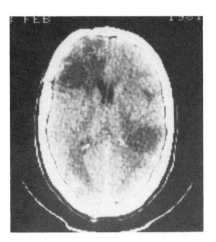

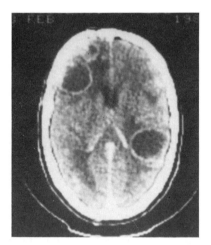

Fig. 6.8 *Multiple cerebral metastases, before and after contrast.*

children, metastasis in adults) cause severe truncal ataxia and early hydrocephalus. Haemangioblastoma may be sporadic or occur as part of a hereditary syndrome with angiomas of the retina (Hippel–Lindau syndrome).

Meningiomas

Rarely, meningiomas may arise in the posterior fossa from the dura over the clivus or foramen magnum, in the cerebellopontine angle, the tentorium cerebelli, or from the internal surface of the occipital bone. They usually present by their local effects, either on lower cranial nerves – particularly with deafness (VIIIth nerve) or facial weakness (VIIth nerve) – or on cerebellum (ataxia), or in long tracts (weakness and sensory change in the limbs).

Acoustic Schwannoma (Fig. 6.9)

Schwannomas can arise on most cranial nerves but the commonest site is in the VIIIth nerve at the internal auditory meatus in the cerebellopontine angle. This tumour causes progressive unilateral deafness, loss of vestibular function, and sensory disturbance (or pain) in the Vth nerve territory with early depression of the corneal reflex. As the tumour expands, facial weakness results from compression of the VIIth nerve, and later a central type of nystagmus, ipsilateral cerebellar ataxia, and corticospinal tract signs are found as the brainstem is distorted. Occasionally, initial symptoms go unnoticed and the patient presents with features of raised intracranial pressure secondary to hydrocephalus.

INVESTIGATION

A thorough general examination is of course essential, with particular attention being paid to the lungs, breasts, thyroid, kidney, liver and lymph nodes. Once the clinical suspicion of an intracranial space-occupying lesion is raised, special investigations are employed, firstly to confirm the presence of a tumour and to exclude abscess or haematoma and secondly, if tumour is disclosed, to plan technical aspects of operative treatment.

Plain Skull X-ray

This remains an important, non-invasive investigation. Any increased ICP may cause erosion of the dorsum sellae, while in some cases, where the pineal gland is calcified, a mid-line shift may be identified. Enlargement of the pituitary fossa (Figs 6.5, 6.7), suprasellar calcification, sclerosis of the bony skull, or enlargement of the internal auditory meatus are features which may be demonstrated, indicating (respectively) pituitary adenoma, craniopharyngioma, meningioma and acoustic schwannoma. Plain x-ray of the chest is also essential, to screen for primary or metastatic bronchial tumours.

CT Scan

Computerised axial tomography of the brain is now the most important single procedure in screening for an intracranial space-occupying lesion. The scan generally shows the tumour directly, as well as its relationships to normal structures and the degree of surrounding

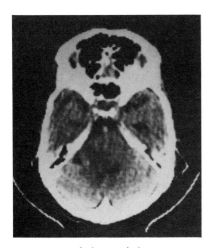 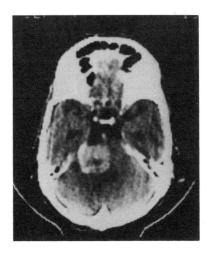

Fig. 6.9 *Acoustic neuroma, before and after contrast.*

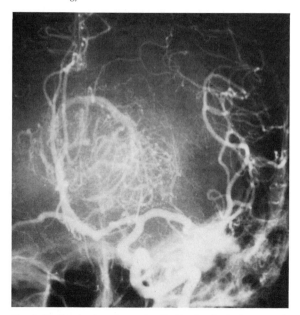

Fig. 6.10 *Cerebral angiography (A-P). Cerebral glioma with pathological circulation.*

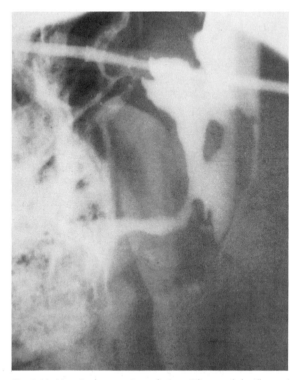

Fig. 6.11 *Ventriculogram. Lateral view. Glioma of the floor of IIIrd ventricle.*

oedema. In the specialist neurosurgical unit other investigations, all of which are 'invasive' to some extent and involve a definite morbidity, may be required to define the nature and site of an intracranial tumour more exactly, prior to surgery. Cerebral angiography may reveal a tumour circulation (Fig. 6.10), as well as showing feeding vessels and the relationship of normal arteries. Ventriculography (Fig. 6.11) and pneumoencephalography (Fig. 6.12) outline with positive contrast or air the CSF-filled spaces in and around the brain, and are important in delineating space-occupying lesions in the suprasellar and pineal regions, in the cerebellopontine angle, and within the 3rd ventricle. Nuclear magnetic resonance scanning seems likely to be of importance in future in defining certain tumours, particularly in the posterior fossa.

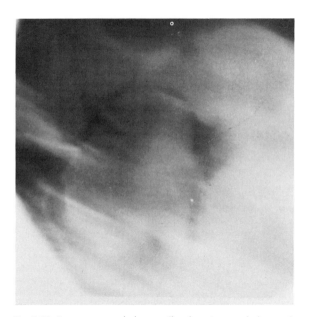

Fig. 6.12 *Pneumoencephalogram (lumbar air encephalogram). Coned lateral view. Pituitary adenoma with large suprasellar extension.*

Other Investigations

Isotope scanning is an alternative non-invasive imaging technique (Fig. 6.13), though rather less reliable than CT scan. The erythrocyte sedimentation rate may be raised in metastatic carcinomas and endocrine assessment is relevant in pituitary tumours. Occasionally,

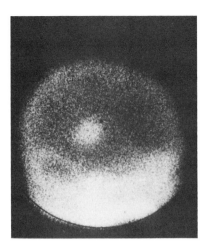

Fig. 6.13 *Isotope scan. Lateral. Cerebral glioma (posterior temporal).*

specific chemical markers, such as α-fetoprotein or chorionic gonadotrophin, are assayed if a teratoma is suspected.

TREATMENT OF CNS SPACE-OCCUPYING LESIONS

Medical Management

In some patients with intrinsic brain tumour (glioma, metastases), a conservative approach may be indicated. In cases of presumed low-grade gliomas, causing epilepsy only, it may be reasonable to await the development of other signs before considering surgery, particularly if biopsy or attempted removal carries a major risk of causing neurological deficit. In cases of multiple cerebral metastases, where diagnosis is not in doubt, it may not be desirable to offer surgical treatment. However, the patient may respond very well, in the short term, to removal of solitary metastases.

Surgery

There are two purposes of surgery for brain tumour. The first is to establish a conclusive histological diagnosis. The second is to remove as much tumour as safely as possible in order to relieve raised ICP and neurological dysfunction, as well as, in the optimum case, achieving radical removal and cure. Once preoperative radiological investigations have localised the site of an intracranial space-occupying lesion, the surgeon plans operative exposure, biopsy and, when possible, removal of the mass. Scrupulous asepsis and minimal trauma to normal tissue are particularly important in neurosurgery, where additional postoperative cerebral oedema or infarction may greatly increase the morbidity of a procedure.

In the supratentorial compartment, craniotomy (i.e. removal and replacement of a bone flap) is used for extensive exposure and radical curative resection of benign tumours like meningioma or pituitary adenoma with suprasellar extension, as well as for partial palliative removal of cerebral glioma. In some of the latter cases a 'lobectomy' – frontal, temporal or occipital – will be performed. In the posterior fossa, craniectomy (i.e. piecemeal removal of the occipital bone) is carried out to expose the cerebellum, 4th ventricle or cerebellopontine angle for intrinsic tumours (astrocytoma, medulloblastoma, ependymoma, haemangioblastoma) or for acoustic schwannoma or meningioma.

Other surgical procedures commonly employed are burrhole exploration for simple biopsy or cyst aspiration and shunting of the ventricular system to relieve hydrocephalus. The transnasal–transphenoidal approach to certain pituitary tumours is also commonly used.

In the last 15 years there have been major improvements in neurosurgery due to the use of the operating microscope and the control of cerebral oedema at the time of surgery by treatment with synthetic glucocorticoids (dexamethazone) and osmotic diuretics (mannitol). The availability of replacement therapy for anterior and posterior pituitary hormones has also transformed the management of patients undergoing hypophysectomy for pituitary tumours. Neuroanaesthesia has also improved, with a better physiological understanding of the changes in ICP and blood flow during anaesthesia. Hypoxia, CO_2 retention and straining at intubation are all factors which can increase ICP dramatically during induction of anaesthesia in a patient with an intracranial mass lesion. General anaesthesia, particularly with volatile agents such as halothane, increases cerebral blood flow and may increase ICP. Anaesthetic techniques have been modified to avoid, as far as possible, surges of raised ICP and brain herniation at operation.

Radiotherapy

With malignant tumours, such as glioma in the cerebral hemisphere or medulloblastoma and ependymoma in the posterior fossa, residual tumour remains after surgery. Radiotherapy is performed postoperatively, to a level limited to about 5 500 rads over 5–6 weeks. It is delivered to the tumour bed and whole brain. It is extended over the spinal canal if the particular tumour is known usually to spread through CSF pathways. In the most malignant tumours adjuvant radiotherapy can double median survival, although this may still be measured in months rather than years. Higher doses cause severe damage to the whole brain. Certain benign tumours, especially for example pituitary adenoma and craniopharyngioma, also benefit from postoperative radiotherapy in diminishing residual tumour bulk and decreasing the risk of late recurrence.

Chemotherapy

Cerebral glioma and medulloblastoma respond to a modest extent to chemotherapy with nitrosoureas and with procarbazine. These drugs may be administered as adjuvants following surgery and radiotherapy or, in malignant tumours, at the time of recurrence. Cerebral metastases may also respond favourably to chemotherapy with cytotoxic drugs or with hormones, including synthetic steroids.

RESULTS

The operative mortality for intracranial tumours is in the range of 1–10% depending on the type of lesion and surgery required. The worst prognosis is in malignant cerebral glioma where the one-year survival is 20–50% depending on grade and in spite of treatment, and in cerebral metastasis where the one-year survival is 10–25%. In meningioma there is a recurrence rate of 2–25% at 10 years, depending on site, while in pituitary adenoma and acoustic schwannoma the 10-year recurrence is less than 10%.

7

Epilepsy, Migraine and Headache

The epilepsies are a group of disorders in which there are recurrent episodes of abnormal cerebral function characterised by excessive discharge of neurones. Clinical manifestations range from brief lapses of awareness to prolonged violent jerking of the limbs with unconsciousness and incontinence. Epilepsy is relatively common, affecting about 0.5% of the UK population. The incidence is highest in childhood and lowest in middle life.

PATHOPHYSIOLOGY

Cerebral cortical neurones are interconnected via dendritic arborisations and collateral fibres, but spread of electrical activity is normally restricted by recurrent and collateral inhibition. Cortical cells tend, therefore, to be held in a state of inhibition and discharge synchronously in small groups only. This limited amount of synchronisation is responsible for the rhythmical potential changes which are recorded in the normal electroencephalogram (EEG, see p. 112). During an epileptic seizure large groups of neurones undergo repetitive and hypersynchronous activation. Micro-electrode studies show that, under these conditions, single neurones fire rapid runs of action potentials and there is a transient reduction in the base-line resting trans-membrane potential (paroxysmal depolarisation shift). These functional changes probably involve both abnormal excitation and failure of inhibitory synaptic contact. Epileptic activity limited to one part of the cerebral cortex is associated with symptoms and signs of dysfunction in that area (focal or partial seizures). Seizure activity may remain localised or may spread over the same and opposite sides of the brain. Seizures

associated with widespread paroxysmal activity of both hemispheres are termed 'generalised' and either arise by spread from a focus or may be generalised from their onset.

Generalised epilepsy without focal onset has in the past been regarded as arising from deep mid-line structures such as the thalamus ('centrencephalic epilepsy'). Recent animal studies using penicillin to induce epilepsy show that generalised epileptic activity can be produced if the whole cerebral cortex is treated with the drug, but not if it is injected into the thalamic nuclei. This suggests that seizures which are generalised from onset arise in a cerebral cortex whose overall level of excitability is increased, and not as projections from deep mid-line structures.

AETIOLOGICAL FACTORS

Genetic

Many patients with epilepsy have no definable cause for their seizures, either in terms of past history or on investigation. This type of epilepsy may be familial (see p. 218) and is often generalised in type (idiopathic or primary generalised epilepsy). However, generalised epilepsy may be secondary to a definable cause (e.g. hypocalcaemia). Partial (focal) seizures are more likely to have a detectable cause, but primary forms of focal epilepsy are also recognised.

Thirty to forty per cent of patients with epilepsy have a family history of seizures. Some forms of primary generalised epilepsy (e.g. petit mal) appear to be transmitted as an autosomal dominant gene with variable penetrance. When other causes can be identified (e.g. head injury) inheritance is less important, but may still contribute.

Trauma

Perinatal cerebral trauma is believed to be a common cause of childhood epilepsy and may sometimes be inferred from a history of a particularly difficult delivery. Cerebral contusion or haemorrhage may occur, and fetal anoxia during birth may cause cerebral oedema and secondary damage to the temporal lobes at the tentorium (mesial temporal sclerosis). Head injury in postnatal life can cause epilepsy described as early (within a week of injury) or late. An injury sufficient to cause epilepsy is almost always associated with loss of consciousness, and fits are more likely after depressed fractures, dural tears and intracranial haematomata. In 50–60% of cases, seizures begin in the first year after injury, but they may be delayed by a decade or more in some cases. Interestingly, although seizures which start within the first week after injury may become recurrent, this is more likely to happen when the onset of the fits is delayed.

Pyrexia

Pyrexia from any cause may trigger seizures in susceptible individuals, but 'febrile convulsions' are particularly common in infancy. A rectal temperature of 38°C is regarded as the minimum to fulfill this diagnosis. Children between the ages of 6 months and 5 years are usually affected, and there may be a family history of febrile convulsions. In the majority of these children the seizures cease with advancing maturity, but some (4–20%) will go on to have afebrile seizures. Of the latter group, some will have primary generalised epilepsy, while in others prolonged febrile seizures may cause cerebral anoxia, mesial temporal sclerosis, and resultant temporal lobe epilepsy.

Tumours and Raised Intracranial Pressure

Cerebral tumour should always be considered, especially if seizures are of focal origin or presentation is in adult life. Ten to fifteen per cent of late-onset epilepsy is due to this cause. Raised intracranial pressure can present with seizures, especially in children.

Vascular Lesions

Cerebral vascular disease accounts for a significant proportion of epilepsy presenting after the age of forty. Cerebral infarction (especially embolic), haemorrhage and subdural haematoma may all be associated with seizures. Cerebral arteriovenous malformations are often associated with epilepsy, and it is also a recognised complication of large cerebral aneurysms.

Acute Cerebral Anoxia

Acute failure of the cerebral circulation, due to postural or reflex syncope or cardiac arrhythmia, commonly causes loss of posture and consciousness (see p. 53). In some cases of acute cerebral anoxia, tonic or clonic movements may occur (convulsive syncope) and it may be difficult to distinguish such attacks from epilepsy of entirely cerebral origin. This point is discussed more fully in the section of differential diagnosis.

Other Causes of Epilepsy

1. *Drugs*
   Phenothiazines
   Monoamine oxidase inhibitors
   Tricyclic antidepressants
   Amphetamines
   Nalidixic Acid
   Lignocaine
   Withdrawal from long-term barbiturates and benzodiazepines.
2. *Alcoholism*
   2–5 days abstention
   Hypoglycaemia during acute alcoholic bouts
3. *Metabolic*
   Hypoglycaemia
   Hypocalcaemia
   Hyponatraemia
   Hypoxia
   Porphyria
   Renal and hepatic failure

4. *Inflammatory Conditions*
    Meningitis
    Encephalitis
    Cerebral abscess
    Subdural empyema
    Cortical thrombophlebitis
5. *Degenerative Conditions*
    Cerebral lipidoses
    Leuko-dystrophies
    Alzheimer's and Pick's diseases
    Subacute spongiform encephalopathy
    Multiple sclerosis (uncommonly)
6. *Haematological Conditions*
    Polycythaemia
    Hyperviscosity
    Leukaemia
    Lymphomas

CLINICAL FEATURES: SEIZURE PATTERNS

Classification of the epilepsies is summarised in Fig. 7.1.

Generalised Tonic-Clonic Seizures (Grand Mal)

Prodromal malaise and irritability may be reported hours or days before an attack. Seizures generalised from onset usually begin without warning, but if the fit starts focally the patient may experience an aura. The aura often lasts only a few seconds; it reflects the site of origin. It may consist of sensory phenomena (parietal), motor activity (motor cortex), versive movements of the eyes and head (frontal), but is commonly psychic in nature (temporal). Temporal lobe auras are variable; patients describe nauseating epigastric sensations, hallucinations of smell, taste, vision or sound and distortions of perception such as *déjà-vu* (see p. 50). As the seizure becomes generalised, a tonic phase of 10 to 30 seconds occurs. The legs are extended and arms adducted, flexed at the elbows and wrists. Consciousness is lost and the patient falls. Clonic jerking of muscles – initially rapidly and later slowing – follows, usually lasting 1 to 5 minutes. It is followed by a post-ictal phase of deep unconsciousness and flaccidity, with absence of corneal and tendon reflexes and

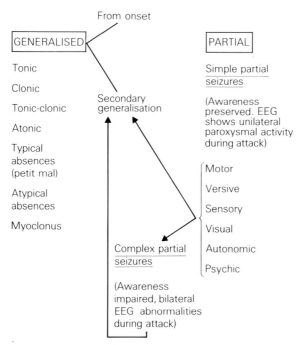

Fig. 7.1 *Clinical classification of the epilepsies (based on the International League Against Epilepsy classifications 1969 and 1980).*

with extensor plantar responses. This state may last for a few minutes up to several hours, during which time consciousness gradually returns. On waking, the patient may have a headache, feel dazed, and find that he has bitten his tongue or cheek or been incontinent of urine. Aching pains in the muscles are common after a tonic-clonic seizure and some patients show periods of post-ictal confusion and automatic behaviour (occasionally violent) of which they may have no recall later.

Partial Seizures

Simple partial seizures

During a simple partial seizure the EEG shows epileptic activity limited to one part of the affected hemisphere; consciousness is preserved during the attack. Epilepsy arising in the primary motor area of the frontal cortex causes jerking or tonic spasms of the contralateral face and limbs. Often movement begins at the angle of the mouth or thumb and index finger and then spreads progressively to the arm, trunk, and then leg and foot. This 'march' pattern is called Jacksonian epilepsy. After a partial motor seizure or a seizure which has generalised from a focal motor origin, weakness of the affected limbs may be present for several hours after the fit (Todd's paralysis). If the post-central gyrus is the site of origin, paraesthesiae of 'electric' sensations spread in a similar way to Jacksonian epilepsy. Seizures arising in the frontal lobe may involve the frontal eye field, causing turning of the eyes and head to the contralateral side (versive seizure). Occipital foci may cause crude visual images (e.g. balls of light or geometric shapes). Temporal lobe simple partial seizures may be associated with olfactory hallucinations, usually of unpleasant odours (e.g. burning rubber), feelings of unreality (*jamais-vu*) or undue familiarity with events and surroundings (*déjà-vu*). Sexual sensations and autonomic activity (e.g. piloerection, flushing) may also be reported. Less commonly temporal lobe seizures are associated with formed visual hallucinations of scenes or faces, or there may be auditory hallucinations of crude noise, music, or voices.

Complex partial seizures

This term implies loss of awareness during a partial seizure. EEG records during this type of attack show bilateral abnormalities and it is likely that mid-line structures (e.g. thalamus) are involved. Complex partial seizures usually arise from temporal lobe foci, but those from other areas (e.g. frontal) may cause similar effects. The patient may experience an aura similar to those described for simple partial temporal lobe seizures, but awareness becomes diminished and many patients enter a trance-like state and are amnesic for the attack. Motor activity may occur and varies from small fidgeting automatisms, lip smacking and chewing, to running, laughing or undressing. Aggressive and purposeful behaviour is rare.

Typical Absence Seizures (Petit Mal)

This is a form of primary generalised epilepsy seen mostly in children. There is often a family history of epilepsy. Attacks usually last only a few seconds but may recur many times a day. The child stops activity, stares blankly and fails to respond to questions. The eyelids may flutter and the face become flushed or pale. The patient usually has no recall of the attack. Occasionally, prolonged or rapidly recurrent absences cause a trance-like state (petit mal status). During a typical absence the EEG shows generalised bilaterally synchronous spike and slow wave complexes repeating at three per second. Less frequently, similar paroxysms are associated with simple automatisms (complex absences), a single myoclonic jerk, or akinetic attacks causing sudden falls. Petit mal often ceases after childhood, but may persist into adult life or be replaced by tonic-clonic seizures.

Infantile Spasms (Salaam Attacks)

These attacks are limited to children under the age of 1 year, being more common in boys than girls. The seizure pattern – the salaam attack – is characteristic, but the clinical picture may be due to many different forms of preexisting or progressive cerebral degeneration. The combination of characteristic spasms, mental retardation or deterioration, and severe EEG abnormalities are known as West's syndrome. The spasm consists of sudden flexion of the head, abduction of the arms, and flexion of the elbows and knees lasting no more than a few seconds. The EEG between attacks shows chaotic high-amplitude slow waves and multi-focal spike complexes (hypsarrhythmia). During attacks the EEG tends to become flattened or show low-amplitude fast activity.

CLINICAL ASSESSMENT

History

Blackouts are common and their diagnosis depends largely on an accurate and detailed history. Epileptic episodes need to be differentiated from several other categories of 'blackout' (see differential diagnosis, p. 117). An eyewitness account of the attacks is most helpful. Details should be sought about the physical circumstances of the attack (e.g. lying, sitting, standing) and possible precipitants (e.g. flashing lights or emotional upset). Witnesses should be asked to describe or possibly simulate any limb movements which they observed, and the occurrence of cyanosis, laboured breathing, salivation, incontinence, and tongue trauma should be sought. The patient's own recollections of the attack, especially of any aura, may indicate a focal onset or provide evidence of tongue or lip trauma, incontinence, post-ictal confusion, headache or limb pains. Specific enquiry is made about perinatal injury, intracranial infection, febrile convulsions in infancy and head injuries, together with possible trigger factors which may include flickering lights, proximity to television screens or video games, menstruation, alcohol ingestion or withdrawal, sleep deprivation and physical or mental stress. Some patients with primary generalised epilepsy may have noticed brief myoclonic jerks of their limbs in the mornings (matinal myoclonus). A family history is taken, asking specifically about any relative with epilepsy.

Examination

Asymmetries of the skull, face or limbs may be associated with longstanding or congenital intracerebral lesions. Cutaneous and retinal abnormalities may give a clue to some disorders associated with epilepsy, e.g. neurofibromatosis, tuberose sclerosis (see Chapter 12), Sturge–Weber syndrome (facial capillary haemangioma – port-wine stain – and leptomeningeal angiomatosis): a bruit over a head or orbit may suggest an arteriovenous malformation. Focal neurological signs or evidence of raised intracranial pressure are of obvious importance and particular attention is given to examining the vascular system and heart.

Investigations

The details of the individual patient will dictate the level of investigation required. A child or teenager is less likely to have an underlying structural cause for epilepsy than an adult presenting with seizures for the first time. Similarly, a history of petit mal attacks in childhood leading to major seizures later requires less intensive investigations than focal seizures presenting in adult life.

Haematological tests

Polycythaemia and hyperviscosity may cause seizures by reducing cerebral blood flow and causing areas of cerebral infarction. An elevated ESR may suggest the presence of a vasculitic connective tissue disease (e.g. systemic lupus erythematosus) or chronic granulomatous disorders (e.g. sarcoidosis). Unexplained macrocytosis may be a feature of alcoholism and hypothyroidism, both of which may lead to seizures.

Biochemical tests

Plasma electrolytes, urea, calcium and glucose (preferably fasting) should be tested. In patients whose history raises the possibility of hypoglycaemic attacks, appropriate provocative tests such as prolonged fasting for 72 hours (spontaneous hypoglycaemia) or a glucose tolerance test (reactive hypoglycaemia) may be indicated.

Serological tests for syphilis (VDRL and TPHA) should be carried out in all cases.

A routine electrocardiogram (ECG) should be carried out in all patients suspected of epilepsy, and ambulatory ECG recording should be considered particularly in elderly patients or where there is a suspicion of cardiac dysrhythmic attacks. It has been estimated that up to

20% of patients presenting as possible cases of epilepsy may have a potential cardiac cause (see also p. 108).

Radiology

X-ray of the chest may show evidence of relevant cardiac or pulmonary disease and of the skull will rarely show evidence of raised intracranial pressure or intracranial calcification suggesting tumour, aneurysm or vascular malformation (see Chapter 3).

Computerised axial tomography of the brain (CT scanning) is carried out if there are focal features in the history, on examination or in the EEG record: it is not regarded as routine if there are strong reasons (e.g. family history, EEG evidence of generalised epilepsy) to suggest primary generalised epilepsy. Any patient presenting with epilepsy after adolescence should have a CT scan as a routine procedure, since the chance of finding an underlying lesion is relatively high.

Electroencephalography (EEG)

Electroencephalography consists of the detection of electrical potential changes originating from the cerebral cortex. An array of silver/silver chloride electrodes is glued to the scalp or held in place with elastic bands so that all the major areas of the cerebral cortex are represented. Electrical potential changes, usually between pairs of adjacent electrodes, are amplified and displayed on a moving paper trace. In most laboratories, eight- or sixteen-channel machines are available.

Normal subjects show variable amounts of rhythmical activity at various frequencies: alpha (8–13/second), beta (> 13/s), theta (4–7/s), delta (< 4/s). Children tend to show more slow activity than adults and this declines with increasing maturity. A routine twenty-minute recording may provide diagnostic information, but a normal EEG does not exclude epilepsy, nor are paroxysmal abnormalities diagnostic of epilepsy without an appropriate history. EEG abnormalities may be generalised or focal. In primary generalised epilepsy, paroxysmal activity is usually generalised and synchronous, often consisting of spike and slow-wave complexes in single bursts or in runs with a frequency usually 2–4/s (Fig. 7.2).

Generalised paroxysmal activity of this type can sometimes be activated by flickering photic stimulation and this technique is often employed as a routine provocative procedure. Partial or secondarily generalised tonic-clonic seizures are often associated with focal spikes, sharp waves or spike and slow-wave complexes (Fig. 7.3). Routine EEG recordings usually detect only interictal disturbances, but petit mal absences are often frequent enough for a typical three-per-second spike-and-wave paroxysm to be detected. The chance of capturing a seizure increases with prolonged recordings and these can now be performed on ambulant patients using a portable miniature tape-recorder with head mounting amplifiers to reduce movement artefact. In special centres, facilities are available for prolonged telemetric monitoring of the EEG together with simultaneous video-

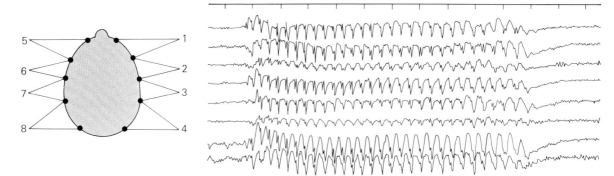

Fig. 7.2 *Portion of EEG tracing from patient with petit mal epilepsy showing a 10-second burst of generalised 3/sec spike-and-wave activity. Discharges of this type are seen mostly in primary generalised epilepsy.*

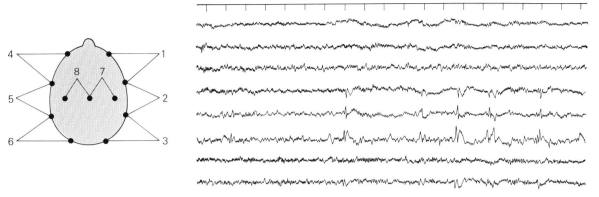

Fig. 7.3 *Portion of EEG from a patient with temporal lobe epilepsy recorded during light sleep. Note the spike-and-slow-wave complexes occurring intermittently on the left side and showing phase reversals between the anterior and mid-temporal channels.*

recording of the patient. Less sophisticated laboratories may improve the yield of abnormalities in routine EEG recording by depriving the patient of sleep and allowing a period of natural sleep during recording, or by promoting sleep with phenothiazine/barbiturate administration.

MANAGEMENT OF EPILEPSY

When to treat

Since epilepsy implies a tendency to recurrent seizures, a patient who had had a single fit should not be regarded as epileptic; most neurologists would not give treatment unless obvious risk factors were apparent, further attacks occurred, or the EEG showed gross epileptic disturbances. A single seizure is, therefore, an indication for investigation and observation but not necessarily for treatment. A significant proportion of patients will go on to have subsequent attacks and will require prophylaxis with drugs.

Anticonvulsant drugs (Table 7.1)

Seizure frequency can usually be reduced by anticonvulsants. How these agents work is unclear; stabilisa-

tion of neuronal and axonal membranes and alteration of neurotransmitter systems are probably involved. Treatment should start with one drug, and be changed only if fits continue in the presence of adequate serum levels of the drug. In this case, the drug should be withdrawn gradually while alternative medication is slowly introduced. Sudden withdrawal of drugs, especially barbiturates, may exacerbate seizures. Drug combinations should be avoided, but are sometimes necessary. Many patients with epilepsy fail to take their prescribed regime regularly, which leads to poor seizure control. Measurement of serum drug levels has improved the treatment of epilepsy. For most drugs in common use a range of plasma levels associated with seizure control without acute toxic symptoms ('therapeutic range') can be defined. It must be remembered that these ranges are approximations and patients may show individual variations of tolerance and response. Total plasma levels measure both free and protein-bound fractions of drugs. In circumstances where protein binding is altered (e.g. pregnancy, liver disease, combination of phenytoin and valproate), salivary levels may be helpful. Salivary levels of drugs reflect the free plasma concentrations but, being much lower than blood levels, are technically more difficult to perform. The measurement of anticonvulsant levels in blood or saliva helps to establish a correct dose, particularly for phenytoin where the useful dosage range may be very narrow. With combined drug treatment, drug level

Table 7.1
Anticonvulsant Drugs, Doses and Side-effects

Drug	Adult daily dose mg	Serum half-life hrs	Dose frequency ×/Day	Therapeutic serum levels μmol/l	Side effects Dose related	Idiosyncratic	Long-term
Phenytoin	200–500	24–48	2 (1)	40–80	Ataxia, diplopia nystagmus dysarthria dystonia confusional state	skin rashes blood dyscrasias lymphadenopathy systemic lupus	gum hypertrophy hypertrichosis osteomalacia folate deficient anaemia polyneuropathy
Carbamazepine	200–1500	12–15	3	20–50	drowsiness ataxia, diplopia nystagmus water intoxication	skin rashes blood dyscrasias	
Phenobarbitone	60–180	24–48	2 (1)	50–150	drowsiness ataxia dysarthria nystagmus	skin rashes systemic lupus	osteomalacea folate deficient anaemia polyneuropathy
Primidone	250–1000	24–48	2 (1)	Measure as Phenobarbitone 50–150	,,	,, nausea	,,
Sodium valproate	600–3000	5–8	3	Poorly defined ? 200–700	postural tremor involuntary movements thrombocytopenia	nausea, vomiting anorexia hair loss liver damage	weight gain (females)
Ethosuximide	500–1500	20–36	2	200–700	drowsiness	blood dyscrasias nausea, vomiting anorexia	
Clonazepam	1–6	16–40	2–3	Poorly defined ? 50–300 nMol/l	drowsiness irritability ataxia		diminished effect due to receptor tolerance

see p. 116 for status epilepticus

measurements help to establish which of the drugs is likely to be causing toxic symptoms. Monitoring also helps improve patient compliance if levels are found to be persistently low despite apparently normal doses.

Phenytoin (diphenylhydantoin)

This is potent in the prevention of tonic-clonic seizures of both generalised onset or secondarily generalised type. It is also useful in controlling partial seizures, but has little effect on petit mal or myoclonus. Since its plasma half-life is long (24–48 hours) phenytoin needs to be given only twice or even once daily. When oral administration is not possible, the drug can be given intravenously (e.g. 100 to 250 mg at ≤ 50 mg/minute in an adult). The parenteral preparation is strongly alkaline and may crystallise out in tissues; the intramuscular route is therefore painful and associated with unreliable absorption. Because the enzyme responsible for phenytoin metabolism is saturable, the serum level/dose curve is exponential (see Fig. 7.4). Daily doses over 300 to 350 mg should be exceeded only cautiously and with frequent monitoring of serum levels: increments in daily dose should not exceed 25–50 mg at this level. Therapeutic serum levels may be associated with lethargy, gum hypertrophy (especially in children) and

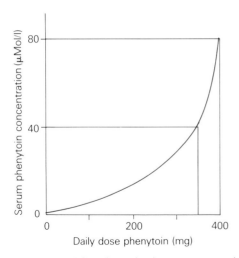

Fig. 7.4 *The shape of the relationship between serum pheny-toin level and daily dose. The absolute position of the curve along the x axis varies widely between patients. The construction lines illustrate how a dosage increment from 350 to 400 mg/day could cause a doubling of serum concentration.*

hirsutism in females. Other long-term side-effects are listed in Table 7.1. Toxic levels of the drug cause ataxia, vertigo, diplopia, nystagmus, dysarthria, drowsiness and, rarely, dystonia. Toxicity may permanently destroy cerebellar cells and must be corrected rapidly.

Carbamazepine

This drug is useful in partial seizures, particularly of temporal lobe type, and in major tonic-clonic epilepsy. Initial drowsiness is common but can be avoided by starting with a small dose (100 to 200 mg/day) and increasing gradually over several weeks. Allergic reactions, especially skin rashes, are not uncommon, and if they occur the drug must be stopped and an alternative used. The serum level/dose curve is linear and dosage can be increased accordingly. Water retention can occur with high plasma levels and may cause hyponatremia, confusion and exacerbation of seizures. Leukopenia may occur and, if this is severe, it may warrant stopping the drug. Fluctuations in the serum level may occur throughout the day and may be associated with intermittent symptoms such as ataxia or diplopia. Monitoring of levels at different times through the day and appropriate adjustment and spacing of doses may avoid these problems.

Barbiturates

Phenobarbitone is effective against tonic-clonic and partial seizures but not petit mal. Barbiturates often cause sedation and depression, and are unsuitable for children because they cause hyperactivity and behavioural problems. Toxicity causes cerebellar dysfunction as with phenytoin, but sedation is more marked with barbiturates. Serum level monitoring is in general less helpful since patients show wide individual variations of tolerance to barbiturates. In general the barbiturates are less effective than phenytoin and carbamazepine for seizure control, and tend to be more sedative. Some patients, however, may be well controlled without difficulty and the drugs are usually safe.

Primidone is used in the same conditions as phenobarbitone. A large proportion of the drug is metabolised to phenobarbitone, but unaltered primidone may have anticonvulsant action too. Combination with phenobarbitone is inadvisable, since toxicity is frequent.

Sodium Valproate

This agent inhibits the breakdown and re-uptake of the inhibitory neurotransmitter gamma aminobutyric acid (GABA). It is mainly useful in the primary generalised epilepsies, particularly petit mal but also in generalised tonic-clonic attacks. Partial seizures respond less well. Side-effects are usually slight; gastrointestinal upset is commonest and can be reduced with enteric coated tablets. Hair loss may occur but is usually transient, and excessive weight gain can be a problem particularly in children and young females. A small number of fatal cases of acute hepatic necrosis have been described. This seems to occur especially in children with progressive cerebral degeneration and in patients who have been taking valproate in combination with other drugs. Monitoring of liver function tests during the first six months of treatment is recommended but may not predict serious hepatic damage.

Ethosuximide

This is used mainly in petit mal, but it is also useful in akinetic and myoclonic attacks associated with generalised EEG spike-and-wave paroxysms. Some workers believe that the drug lowers the threshold for tonic-clonic seizures. It is sometimes necessary to use a combination of valproate and ethosuximide to control complex absences, or in patients with combined absence and tonic-clonic seizures where valproate may fail to control the absences satisfactorily.

Benzodiazepines

Oral benzodiazepines are weak anticonvulsants, but clonazepam may be useful in petit mal, in complex partial seizures, and for suppressing myoclonic jerks. To avoid sedation and irritability, treatment should begin with small doses (0.5 mg twice daily), and increased gradually over several weeks. Newer benzodiazepines like clobazam may be useful adjunctive therapy in severe epilepsy and are claimed to be less sedative than clonazepam.

Status Epilepticus

This occurs when a series of fits follow each other without the patient regaining consciousness. Although the first priority is to control the seizures, a cause for the epilepsy needs to be sought especially if it is occurring for the first time. Common causes are withdrawal of drugs, especially anticonvulsants or alcohol. Electrolyte imbalance, hypoglycaemia, hypocalcaemia should all be excluded, and evidence of acute meningitis, encephalitis or a cerebral tumour should be sought.

Status epilepticus is a medical emergency, as the patient may become anoxic, suffer brain damage, or die. The drug of first choice is diazepam; in adults, 10 mg is given intravenously over 1–3 minutes. If seizures persist or recur, this dose can be repeated and an infusion set up to give 10–50 mg per hour. Respiration and pharyngeal reflexes may be depressed by medication or repeated fits and, in all patients with status epilepticus, close attention must be paid to the airway and to arterial oxygenation; facilities for artificial ventilation should be available. The patient should ideally be cared for in an intensive-care area, where blood pressure, arterial blood gases, ECG and, if necessary, EEG can be monitored. The EEG record may be valuable in assessing patients undergoing artificial ventilation since convulsions may not be evident due to the use of muscle relaxant drugs.

If diazepam fails, an infusion of chlormethiazole, 0.5 to 0.7 g/hour, may be effective. Paraldehyde, 10 mg intramuscularly, is a safe alternative if venous access or ventilation facilities are limited, but muscle abscesses often result. If other methods fail, a thiopentone infusion is usually effective. This is given under the supervision of an anaesthetist, since artifical ventilation is usually required. The serum levels of the patient's usual anticonvulsants should be assayed and their usual dosage administered by nasogastric tube or parenterally until the results are available. If status epilepticus is the presenting feature of epilepsy then phenytoin may be started intravenously and, as the fits come under control, the patient can be changed to oral administration later. Intravenous preparations of sodium valproate are not yet freely available but are undergoing trials and may prove useful.

Surgery

Cerebral tumours, arteriovenous malformations, aneurysms, cysts, or hydrocephalus may warrant surgery for reasons other then intractable epilepsy. Surgery is considered for the control of epilepsy only if a focal (usually temporal) abnormality can be demonstrated on EEG, and when medical treatment has been well tried without success. Such cases make up only a small fraction of all patients with epilepsy, but careful selection of cases for temporal lobectomy can result in improved seizure control and behaviour.

Day-to-day Life

There is still public ignorance about epilepsy, and the sight of an epileptic seizure produces considerable anxiety and fear in those nearby. As a result of public attitudes and the restrictions placed on employment, driving, and daily activities, patients with epilepsy may feel a resentment towards society in general. Personality disorders and depression are not uncommon and, in temporal lobe epilepsy, psychotic states resembling schizophrenia may occur.

Restrictions on living depend on the type and frequency of seizures. A change in occupation may be sensible if the patient works with machinery or above ground level. The police and armed forces exclude those with epilepsy. Children whose seizures are well controlled should attend normal schools, but specia schooling may be indicated when frequent seizures make this impossible. Patients should be advised against recreations in which a fall would be dangerous (e.g. rock climbing), but swimming can be permitted under supervision. Sensible restrictions of this type should be carefully balanced against the likelihood of seizures occurring.

Driving

Anyone who has had a seizure after the age of three years cannot hold a public service or heavy goods vehicle or aircraft pilot's licence. A private vehicle licence is revoked until no fits have occurred for two years, or if seizures have been only during sleep for three years. If anticonvulsants are stopped, driving must be resuspended for a trial period. It is the patient's duty to inform the driving licensing authorities and his insurance company about the occurrence of seizures. The doctor has a duty to ensure that the patient understands the regulations and the possible consequences of ignoring them.

Triggering of Seizures

Patients should be warned that alcohol may induce seizures and exacerbate the sedative side-effects of anticonvulsant drugs. In some cases fits are triggered by flickering light, which may be encountered in discotheques or more commonly from television sets. Close proximity to the screen reveals a 25 Hz flicker which may trigger a fit, but the risk can be reduced if the patient sits far from the screen and covers one eye while viewing.

Pregnancy and Contraception

Patients with epilepsy often ask if they will pass the disorder on to their children. With one parent affected, the overall risk is low (2.5–6%). The risk is highest in patients with primary generalised epilepsy, in particular petit mal, and lowest in those with partial seizures particularly if there is evidence of a local lesion. If both the parents have epilepsy the risk of transmission to offspring is much higher (25%). During pregnancy, blood anticonvulsant levels may fall and require more frequent monitoring. There is an increased incidence of congenital abnormalities (especially cleft lip and palate) in babies born to epileptic mothers taking anticonvulsants. The risk is relatively low and no single anticonvulsant drug is free from suspicion. Therefore, most neurologists do not change an effective anticonvulsant regime in pregnancy, particularly since the risk of uncontrolled seizures is potentially more harmful to the developing fetus than continuing with anticonvulsant medication. The concentrations of anticonvulsant agents in breast milk are generally low and breast feeding can be encouraged as usual in most cases. With ethoxusimide the baby may acquire a low dose from breast milk. If the mother is taking phenobarbitone the neonate may develop a barbiturate withdrawal syndrome after some days and breast feeding may actually help to prevent this.

Phenytoin, barbiturates and carbamazepine induce hepatic enzymes which break down the hormonal components of oral contraceptives, thus rendering them less effective. Unplanned pregnancies may occur and are usually heralded by the presence of breakthrough bleeding in mid-cycle. This problem may be overcome by using an anticonvulsant which does not induce enzymes (e.g. sodium valproate), by recommending alternative contraceptive methods, or by prescribing a higher-dose oestrogen preparation.

Differential Diagnosis of Epilepsy

Syncope (fainting)

Loss of consciousness due to impaired cerebral perfusion is a common phenomenon and may effect people of all ages, but is especially common in adolescence. Prolonged standing, especially in a warm environment, promotes peripheral venous pooling of blood, impaired cardiac output, and reduced cerebral blood flow. At a critical level of reduced cerebral perfusion. bradycardia and reflex vasodilatation in muscle occur, causing a sudden fall in the blood pressure with loss of consciousness and posture. Syncopal attacks are often preceded for several minutes by premonitory symptoms of nausea, lightheadedness, vertigo, visual blurring and darkening, tinnitus and sweating. The patient looks pale and falls limply, usually without movement, and regains consciousness within a minute or two. If falling is impeded (e.g. in a confined space) then the reduction in cerebral blood-flow may be severe enough to induce convulsive movements. These are usually briefer than in an epileptic attack of primarily cerebral origin (convulsive syncope). Reflex forms of syncope should also be considered. Sudden pain or unpleasant sights may induce fainting, as may exaggerated physiological reflexes (e.g. carotid sinus hypersensitivity, micturition syncope, and cough syncope).

Cardiac dysrhythmias

Disorders of cardiac rhythm due to degeneration of the cardiac conducting system or myocardium are a common cause of syncope, especially in the elderly. A history of palpitation, with pallor during attacks and flushing thereafter, should raise this possibility. Reflex bradycardias may occur in carotid sinus hypersensitivity, and periods of asystole have been described in children after minor head injuries. As with postural syncope, convulsive movements are rare but can occur.

Hypoglycaemic attacks

Spontaneous or reactive hypoglycaemia may cause loss of consciousness and sometimes convulsions. There is often a prolonged warning of unease, tremulousness, sweating, tachycardia and hunger. The duration of loss of consciousness is usually longer than in syncope or epilepsy – sometimes up to an hour or more. Suspicion of spontaneous hypoglycaemia should be aroused if attacks occur after fasting or early in the morning. Reactive hypoglycaemic attacks tend to appear $1\frac{1}{2}$–2 hours after a meal, particularly in patients who have undergone gastric surgery involving gastro-enterostomy or pyloroplasty.

Psychogenic (hysterical) attacks

These are not uncommon in adolescence, particularly in females. Attacks are often frequent and variable in type. They may be triggered by emotionally tense situations, but often seem to arise as attention-seeking behaviour. In some cases hyperventilation with symptoms of alkalosis (paraesthesiae in the face and hands, carpo-pedal spasm) may be linked to the attack which can be reproduced by voluntary hyperventilation. Hysterical fits may occur in isolation or sometimes in patients with established epilepsy. The attacks often consist of bizarre and irregular limb movements, without a clear pattern or the typical time-course of an epileptic attack. The attack may often be altered by external intervention but usually the patient denies awareness of the episode itself. Incontinence and injury are unusual in hysterical attacks but do sometimes occur and it may be possible to distinguish an hysterical from a genuine epileptic attack on clinical grounds alone.

Narcolepsy/cataplexy syndrome

Narcolepsy is a rare disorder of unknown cause. Some cases may have a familial basis but the majority are sporadic. In full-blown form the patient may suffer from a tetrad of sleep attacks (narcolepsy), attacks of loss of posture and limb weakness but preservation of consciousness (cataplexy), frightening hallucinations on falling asleep or waking (hypnagogic hallucinations), and periods of inability to move whilst falling asleep or waking (sleep paralysis). Single features may occur alone, but the combination of narcolepsy and cataplexy is the most frequently seen. The pathophysiology is very poorly understoood but is believed to be a dysfunction of that part of the brainstem reticular formation responsible for the generation of rapid eye movement (REM) sleep. Narcoleptic attacks are irresistible periods of sleep, often induced by lack of external stimulation but sometimes occurring during meals, riding in vehicles or even on horseback. The attacks are characteristically brief (10 to 20 minutes) and the patient awakes feeling refreshed. The usual hallmark of narcolepsy is a period of sleep which begins with rapid eye movements (REM onset sleep).

Cataplectic attacks may occur because the descending inhibition of spinal motor neurones (which normally accompanies REM sleep) arises inappropriately. The EEG remains of low amplitude during the attack and consciousness is preserved. Attacks are often set off by surprise, by emotional events (e.g. laughter or crying), or by apprehension. During cataplexy, tendon reflexes are diminished and the plantar responses may be extensor. Most attacks last only a minute or so and can sometimes be terminated by touching the patient lightly.

Narcoleptic attacks may be reduced by methylphenidate or other amphetamine-related drugs, e.g. mazindol. Since these may be addictive, it is essential that a precise diagnosis is made before treatment is started. Cataplexy usually responds to tricyclic antidepressants (e.g. clomipramine), but these do not help the narcoleptic symptoms.

MIGRAINE AND OTHER FORMS OF HEADACHE

Patients with recurrent headache constitute a substantial proportion of neurological out-patient referrals. The majority of such cases are due to migraine or tension headache, but a small minority are caused by a sinister lesion causing raised intracranial pressure (e.g. cerebral tumour). The two common causes of headache are discussed here and other forms are illustrated in Fig. 7.5.

Migraine

Migraine consists of a group of disorders in which there are recurrent attacks of headache, often unilateral, frequently preceded by visual or other symptoms and accompanied by nausea. About 10% or more of the population suffer from migraine at some time and there is often a family history of similar disorder. The female to male ratio is 3:2. Although the conscientious may be more prone, migraine may affect people of widely different personality and intelligence.

Pathophysiology

Studies of regional cerebral blood flow (rCBF) using the intracarotid Xenon clearance method, have shown reduced rCBF in the affected hemisphere during the aura and headache phases of classical migraine. Reductions in cerebral blood flow have not been found during attacks of common migraine (see p. 121). Recent studies suggest that in some cases a migraine attack may start with a localised cerebral hyperaemia which is then followed by spreading oligaemia, not confined to

strict arterial zones, which may spread to the opposite hemisphere. The occipital cortex is often the initial site of oligaemia and, although spread of reduced cerebral blood flow matches the clinical symptoms, the degree of reduction in rCBF is probably insufficient to account for the symptoms in most cases, and also tends to outlast them. This has caused some workers to suggest that the initial event in migraine may be neuronal rather than vascular. 'Spreading cortical depression' (electrical silence induced in experimental animals by application of potassium chloride to the exposed cortex) advances at a rate of 2–3 mm/minute – a rate similar to that estimated for the area of cortex involved as a migrainous aura spreads. Although 'spreading depression' has been shown experimentally to cause hyperaemia followed by long-lasting oligaemia, it has not yet been observed in the human brain. Thus, although the focal or general hemispheric reduction in rCBF which has been found during the migrainous aura might suggest that the symptoms at that time are caused by neuronal ischaemia, the time relationships between rCBF changes and symptoms do not match well.

The headache of both classical and common migraine (see below) is believed to be due to painful dilatation of extracranial arteries. Some patients do show an increase in the pulse amplitude in the superficial temporal arteries on the painful side; but this is not always true, and increased pulse amplitude may be present without headache. In addition to arterial dilatation it is likely that a sterile inflammatory process in and around the artery is required to cause the headache. Some authors have argued that meningeal vessels may also be involved in this painful dilatation.

The mechanisms underlying these vascular changes are poorly understood. Cerebral arterial tone is known to be influenced by both neural and chemical factors: biogenic amines, catecholamines, 5-hydroxy-tryptamine (5-HT), histamine, kinins, and prostaglandins may all affect the cerebral arteries. Although increased urinary excretion of catecholamine products has been reported during migraine attacks, changes in 5-HT have been the most consistent. The concentration of 5-HT in blood rises slightly at the onset of a migrainous aura and then falls to about 45% of resting levels in the headache phase. Since 5-HT is known to cause constriction of large cerebral arteries, these changes could underlie the initial vasoconstriction and later

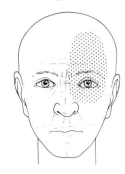

Periorbital

Orbital, ocular,
sinus disease
Carotid artery, ⎫ disease
Cavernous sinus ⎭ (aneurysm)
Involvement V_I
Migraine
Migrainous neuralgia
Depression

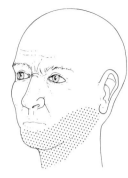

Lower jaw

Dental, bone disease
Disease of parotid,
tongue, floor of mouth.
Claudication of masseter
(temporal arteritis)
V_{III} pathology
Trigeminal neuralgia
Cardiac pain

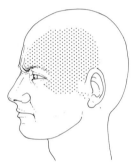

Side of head

Temporal arteritis (> 55 yrs)
Migraine
Post traumatic
Temporomandibular neuralgia
Ear disease
(Parotid gland)

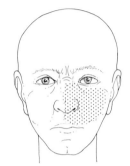

Cheek, central face

Dental, sinus,
nasopharyngeal disease
V_{II} involvement
Trigeminal neuralgia
Depression

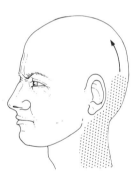

Back of neck, occiput

Local bone, joint disease
of neck
Retropharyngeal mass
Meningism
Tonsillar herniation
Muscle contraction
$C_{2/3}$ root irritation

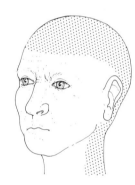

'Whole' head (and neck)

Muscle contraction headache
Migraine
Other vascular headache
− malignant hypertension
− phaeochromocytoma
Post traumatic
Raised intracranial pressure
Meningitis

Fig. 7.5 *Nature of headache related to site of pain.*

vasodilatation of the classical attack. About 98% of the 5-HT in blood is stored in platelets and can be released by drugs (e.g. reserpine), or other amines (catecholamines and tyramine), all of which may precipitate migraine in susceptible individuals. Blood platelets have been shown to be more likely to aggregate during migraine attacks, and the release of a platelet-specific protein (beta-thromboglobulin) increases during attacks. It may be that kinins and prostaglandins are formed in the dilated extracranial arteries and are responsible for the pain and arterial oedema during the headache phase.

Aetiological and trigger factors

Inheritance: Genetic factors are important; many migraine sufferers have affected relatives. The inheritance may be autosomal dominant.

Hypertension: The onset of arterial hypertension in middle adult life may be associated with late-onset migraine, especially when the hypertension is paroxysmal.

Head Injury: Migraine may appear for the first time following head injury, and mild head trauma may trigger an attack (see p. 92).

Intracranial Lesions: Very rarely typical migrainous symptoms appear in association with cerebral arteriovenous malformations, aneurysms and tumours. Such associations may be no more than coincidence, but suspicion of an underlying lesion should be raised when symptoms always recur on the same side.

Trigger Factors: Some patients can recognise a variety of triggers. Emotional stress is a common precipitant, when the migraine usually comes on when the stress is over.

Attacks are more common at weekends and holidays and before or during menstruation. Pregnancy may improve or exacerbate migraine. Oral contraceptives often induce or exacerbate migraine and may provoke alarming focal features. About 20% of patients relate attacks to eating specific foods or drink, when the migraine usually follows some hours later. Foods which are commonly implicated contain the amines tyramine and phenylethylamine. The foods most frequently reported are cheese, chocolate, bananas, onions, strong coffee, citrus fruits, dairy produce and red or fortified wines. There is no good evidence that true allergy plays a part in the genesis of migraine.

Other factors which may trigger migraine attacks include: strong stimuli such as bright light, vivid visual patterns, loud noise, strong smells and excessive emotion; missed meals, lack of sleep, and physical exercise, especially when related to mild head trauma (e.g. footballers' migraine). Roughly 50% of patients can relate their migraine to changes in the weather, with dull cloudy days being the most often cited.

Syndromes of Migraine

Classical migraine

The attack itself may be preceded for several hours by prodromal symptoms of mood-change, coldness or warmth, anorexia or increased appetite, or by heightened sensitivity to light, sound or smells. Elation or unusual energy may herald an attack. The classical attack begins with an aura, probably originating in the occipital cortex, consisting of bright specks of light (teichopsia) or crenated patterns (fortification spectra) in the visual fields. Hemianopias, expanding scotomata, constricted visual fields or total blindness can all occur. Less often there is numbness and paraesthesiae in the face, hand or arm on one side, presumably relating to oligaemia which has spread to the parietal cortex. Occasionally dysphasia occurs, but limb weakness is very rare (see below). The aura usually precedes any headache but may accompany it; and typically it lasts 15–20 minutes but occasionally persists for up to an hour. As it passes off, it is replaced by a throbbing headache usually lateralised over one eye, but sometimes occipital or generalised. The attack is often accompanied by malaise, nausea, vomiting, photophobia, pallor and later diuresis. The headache may last from several hours to two days or more.

The focal symptoms of a migraine attack may be confused with those due to transient cerebral ischaemia, thromboembolic disease, or sometimes those of sensory epileptic seizures. Embolic transient cerebral ischaemic attacks begin abruptly and tend to resolve over minutes or hours; the features are restricted to the territory of one major cerebral artery; headache may be present but is often absent. Migrainous symptoms, by contrast, spread slowly over minutes and may cross vascular boundaries. Headache usually follows the resolving focal features and nausea is common. In focal epilepsy, symptoms are abrupt in onset and usually brief (seconds) in duration. They are usually stereotyped, sometimes accompanied by loss of awareness and myoclonic movements.

Common migraine

This is more frequent than the classical variety and particularly affects women. There is no true aura, but prodromal symptoms as listed above may be present and there may be vague light headaches, photophobia and anorexia. The headache is often present on waking and has the same features as that in classical migraine. Nausea and vomiting are prominent. Attacks usually last one or two days.

Basilar artery migraine

This is a variety of classical migraine seen most commonly in young women. The aura is thought to be due to vertebro-basilar ischaemia and may comprise vertigo, dysarthria, ataxia, diplopia, and bilateral visual impairment or sensory symptoms. Occasionally syncope or drowsiness occur. The succeeding headache is usually occipital. A variant of this form in which nausea and drowsiness may be prominent is sometimes seen following head trauma in children.

Hemiplegic migraine

Although vague heaviness of the limbs on one side occurs frequently in classical migraine, true hemiplegic migraine is very rare. The headache precedes the hemiparesis by a day or more, and the weakness subsides gradually over several days. There is usually a strong family history of this type of migraine. An underlying lesion should always be excluded.

Ophthalmoplegic migraine

This is also rare and usually begins in childhood. The headache localises around one eye and is followed hours later by a IIIrd or VIth nerve palsy on that side, which gradually improves over several days or weeks. Oedema of the internal carotid artery is thought to compress the IIIrd or VIth nerves in the cavernous sinus. An aneurysm should always be considered when these features present for the first time.

Migrainous Neuralgia (Cluster Headache)

This variety of headache may appear with or without other forms of migraine in the same patient. Men are particularly prone. Typically, attacks occur one or more times daily for several months and then subside for months or years. Attacks are usually brief (30–120 minutes), often waking the patient at night with excruciating throbbing pain in or around one eye, and always recur on the same side. On the affected side there may be dilatation of the conjunctival and facial vessels, nasal congestion, epiphora and sometimes a Horner's syndrome. Attacks are often triggered by small amounts of alcohol. Occasionally a chronic

variety is seen in which the typical periodic clusters are absent.

Clinical assessment

History

The diagnosis of migraine rests almost entirely on the patient's account. Attention should be paid to the periodicity of attacks. Migraine usually lasts 1–3 days and then disappears for a week or more; some patients have only one or two headaches a year, while others may have several a week. Headache recurring daily for weeks is unlikely to be migraine. Details of any aura or associated systemic upset should be noted. There may be a family history of migraine and, although attacks usually begin in puberty, there may have been cyclical vomiting or travel sickness in childhood.

Examination

Examination is usually normal. Hypertension should be excluded, and the head and eyes examined for bruits which might suggest an underlying vascular malformation. Focal signs are rare unless there has been migrainous cerebral infarction or there is an underlying lesion. Horner's syndrome may be found in migrainous neuralgia and sometimes persists between attacks. Ophthalmoplegia and cycloplegia may persist in ophthalmoplegic migraine.

Investigation

Routine haematological tests are worthwhile since anaemia and polycythaemia may exacerbate migraine. Thrombocytopenia has been shown to be associated with the appearance or exacerbation of migraine, possibly because of the excessive release of 5-HT from platelets which are being destroyed. Plain skull X-rays may show calcification in vascular malformations or tumours, and occasionally provide evidence of raised intracranial pressure. Specialised neuroradiology is not indicated unless headache or focal features always recur on the same side or there are persistent neurological signs.

Management of migraine

General measures

Patients should be encouraged to live with their migraine, learning to identify and avoid precipitating factors such as foods, alcohol or visual stimuli. Stopping oral contraceptives is often indicated. Irregular eating habits, lack of sleep or excessive periods of sleep often exacerbate the condition and should be avoided. Some patients with clear stress factors may benefit from psychological measures to help avoid stress, or from learning physical relaxation techniques.

Acute attacks

Most migrainous headaches respond to simple analgesics (e.g. soluble aspirin 600–900 mg., or paracetamol 1 g) combined with anti-emetics (e.g. metoclopramide or prochlorperazine). Some patients with classical migraine derive benefit from ergotamine tartrate, 0.5–3 mg (sublingually, by inhalation or suppository), taken at the onset of the aura. Ergotamine is a vasoconstrictor and may prevent the headache phase but can itself cause vomiting and some patients find this intolerable. It should be avoided in patients with ischaemic heart disease or peripheral vascular disease and should not be used in pregnancy. Patients should be limited to about 10 mg of ergotamine a week since chronic intoxication with this drug may cause peripheral limb ischaemia and, paradoxically, headache.

Prophylactic drugs

If migraine is recurring more than approximately once every two weeks, drug prophylaxis may be justified. A single agent should be tried for two to three months and, if successful, can often be withdrawn gradually without recurrence of frequent attacks. A beta-blocking drug (e.g. propranolol 20–80 mg three times daily) is often effective, particularly when there is associated hypertension. Propranolol is also a 5-HT-receptor antagonist and this property may underlie its effectiveness. Pizotifen 0.5–1 mg three times daily, or 1.5 mg at night, is also useful. It has antagonistic activity against several vasoactive amines, including 5-HT, and seems free of long-term side-effects, but may cause drowsiness and weight gain. Clonidine 25–50 μg three times daily is a weak agent and seems to help only a small proportion of patients. The most potent prophylactic drug is methysergide, a strong 5-HT antagonist. A dose of 0.5–1 mg three times a day is frequently effective in resistant cases, but must be given in short courses of two to three months to avoid development of retroperitoneal fibrosis.

Some patients suffer from a mixture of chronic tension headache and migraine attacks. There is often an element of anxiety and depression, and such patients may be helped by antidepressants such as amitriptyline, 25–75 mg at night (see p. 271).

In *migrainous neuralgia*, individual attacks are usually too brief to respond to treatment and so the basis of drug therapy is prevention. Ergotamine tartrate, 2 mg by suppository at bed-time or before a predicted attack, is usually effective. Administration of the drug by mouth or inhaler is less effective. Propranolol is also useful in the prophylaxis of this condition while methysergide, pizotifen, clonidine and antihistamines are less often helpful. Lithium carbonate is sometimes effective in chronic migrainous neuralgia and, if used, it should be accompanied by the monitoring of serum lithium levels. Resistant chronic migrainous neuralgia may be treated with a short course of corticosteroids and, very occasionally, with radio-frequency coagulation of the trigeminal ganglion.

TENSION HEADACHE

As its name suggests, this type of headache is thought to arise from excessive contraction of muscles situated over the head and neck. Electromyographic activity has been shown to be increased over the temporalis and frontalis muscles of some patients reporting tension headache, but the association is not precise. This has led to the suggestion that the pain of tension headache arises because of muscle ischaemia due to vasoconstriction rather than being due primarily to muscle contraction.

Although muscle-contraction headache is often seen in patients with anxiety or depression, and can often be associated with periods of emotional stress, it can sometimes be secondary to physical disorders. Dental malocclusion may be associated with dysfunction of the temporalis, masseter and pterygoid muscles resulting in unilateral pain around the temporomandibular joint. Cervical root irritation, due for example to cervical spondylosis, can also cause secondary muscle contraction and pain.

Tension headache is often a daily occurrence and may be present for brief periods (especially as the stresses of the day mount up) or in some cases may be virtually continuous. Patients may report exacerbation of pain with periods of stress and relief during relaxation. The site of pain is typically bitemporal, frontal, occipital, or localised to one parietal area. Description of the pain ranges from a dull pressure, a tight feeling, a band stretched round the head or sharp localised stabs of pain. Some patients describe throbbing ('tension–vascular headache'), but nausea is rare. Localised tenderness may be evident when pressure is applied to the scalp and neck muscles and, when dental malocclusion is involved, pain may be noted when the mouth is open and closed or pressure applied over the temporomandibular joints. Features of anxiety or depression are often present.

Treatment of tension headache should be based on exclusion of any local causes of muscle contraction. Reassurance that no sinister disorder is present is often helpful. This may be combined with simple analgesics, with or without minor tranquillisers. Chronic tension headache may be resistant to this type of treatment but amitriptyline, 25–100 mg at night is often effective and may be combined with propranolol, 20–80 mg three times daily, if migrainous features are also present. Psychological methods of stress management and muscle relaxation exercises, with or without biofeedback techniques, may also help some patients.

Raised intracranial pressure headache is described in Chapter 4 and 6.

OTHER CAUSES OF HEADACHE

These are illustrated in Fig. 7.5.

Periorbital pain

This may be due to orbital disease (e.g. tumours) and sinus disorders (e.g. sinusitis or tumours). Disorders of the carotid artery, particularly intracavernous aneurysm or carotico-cavernous fistula may, in addition to periorbital pain, cause numbness in the distribution of the first division of the Vth nerve and sometimes diplopia due to ocular motor nerve compression. Ocular disease (e.g. glaucoma) should be excluded. Migraine, particularly migrainous neuralgia, frequently produces periorbital pain.

Temporal pain

Pain over the temple is often due to migraine. In patients over the age of 55, giant cell arteritis (see Chapter 8) should be considered and the ESR checked. Temporomandibular joint dysfunction and malocclusion may also cause recurrent unilateral temporal pain. Disease in the ear or parotid gland may also cause pain referred to this area.

Pain at back of neck or occiput

This may be due to muscle contraction in tension headache or may be caused by cervical spondylosis or other bony or joint disorders in this region. Posterior fossa tumours and cerebellar tonsillar herniation may also produce pain at this site. Basilar artery migraine (throbbing pain) and meningeal irritation from subarachnoid haemorrhage or meningitis (severe constant pain) are further important causes to consider.

Whole head pain

This is fairly common in tension headache and migraine; but is also a feature of raised intracranial pressure, hypertension, and meningitis. Pain localised to the top of the head which has a dull pressing feeling is often psychogenic in origin and reported by patients with depression.

Pain in the centre of the face

Pain around the cheek on one side may be due to dental disease or disorders in the maxillary sinus or nasopharynx. Tumours in these regions may cause objective evidence of sensory disturbance in the distribution of the maxillary nerve. Trigeminal neuralgia affecting the second division of the Vth nerve causes sharp lancinating pain radiating into this area; there is not objective sensory deficit, but 'trigger spots' (areas which induce pain when touched) may be detected.

Persistent pain in the central face for which no cause can be found is seen mostly in middle-aged women and is often associated with depression (atypical facial pain).

Pain in the lower jaw

This may be due to dental or bony disease in the mandible. Disorders of the parotid gland, tongue or floor of the mouth may be responsible. In giant cell arteritis, ischaemia of the masseters may be induced by chewing or talking, causing pain in the jaw which is relieved by rest. Lesions of the mandibular nerve due to disease in the infratemporal region may cause pain radiating to the jaw. Trigeminal neuralgia involving the mandibular branch of the Vth nerve can cause lancinating pain radiating downwards towards the chin. Trigger spots may be present as above. Ischaemic heart disease occasionally causes jaw pain, which is usually bilateral and induced by exercise or associated with breathlessness.

8

Cerebrovascular Disease

Cerebrovascular disease accounts for approximately one hundred thousand deaths per annum in the UK; it ranks third behind heart disease and cancer as a cause of death. 'Stroke' or 'apoplexy' are popular terms for an acute neurological disturbance involving paralysis and, frequently, loss of speech; it is usually considered under three categories: thrombosis, embolism, haemorrhage.

CEREBRAL BLOOD FLOW

The supply vessels comprise the two internal carotid and two vertebral arteries, connected at the base of the brain by the circle of Willis (Fig. 8.1). These large muscular arteries have a relatively low resistance and the circle of Willis can function as an effective collateral channel. If one of the supply arteries is occluded, the flow through the other vessels immediately increases.

The pial network covers the convoluted surface of the brain and is fed by three main arteries: the anterior, middle and posterior cerebral arteries (Fig. 8.2). Adjacent vascular territories are connected on the surface of the brain by small anastamotic vessels. The pial or distribution vessels are richly innervated by both adrenergic and cholinergic nerve fibres and also respond directly to CO_2. Mean blood pressure in the pial network is 75% of aortic pressure.

The resistance vessels are the penetrating intracerebral arteries to grey and white matter. Each vessel is surrounded by a sleeve of CSF. These vessels are poorly supplied with nerves, but the vascular smooth muscle contracts in response to variations in wall tension and to biochemical changes in the perivascular fluid. There are no significant anastomoses between the penetrat-

ing vessels and they connect directly with the capillary plexus.

The brain requires a relatively constant blood supply (one-fifth of the cardiac output at rest). Grey matter receives twice the blood-flow of white matter and has a denser capillary network. A number of homoeostatic systems protect the brain from reduction in its blood supply and also adjust the cerebral blood-flow to metabolic demand. Thus when cerebral metabolism is increased, as during an epileptic seizure, cerebral blood-flow increases. Conversely in states of coma or barbiturate anaesthesia total cerebral blood-flow is decreased. Any regional increase in cortical activity, e.g. resulting from a sensory stimulus such as flashing light, produces a focal increase in metabolism and blood-flow in the appropriate occipital and parietal lobe.

This coupling of blood-flow and metabolism is probably mediated by the resistance vessels, which change their calibre in response to biochemical changes in the surrounding perivascular fluid. The stimulus is uncertain, but it may be hydrogen, bicarbonate or potassium ions or possibly adenosine. These humoral changes can be modified by neurogenic influences.

Systemic blood pressure varies greatly during each 24-hour period and the brain must be protected against possible damage from excessively high or low pressures. Two mechanisms exist:

1. The baroceptor reflexes adjust the peripheral resistance and heart rate in response to changes in tension in the walls of the carotid sinus. The effect of this is to maintain a steady perfusion pressure to the brain.

2. The vascular smooth muscle of intracerebral resistance arteries responds to changes in the pressure

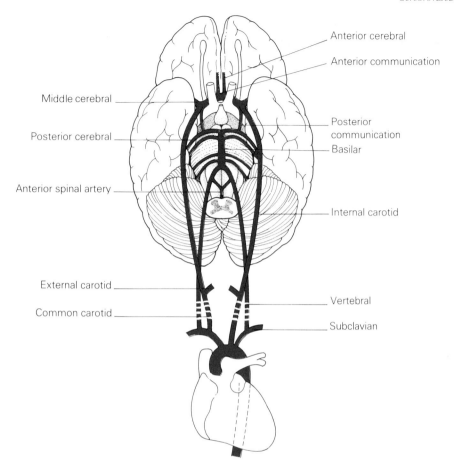

Fig. 8.1 *Arterial supply to the brain.*

gradient across the vessel wall (autoregulation). Thus a rise in blood pressure (or a decrease in CSF pressure) increases the pressure gradient and causes contraction of the smooth muscle and so a decrease in the size of the lumen. (Fig. 8.3). There is a range over which cerebral blood-flow is independent of perfusion pressure. This range can be modified by neurogenic tone, but autoregulation can function even in denervated vessels.

PATHOPHYSIOLOGY

Cerebrovascular homoeostasis may be disturbed in a number of conditions.

Hypotension

If the perfusion pressure falls below the autoregulatory range, the resistance vessels are already fully dilated: the circulation becomes passive and further reduction in blood pressure leads to a fall in blood-flow. When this affects the whole brain, ischaemia affects preferentially the border zones between vascular territories, where the perfusion pressure is normally at its lowest.

Hypertension

If the systemic blood pressure exceeds the autoregulation range, 'breakthrough' occurs and cerebral blood-flow increases. The blood–brain barrier may be

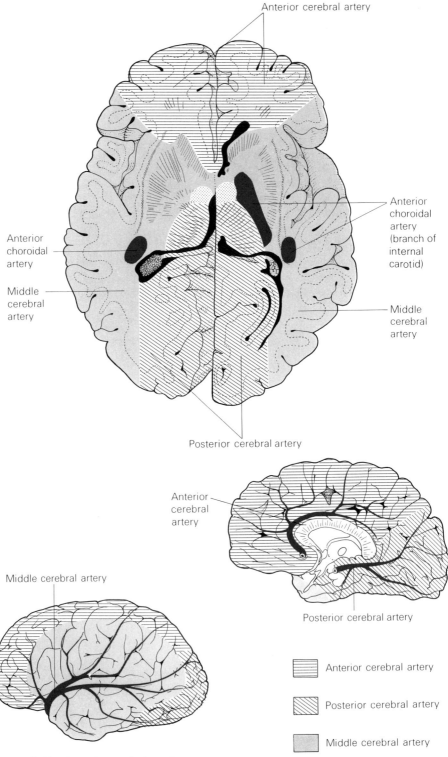

Anterior cerebral artery

Anterior choroidal artery (branch of internal carotid)

Anterior choroidal artery

Middle cerebral artery

Middle cerebral artery

Posterior cerebral artery

Anterior cerebral artery

Posterior cerebral artery

Middle cerebral artery

Anterior cerebral artery

Posterior cerebral artery

Middle cerebral artery

Fig. 8.2 *Territories supplied by the major cerebral arteries.*

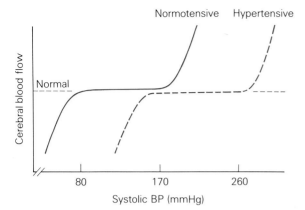

Fig. 8.3 *Autoregulation range in normotensive and hypertensive subjects.*

damaged and cerebral oedema may occur. This condition is reversible if the blood pressure is rapidly lowered (Fig. 8.3).

Raised Intracranial Pressure

Slight increases in CSF pressure are compensated for by autoregulation, and flow is unchanged. If CSF pressure is very high, a reflex rise in systemic blood pressure occurs (Cushing effect), but even this may be insufficient to prevent a fall in cerebral blood-flow. Flow eventually ceases when ICP exceeds systolic blood pressure.

Hyper- and Hypocapnia

Carbon dioxide is a highly efficient 'physiological' vasodilator, and an increase in CO_2 causes an increase in blood-flow (Fig. 8.4). However, in vascular disease or cerebral ischaemia, the vessels may fail to respond to this stimulus either because the walls are too rigid or because they are already maximally dilated. Hypocapnia causes vasoconstriction, with a decrease in cerebral blood-flow, vascular volume and intracranial pressure. This property is useful in neurosurgery since the anaesthetist may, by adjusting ventilation, reduce blood-flow and ICP at appropriate times.

Hypoxia

There is a close relationship between the oxygen content of arterial blood and cerebral blood-flow (Fig. 8.5). When haemoglobin concentration increases, cerebral blood flow falls, and vice versa. Because of the shape of the haemoglobin dissociation curve, variations in PO_2 have less effect on cerebral blood-flow and no significant change occurs until PO_2 is less than 60 mm (8 kPa). Below that level a steep rise in blood-flow occurs.

Vascular Occlusion

The effects of vascular occlusion on cerebral blood-flow depend on the arteries available for collateral flow. In obstruction of the internal carotid artery, sufficient blood is available via the other supply vessels of the circle of Willis and, in 80% of patients, no cerebral infarction occurs. In middle cerebral artery occlusion, the pial anastamoses are usually insufficient to prevent infarction, which affects the centre of the vascular territory; the border zones are usually spared (Fig. 8.6). Occlusion of an intracerebral penetrating artery results in a small deep infarct (lacunar infarct).

Vascular Steal

If occlusion occurs in the first part of the subclavian artery, the pressure beyond the occlusion may be less than in the basilar artery. If this occurs, blood flows in a retrograde direction down the vertebral artery and into the arm. This usually produces no symptoms, but occasionally transient ischaemia occurs during exercise of the arm (subclavian steal) (Figs 8.7a, 8.7b).

PATHOGENESIS

Thrombosis

Thrombosis is usually superimposed upon an atheromatous plaque and, although thrombosis may occur in any major cerebral vessel, parts of the internal carotid and basilar arteries are especially susceptible. In hyper-

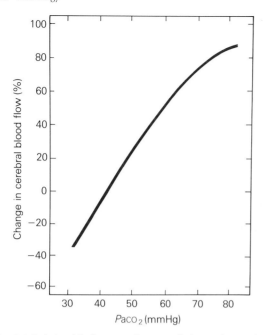

Fig. 8.4 *Relationship between PaCO$_2$ and change in cerebral blood flow.*

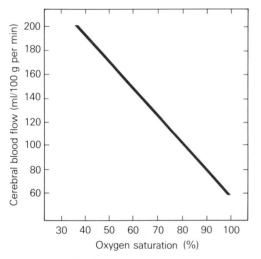

Fig. 8.5 *Relationship between oxygen saturation of arterial blood and cerebral blood flow.*

tensive vascular disease the severity and extent of atheroma is increased in all vessels. In addition, lipohyaline change with microaneurysms tends to occur in the deep penetrating arteries of the internal capsule, thalamus and pons (Fig. 8.8). Although hyper-

tension is the major risk factor for cerebral arterial thrombosis, there are a number of other predisposing causes, including indirect trauma to the carotid artery in the neck.

Infarction follows thrombosis if the collateral circulation is inadequate. A central zone of necrosis develops, but around this there is an ischaemic 'penumbra' which is functionless but viable for a time. Normal CBF is 60–70 ml/100 g/min; electrical function ceases at about 20 ml/100 g/min, and death of neurones occurs below about 10 ml/100 g/min. If CBF can be restored to the penumbra, some tissue may recover function. Normal vascular reactivity to CO$_2$ and autoregulation to pressure may be disturbed in the region of an infarct, and CBF may become passively dependent on blood pressure (Fig. 8.3).

Damaged cerebral tissue tends to swell due to accumulation of water in glial cells (cytotoxic oedema). In addition, if breakdown of the normal blood–brain barrier occurs, extracellular (vasogenic) oedema may occur. Ischaemic oedema is a mixture of early cytotoxic oedema and, after a few days, vasogenic oedema. The combined effect is to cause substantial brain swelling with herniation and compression of adjacent structures, leading to clinical deterioration.

Embolism

Cerebral emboli also cause vascular occlusion and cerebral infarction, but there are some important differences from thrombosis *in situ*.

    a. A source of embolism is usually present in the heart or major vessels.

    b. The site of occlusion is often different; the middle cerebral artery is frequently affected by embolism, rarely by thrombosis.

    c. The infarct is often haemorrhagic. This is caused by movement of the embolus as it fragments and is pushed distally into smaller arteries, thus allowing blood to reenter the damaged tissue.

    d. Infarcts are often multiple and in different vascular territories.

Haemorrhage

There are three main causes of haemorrhage in or around the brain.

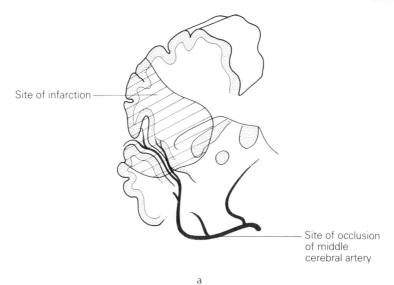

Site of infarction

Site of occlusion
of middle
cerebral artery

a

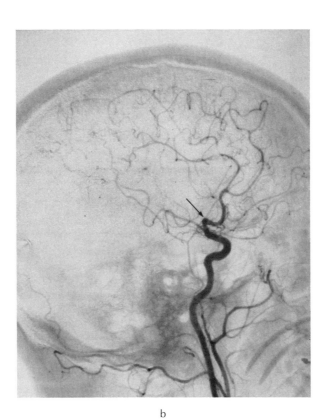

b

Fig. 8.6 (a) *Occlusion of branches of the middle cerebral artery.*
(b) *Angiogram: occlusion of middle cerebral artery (arrow).*

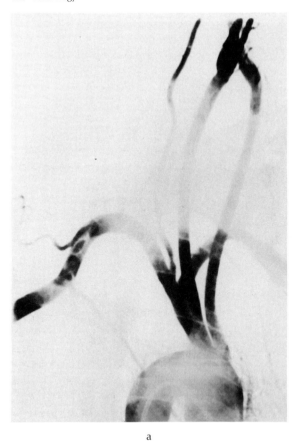

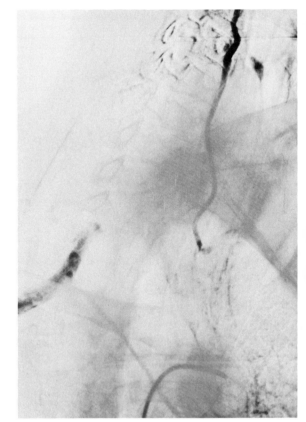

a

b

Fig. 8.7 (a) *Left subclavian artery stenosis: arch angiogram; note absence of left vertebral artery. (b) Left vertebral artery filling retrogradely from above on later film.*

Spontaneous intracerebral haemorrhage

This originates from small intracerebral arteries affected by lipohyaline degeneration. It occurs in certain well defined sites: basal ganglia, subcortical white matter, cerebellum and pons. Lipohyaline change is caused by plasma permeating into the walls of arterioles which have become weakened through loss of elastic and smooth muscle tissue – a change brought about by chronic hypertension. Intracerebral haemorrhage may cause death from brain swelling, tentorial herniation and brainstem compression (Fig. 8.9). If the patient survives, the haemorrhage usually absorbs, leaving a cystic cavity. There is often considerable recovery of function.

Subarachnoid haemorrhage

This usually originates from rupture of berry aneurysms arising on large extracerebral arteries in relation to the circle of Willis (Fig. 8.11). Berry aneurysms may arise at sites of congenital defect in the walls of these arteries, but are aggravated by atheroma and hypertension. Aneurysmal bleeding may also extend into the brain, especially into the frontal or temporal lobes. Subarachnoid haemorrhage may cause death from acute raised intracranial pressure and medullary ischaemia. If the patient survives, blood-clot may organize around the tentorial opening and cause a communicating hydrocephalus (see p. 81).

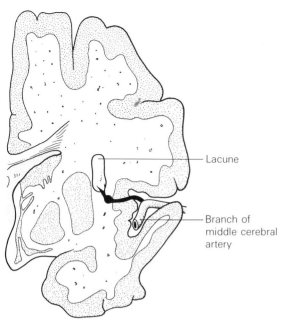

Fig. 8.8 *Occluded microaneurysm on penetrating artery from middle cerebral causing lacunar infarct (After Fisher C.M. 1969, Acta Neuropath.,* **12:** *1).*

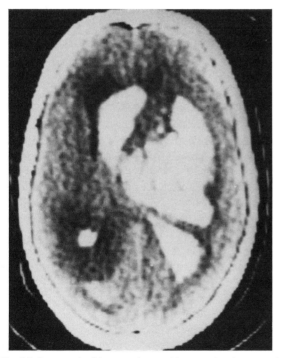

Fig. 8.9 *Intracerebral haemorrhage with extension into ventricular system.*

Angiomas (arteriovenous malformations)

These are another type of congenital defect, and consist of a tangled mass of arteries and large veins. These slowly enlarge during adult life and present with haemorrhage (subarachnoid or intracerebral) or epileptic seizures. Angiomas are usually situated in the hemispheres. The bleeding is less profuse and dangerous than from berry aneurysms.

Other causes of cerebral or subarachnoid haemorrhage are trauma, haemorrhagic disease and anticoagulant overdose.

Clinical Syndromes and Management: Vascular Occlusion

Anterior cerebral artery

The anterior cerebral artery passes forwards and over the corpus callosum, supplying the medial part of the cerebral hemisphere, including the entire motor and sensory cortex controlling the leg. Ischaemia initially causes a flaccid paralysis of the contralateral leg, an extensor plantar response, and cortical sensory loss. The limb may be hypotonic, but increased tone and brisk reflexes commonly supervene within a few weeks. Urgency or incontinence of micturition may occur because the area anterior to the 'leg area' of the cortex is concerned with the voluntary control of bladder function. There is also disturbance of intellect, judgement, and emotional control.

Middle cerebral artery

The middle cerebral artery passes laterally and upwards in the sylvian fissure, and its branches spread over to supply almost the whole of the lateral surface of the cerebral hemisphere (Fig. 8.2). Near its origin it also gives off pentrating branches (striate arteries) which supply the basal ganglia and internal capsule.

Occlusion results in a hemiplegia affecting the face and arm and, to a lesser extent, the leg. Hemi-anaesthesia and homonymous hemianopia often accompany the hemiparesis. Changes in tone and reflexes follow a similar pattern to that described in anterior cerebral artery occlusion.

In addition, if the left (dominant) hemisphere is

affected, dysphasia occurs, its type depending on the major site of damage (see p. 49). Infarcts in the right (non-dominant) middle cerebral artery territory produce topographical disorientation, with inattention and neglect of the left side and difficulty in route-finding; sometimes there is also difficulty with dressing (right parietal lobe syndrome). The patient appears less aware of his symptoms and, in spite of preservation of speech, a left-sided hemiplegia is often more disabling than a right.

Internal carotid artery

This produces a clinical picture resembling a combined anterior and middle cerebral artery occlusion. The first branch of the internal carotid artery is the ophthalmic artery; the presence of retinal ischaemia with a contralateral hemiplegia strongly suggests carotid artery disease. More frequently, however, episodes of fleeting visual loss (amaurosis fugax) occur due to emboli. Cholesterol and platelet emboli become lodged in the ophthalmic and retinal arteries, producing either transient uniocular loss of vision or altitudinal

field loss if only the upper or lower half of the retina is involved. These emboli often arise from atherosclerotic plaques at the origin of the internal carotid artery (Fig. 8.10).

In addition, an ipsilateral Horner's syndrome may be present because of involvement of the sympathetic fibres in the carotid sheath. Because of increased collateral blood flow, the arteries of the scalp may be more prominent on the side of an internal carotid artery occlusion.

Posterior cerebral artery

These paired vessels are formed by the bifurcation of the basilar trunk (Fig. 8.1). The posterior cerebral arteries pass backwards around the brainstem and supply the upper part of the brainstem, the occipital lobes (calcarine and parieto-occipital branches), and the medial surface of the temporal lobe (posterior temporal branch) (Fig. 8.2).

A right or left homonymous field defect is the principal result of ischaemia in the posterior cerebral territory. Simultaneous lesions on both sides may result

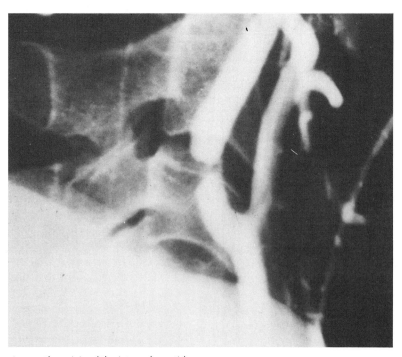

Fig. 8.10 *Severe stenosis near the origin of the internal carotid artery.*

in cortical blindness. Pupillary responses are spared since the pupillary fibres travelling to the midbrain are not involved. The patient may confabulate or have hallucinations, and lacks insight even to the extent of denying his blindness. Transient amnesia can result from ischaemia of the medial aspect of the temporal lobes. The posterior cerebral artery also supplies part of the thalamus. Infarction may result in sensory impairment over the contralateral side of the body, accompanied by a very unpleasant pain which may be spontaneous or induced by light contact with the skin (thalamic syndrome).

Vertebrobasilar occlusion

The symptoms and signs following infarction in the vertebrobasilar territory depend on the level of the lesion in the brainstem. Occlusion of the terminal basilar artery may produce signs of posterior cerebral artery occlusion. There are a number of rare syndromes which may follow ischaemia to a localised region of the brainstem. The most widely recognised of these, thrombosis of the posterior inferior cerebellar artery (Fig. 8.11), produces ischaemia of the dorsolateral medulla with palsies of cranial nerves V–VII, IX and X, cerebellar ataxia and a Horner's syndrome on the same side as the lesion, and contralateral spinothalamic loss in the arm and leg. Additionally, pain and temperature loss may occur over the ipsilateral face due to damage to the descending tract and nucleus of V. Hemiplegia is rare because the corticospinal tracts lying ventrally are spared.

In other syndromes there is a general pattern consisting of ipsilateral cranial nerve palsies with contralateral paresis of hemisensory loss which affects either arm and leg or arm, leg and face, depending on the level in the brainstem. Ipsilateral cerebellar signs may also be seen. Pupillary changes with impaired vertical gaze or IIIrd nerve dysfunction are seen in midbrain lesions, and horizontal gaze palsy with facial weakness and sensory loss follow damage to the pons. In either case a hemiparesis or quadriparesis may also occur. Occlusion of the basilar artery itself often results in a fatal coma with ophthalmoplegia, flaccid quadriplegia, and loss of brainstem reflexes. It may also cause the rare 'locked in' syndrome, in which there is limited infarction of pons and midbrain. The clinical picture appears similar; the patient is immobile, seems super-

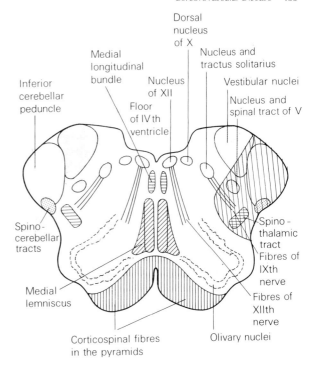

Fig. 8.11 *Cross-section of medulla to show usual area of infarction in lateral medullary syndrome (vertebral or posterior inferior cerebellar artery occlusion).*

ficially unconscious but may be fully alert. The only voluntary movement consists of vertical movements of the eyes and eyelids. It is important to check these movements before accepting that any patient is truly unconscious.

Border zone infarct

The clinical patterns so far described follow occlusion of individual arteries. Sometimes, however, there is a generalised reduction in cerebral blood-flow, e.g. after a cardiac arrest. Ischaemia then is most marked in the border zone between the territories of individual arteries because here perfusion pressure is at its lowest level (Fig. 8.12). This results in border-zone infarction, the clinical picture of which differs from the patterns described for individual vessels. Most commonly it affects the parieto-occipital zone, where it may produce visual field defects, visual disorientation and constructional apraxia. In the frontal border zone, slowing up, grasp reflexes, gait disturbances and incontinence may occur.

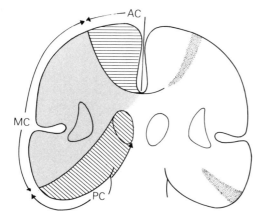

Fig. 8.12 *Cross-section of cerebral hemispheres to show region affected in border-zone infarction (stippled). AC, MC, PC anterior, middle, posterior territories.*

Transient ischaemic attacks

Cerebral infarction is often preceded by minor attacks of ischaemia which recover completely within minutes or hours.

These are most often caused by embolism and are particularly associated with partial occlusions of the internal carotid artery. Small fragments of mural thrombi are detached from the carotid artery and lodge in distal arteries, where they cause a temporary occlusion. Transient ischaemic ataks are important because they often presage a major stroke; the incidence of stroke in patients with transient ischaemic attacks is approximately 5% per year. They also indicate generalised atheromatous vascular disease and patients with transient ischaemic attacks have a higher than normal incidence of fatal or non-fatal myocardial infarction.

Transient ischaemic attacks are of two main types: carotid and vertebrobasilar. Carotid transient ischaemic attacks comprise short-lived attacks of weakness, clumsiness, and paraesthesiae involving the contralateral arm and leg, with or without dysphasia. The patient may temporarily lose sight in one eye on the side of the carotid occlusion (amaurosis fugax). This occurs at a different time from the cerebral symptoms.

Vertebrobasilar transient ischaemic attacks consist of a brief episode of one or more of the following: vertigo, diplopia, dysarthria, visual loss, hemiparesis, perioral tingling and leg weakness.

Differential diagnosis: Transient ischaemic attacks by definition recover in less than 24 hours but may sometimes be difficult to differentiate from migraine, epilepsy, syncope, hypoglycaemia and hypertensive encephalopathy (see p. 142). A careful past history with detailed description of the event, combined with clinical examination and EEG, usually allow these other conditions to be distinguished. Rarely, TIAs occur not on the basis of emboli but as a result of low flow states in patients who have multiple major-vessel occlusions. In these situations the transient ischaemic attacks are often associated with symptoms of generalised cerebral hypoxia, such as dizziness and light headedness, and frequently occur in relation to a slight fall in blood pressure such as may occur on standing up.

Management

Established stroke

Differential diagnosis: Initial assessment of the stroke patient involves confirming the diagnosis. The deficit following cerebral infarction (embolic or thrombotic) is usually of sudden onset but sometimes evolves over a period of hours or days, often in a stepwise manner. This may be caused by propagation of the original thrombus occluding further vessels and reducing collateral flow by additional emboli or by cerebral oedema. Other conditions such as cerebral tumour, subdural haematoma, encephalitis, abscess or an episode of demyelination have to be considered.

More commonly the difficulty is in distinguishing haemorrhage from infarction due to vascular occlusion. There are no completely reliable clinical indicators to this (Table 8.1). A previous history of typical transient ischaemic episodes or the presence of cholesterol emboli in the retinal circulation strongly suggests embolism, whilst early depression of consciousness, vomiting, meningism (suggesting blood in the CSF) or very high blood pressures (e.g. diastolic greater than 130 mmHg) point towards a haemorrhagic episode. Headache may be prominent in both occlusive and haemorrhagic stroke but is generally more acute, severe and generalised in the latter. CT scanning is the most reliable current method of distinguishing an occlusion from a haemorrhagic episode, as well as for excluding other lesions. Acute infarction usually reveals no abnormality on CT in the first 48 hours, whilst haemorrhage is evidenced by a high-density space-occupying lesion.

The patient must be examined for a potential source of embolism, with particular attention being paid to cardiac abnormalities, evidence of other peripheral vascular occlusion, carotid or subclavian bruits, or difference in blood pressure in the two arms (suggesting a subclavian stenosis). In a probably thrombotic stroke particular attention is paid to the retinal vessels, and to palpation of the internal carotid and superficial temporal vessels as well as to other risk factors.

Acute management and investigation: In the acute phase the patient may be drowsy or even unconscious. It is therefore important to check the airway, nurse the patient in the semiprone position, and give regular chest physiotherapy. Passive physiotherapy to all limbs helps to prevent contractures. Care of the bowel, bladder and the prevention of pressure sores by regular turning are all important. It is usually possible to give food and fluid by a nasogastric tube provided there is no ileus. Cases in which a treatable underlying cause for the stroke (e.g. arteritis) is found require the appropriate treatment. Cerebral oedema may be significant in large infarcts and may cause early mortality. However, it is by no means clear whether anti-oedema drugs improve the quality of survival. Clinical trials suggest that steroids are of no long-term value in ischaemic

oedema, although they are sometimes given and occasionally appear beneficial in patients who deteriorate due to brain swelling.

The management of high blood pressure in the acute phase is controversial. As autoregulation in and around the infarct may be lost, lowering the blood pressure may cause a fall in cerebral blood-flow. Unless there is aortic dissection, hypertensive encephalopathy or cerebral haemorrhage, it is prudent not to lower moderately raised blood pressure in the acute stroke. When the diastolic blood pressure exceeds 130 mmHg., it is reasonable to lower the blood pressure acutely, but rapid and profound reduction should be avoided; diastolic pressures below 110 mmHg are usually adequate.

All patients should undergo investigations for major risk factors for stroke (see p. 138). Further investigations are dependent on the initial clinical findings and investigations, degree of recovery, age and other associated medical illnesses. CT scan is desirable, and it is essential if there is doubt about the diagnosis. It need not be performed routinely but only in those cases in which the result is likely to alter management. Angiography is of little value in the acute stage of stroke except where haemorrhage originates from a berry aneurysm. Neurosurgery has no part to play in acute thrombotic or embolic strokes. When a superficial cerebral or cerebellar haemorrhage is present and the

Table 8.1

Differential Diagnosis of Stroke

	Thrombosis	Embolism	Haemorrhage
Clinical setting	Elderly, hypertensive, diabetic	Heart disease at any age; ischaemic or rheumatic; atrial fibrillation	Middle-aged: men > women; chronic hypertension
Onset	Rapid, fluctuating over minutes/hours: preceded by TIA. Noted on waking	Very rapid: diurnal TIA in minority	During activity: no preceding attacks
Progression	Maximum within 12 hrs. Thereafter slow improvement	Maximal within minutes	Steady progression over minutes/hours
Associated features	Headache (variable) Seizures (rare) Loss of consciousness (rare)	Seizures (common)	Vomiting } (common) headache } Seizures may occur: Progressive depression of consciousness
Site	Internal carotid, posterior cerebral, basilar (middle cerebral)	Middle cerebral, Postcerebral	Internal capsule, subcortical white matter, thalamus, pons, cerebellum

patient's neurological state is deteriorating, evacuation of the clot may be beneficial.

Anticoagulants are used prophylactically in embolic strokes where a clear cardiac source of embolism is demonstrated, e.g. mitral stenosis. In theory they increase the risk of bleeding into a necrotic infarct. Some start anticoagulants immediately whereas others wait up to a month after the acute episode. Even where embolism clinically seems likely, haemorrhage should be excluded by CT scan before anticoagulation. Examination of the CSF for blood is unreliable because some haemorrhages are isolated from the subarachnoid space and some infarcts produce a haemorrhagic CSF. Lumbar puncture is also hazardous in the presence of a haematoma or brain swelling.

Long-term prognosis and rehabilitation (see also Chapter 19): Prognosis in stroke depends largely on the level of consciousness when first seen. Between 80–90% of those in coma die within a few weeks of admission, compared with 30% of those who are alert. Over half of those who survive become fully independent. Only a small percentage require long-term institutional care. Recovery tends to be poorest in those who have severe weakness, bilateral signs, incontinence and sensory loss in the arm, and who have difficulty sitting up unaided. Most improvement occurs within the first three months, although recovery can continue for up to a year. Physiotherapy, occupational therapy and speech therapy encourage maximum utilisation of such functions that slowly return in the following weeks and months (see also Chapter 19). The role of specialised stroke units and their influence on the patient's ultimate overall disability remains uncertain. Aids to daily living with home assessment can make life more tolerable in many cases. Spasticity may be helped by physiotherapy, by physical methods of treatment such as ice packs and, occasionally, by drugs such as baclofen, diazepam or dantrolene sodium.

Transient ischaemic attacks and stroke with recovery

Future risks: Patients who make a full functional recovery from their initial attack, whether it is a TIA or stroke, should be considered for full investigation. The risk of a further stroke and perhaps permanent disablement is approximately 5–10% per annum. The risk is higher in the carotid territory than the vertebrobasilar. *Treatment of risk factors*: Hypertension is the most important risk factor in both cerebral haemorrhage and occlusive disease. A diastolic pressure in excess of 110 mmHg should normally be lowered to 90–100. Some evidence suggests that the level of the systolic blood pressure is a better prognostic guide. However, this is liable to fluctuate more and may be more difficult to control. It is important to lower blood pressure gradually because the autoregulatory range in hypertension is set higher (Fig. 8.3). This range, however, may revert back towards normal after prolonged treatment. This is *not* an argument against treating hypertension; it is merely a word of caution regarding the rate at which blood pressure is reduced. Other factors such as diabetes mellitus, anaemia, polycythaemia and thrombocythaemia will require treatment. In severe hyperlipidaemia, cholesterol should be lowered by diet and cholestyramine. Patients must be urged to stop smoking.

Further investigation depends on the patient's age and medical fitness. The younger patient usually requires thorough cardiological investigation including echocardiography.

Angiography using intra-arterial contrast injection is the definitive investigation in many patients with TIA. It is performed on those in whom an operable lesion is considered likely and in whom no other source of emboli has been found. A carotid bruit is an important clinical guide to the presence of carotid stenosis, but at least 30% of all patients who have operable lesions do not have bruits. The procedure is not without risk, having a significant morbidity or mortality of between 0.5 and 1%. Less invasive investigations, such as digital intravenous vascular imaging and Doppler sonography, are useful in deciding when to proceed to conventional angiography. As digital vascular imaging becomes more widespread, the need for invasive angiography will undoubtedly fall. For the 30% of patients with TIA who are found to have stenosis or localised ulceration of the internal carotid artery, endarterectomy is probably the treatment of choice. In experienced surgical hands the combined mortality and morbidity of the operation (approximately 1–4%) is less than the natural history of the condition in patients treated medically. Those patients with severe coronary artery disease or severe hypertension have a higher operative risk and are treated medically.

At the present time, patients who are found to have symptomless carotid stenosis are usually not recommended for surgery.

Patients with complete carotid occlusion cannot be treated by endarterectomy. If they continue to suffer TIA the cause is likely to be a failure of collateral blood supply. In some cases this may be improved by the new operation of superficial temporal to middle cerebral artery anastomosis.

A large group of patients, however, have no major risk factor or operable carotid lesion. The choice therefore lies between antiplatelet or anticoagulant drugs. Antiplatelet agents are extensively used in the prevention of stroke after TIA. Aspirin is probably effective, at least in men, in reducing the incidence of strokes and death. The exact dose is as yet unclear. There is some laboratory evidence which suggests that only a small daily dose (e.g. 60 mg) is needed. The most commonly used current dosage is 300 mg a day. Dipyridamole and sulphinpyrazone have no proven benefit.

There is also some evidence that anticoagulants reduce the frequency of stroke after TIA; unfortunately, most of the trials are open to considerable criticism. As the risk of stroke after a TIA may be highest in the first six months, anticoagulants are not usually given on a long-term basis. However, if there is a continuing cardiac source of emboli, such as rheumatic valvular disease with or without atrial fibrillation, then long-term anticoagulant treatment rather than antiplatelet therapy should be instituted.

Summary

It should be apparent that a diagnosis, in a 60-year-old man with sudden onset of a hemiplegia, of a 'stroke' is not enough. It is important to consider each patient in terms of the clinical presentation, underlying anatomy, vascular pathology and identifiable risk factors. Thus the formulation becomes: 60-year-old man, who smokes 20 cigarettes a day, presents with a mild left hemiplegia. Further questioning reveals two previous episodes of amaurosis fugax in the right eye, each lasting five minutes, suggesting emboli in the territory of the right carotid artery. Investigation reveals mild diabetes but all other routine tests are normal. The patient makes a complete recovery over a month: CT scan shows a small right hemisphere infarct. Angiography demonstrates a right internal carotid stenosis, which is removed at endarterectomy.

Subarachnoid Haemorrhage (SAH)

Principal causes

Most cases of subarachnoid haemorrhage (other than trauma) follow rupture of berry aneurysm. These commonly arise from the circle of Willis at points where the vessel wall is congenitally weak (Figs 8.13 and 8.14). Approximately 30% of berry aneurysms arise from the anterior communicating artery and the middle cerebral artery. Less frequent causes of subarachnoid haemorrhage include cerebral (or spinal) angioma, mycotic aneurysm, and bleeding disorders including anticoagulant treatment.

Clinical presentation and initial investigation of aneurysmal SAH

The patient usually presents with a sudden severe headache, vomiting, photophobia and neck stiffness. The level of consciousness varies from coma to full alertness but most often the patient is obtunded and restless. This is particularly likely to occur in anterior communicating aneurysms. Signs of focal damage, e.g. hemiparesis, may be present especially after middle cerebral artery aneurysm rupture. If the haemorrhage is severe and there is a marked rise in intracranial pressure then retinal haemorrhages and papilloedema may be seen. Transient cardiac arrhythmias are common, and glycosuria is sometimes found.

In the acute phase the diagnosis of subarachnoid haemorrhage may be confirmed by CT scan in approximately 90% of cases; alternatively, lumbar puncture may show uniformly bloodstained CSF under increased pressure. Within three hours the CSF supernatant becomes yellow (xanthochromia) due to breakdown of red cells and, because the blood causes a chemical meningitis, there may also be a slight excess of white cells in the fluid. Xanthochromia lasts approximately 10–14 days. Routine tests for bleeding disorder and an ECG are also indicated.

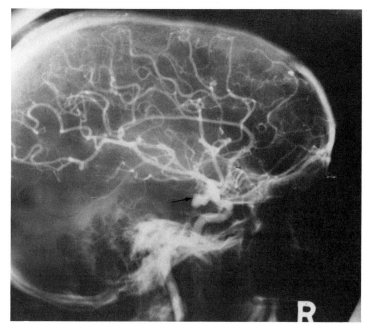

Fig. 8.13 *Aneurysm arising from internal carotid artery at the origin of the posterior communicating artery (arrow).*

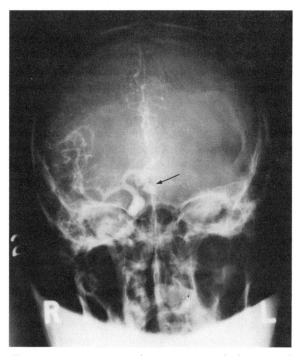

Fig. 8.14 *Aneurysm arising from anterior cerebral artery and extending downwards to compress the optic chiasm (arrow).*

Management

About 30–40% of patients with subarachnoid haemorrhage due to aneurysmal rupture die in the first few days. The greatest incidence of rebleeding occurs two weeks after the first haemorrhage and a major risk exists for almost 6 weeks. Thereafter the risk of further bleeding falls substantially to approximately 5% per annum: management is mainly concerned with reducing the incidence of rebleeding. The definitive test is angiography of all main arteries. Most patients under 65 who are alert or slightly drowsy should be referred for immediate assessment. Angiography is performed when such patients are clinically stable, as soon as possible after the initial event. Approximately 15% of aneurysms are multiple. Surgery appears to improve the prognosis, and posterior communicating artery aneurysms have the best prognosis. The outcome of surgery is directly dependent on the level of consciousness. Those who are in coma almost invariably die after surgery and should not, therefore, be considered for angiography. If surgery is not possible or an aneurysm is not found (10%) then a period of six weeks' bed rest is recommended.

Other complications of aneurysms

Aneurysms occasionally enlarge slowly without rupturing and present as space-occupying lesions. This may occur with internal carotid aneurysms behind the orbit, which can become very large in size, causing visual failure, ophthalmoplegia, pain in the face and reduced sensation in the first two divisions of the Vth nerve. Similar features are seen in caroticocavernous fistulae, which often follow trauma. In these the carotid artery directly communicates with the cavernous sinus and a loud bruit is usually heard over the orbit. The high orbital venous pressure may cause pulsating exophthalmos, chemosis and papilloedema. Posterior communicating artery aneurysms may present as an isolated IIIrd nerve palsy before rupturing. One important complication of subarachnoid haemorrhage, which may occur either in the acute phase or many years later, is hydrocephalus. The blood in the subarachnoid space prevents the absorption of CSF in the arachnoid villae and in view of this there is a progressive increase in the CSF pressure resulting in a communicating hydrocephalus (see p. 81).

Angioma

The mortality from a bleeding angioma is considerably lower than that from an aneurysm. The investigation of migraine by angiography to exclude an angioma is rarely justified, but the finding of a bruit over the orbit or cranial cavity may warrant angiography. The place of surgery in the management of angiomas is dependent on the presentation and site of the lesion. Many patients presenting with epilepsy alone are managed with anticonvulsants, whereas those presenting with subarachnoid haemorrhage would be considered for surgery if the lesion were accessible.

Venous Infarctions

The venous drainage of the brain is chiefly through dural sinuses (Fig. 8.15). Blood from the cortex drains mainly into the superior sagittal or cavernous sinuses. Deeper structures drain into the vein of Galen and thence into the straight sinus. The straight sinus and the superior sagittal sinus drain into the lateral sinuses to leave the skull in the internal jugular veins through the jugular foramina. Emissary veins connect the extracranial veins with the venous sinuses in a number of places, particularly around the orbit and the ear. Because they may facilitate the spread of clot or infection into the head, these are an important cause of venous thrombosis.

Infections of the face, orbits or sinuses may rarely be

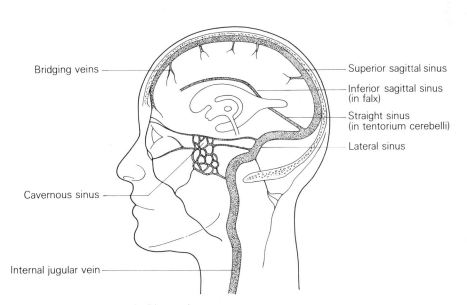

Fig. 8.15 *Principal veins draining the cerebral hemispheres.*

followed by cavernous sinus thrombosis with a swollen red conjunctiva and eyelid, paralysis of the III, IV, VI, V$_1$ and V$_2$ cranial nerves, and marked papilloedema. These patients are often diabetic and should be treated with the appropriate antibiotic: fungal infection, notably with Mucor, is a cause of this syndrome in diabetic ketoacidosis. Veins connect both caverous sinuses and the condition is often bilateral.

Lateral sinus thrombosis may follow ear infections. There is usually raised intracranial pressure due to impaired absorption of CSF; fits, drowsiness, headache, nausea, vomiting and papilloedema are common.

Thrombosis of the superior sagittal sinus also causes raised intracranial pressure. Frequently this is associated with thrombophlebitis of the cortical veins, which often produces focal symptoms. Epilepsy is a frequent occurrence and hemiplegia, dysphasia and hemianopia may also occur. It may be difficult to distinguish the condition from an arterial occlusion although fits, bilateral pyramidal signs and papilloedema are characteristic findings in venous occlusion and infarction. It is associated with a wide variety of clinical conditions including oral contraceptives, haematological disorders such as thrombocythaemia and sickle cell trait, the puerperium, dehydration and cachexia. Treatment of the underlying illness is indicated, but anticoagulants are often withheld because of the high risk of haemorrhagic venous infarction.

Hypertensive Encephalopathy

This refers to an acute disturbance of neurological function which accompanies a sudden severe rise in blood pressure. It may occur in association with glomerulonephritis, phaeochromocytoma, pregnancy or malignant hypertension from any other cause. Severe headache, vomiting, drowsiness, fits, focal neurological deficit and papilloedema are the main features. The diastolic blood pressure is usually in excess of 130 mmHg. The autoregulatory range (Fig. 8.3) is exceeded and there is generalised cerebral hyperaemia. This leads to fibrinoid necrosis of the vessel wall with exudation of fluid. Cerebral oedema follows, with signs of raised intracranial pressure. Petechial haemorrhages may occur in the brain substance.

It is important to lower the blood pressure promptly. However, the autoregulatory curve may have been reset at a higher level if the hypertension is long-standing. One should not, therefore, aim for diastolic pressures of 90 mmHg immediately, since this may be below the lower limit of autoregulation, in which case cerebral blood-flow will fall and cerebral infarction may occur. Values of 100–110 mmHg (diastolic) should be adequate during the acute phase.

Cranial Arteritis

This syndrome usually affects those over the age of 60 years and most commonly involves the temporal artery, causing granulomatous inflammation of the arterial wall particularly affecting the elastic tissue. It causes temporal headaches, often with local swelling and tenderness of the artery which may be so severe that the patient stops brushing his hair and avoids lying his head on the affected side. The headache may be associated with pain and stiffness in the proximal muscles, particularly upon waking (polymyalgia rheumatica), and with weight loss, low-grade fever and anorexia.

Other vessels such as the occipital arteries may be involved, and ischaemia of the jaw muscles or tongue causes pain on chewing. Arteritis in the ophthalmic, vertebral, carotid or systemic arteries may occur. Blindness due to optic nerve infarction on one or both sides, which is the most frequent complication, occurs in approximately 30% of cases. Third or sixth nerve palsy and brainstem stroke also occur.

Elderly patients presenting with headache and other relevant features should have an ESR performed; in cranial arteritis this is invariably greater than 50 mm in 1 hour. Temporal artery biopsy should be performed to confirm the diagnosis.

The headache responds dramatically to steroids (e.g. prednisolone, 60 mg daily), and this should be started immediately the diagnosis is suspected, as it may forestall complications, particularly blindness. The dose can then be reduced as the ESR falls; treatment is usually necessary for 1–2 years. Starting treatment with steroids does not affect the result of the biopsy, provided it is performed within one week.

9

Demyelinating Disease

In the central nervous system (CNS), most neurones have a cell body, short afferent dendritic processes and a long efferent axon (which synapses with neighbouring dendrites). The axon is surrounded by a myelin sheath which is periodically interrupted at the nodes of Ranvier. Neurones are supported in a network of glial cells, of which one variety, the oligodendrocyte, regulates the formation of myelin. The oligodendrocyte corresponds to the Schwann cell in the peripheral nerve, but central and peripheral myelin are not identical and diseases in which there is selective myelin loss (Table 9.1) are usually confined to one system or the other. Demyelinating lesions within the CNS are not uniform: they may be single or multiple, relapsing or progressive, and some are classified by the distribution or age of lesions within the CNS accompanied by inflammatory cells. The underlying cause is sometimes evident; for example, a non-inflammatory focal demyelinating lesion may occur in the pons in patients with hyponatraemia, and acute multifocal inflammatory demyelination is seen in post-infectious encephalomyelitis. However, by far the most prevalent chronic CNS demyelinating disease in man is multiple sclerosis (MS), and here the aetiology is still unclear.

PATHOLOGY

Small multifocal lesions or plaques can be seen macroscopically in the brain and spinal cord of patients dying with MS (Fig. 9.1a–c). Three characteristic abnormalities are seen microscopically. The first is lymphocyte, plasma cell and macrophage infiltration outside vascular channels with no evidence of myelin breakdown (Fig. 9.1d). Secondly there are lesions shelving into normal areas with a peripheral rim of reduced histochemical staining to myelin lipid and protein; in these there is increased staining for proteolytic enzymes surrounding an area of demyelinated axons diffusely infiltrated by macrophage and glial cells and by lymphocytes and plasma cells at the centre (Fig. 9.1e). The third type of lesion is a sharply demarcated area of demyelinated axons and reduced numbers of oligodendrocytes with dense gliosis and no evidence of active lipid destruction or inflammation (Fig. 9.1f). Each type is perivenous and several may be found along the course of a single vein. Clinicopathological correlations suggest that these represent early, recent and chronic lesions due respectively to immunologically-mediated demyelination, phagocytic removal of myelin debris, and glial scarring. In some chronic MS lesions there is continuing myelin breakdown at the edge and others show partial remyelination indicated by thinly myelinated short internodes.

Characterisation of mononuclear cells infiltrating plaques (Fig. 9.1d) indicates that there are ten times more Ig-producing cells in plaques than in non-plaque tissue, and the greatest concentration of Ig is in morphologically recent plaques. There is an overall increase in plasma cell concentration in all chronic plaques, when compared with unaffected white matter, even though myelin damage may no longer be occurring. Both helper/inducer and cytotoxic/suppressor T lymphocyte sub-populations are found in the perivascular cuff extending out into the active lesion and unaffected white matter adjacent to plaques; the relative proportion of each subset varies between plaques of different age.

Table 9.1

Demyelinating Diseases

Disease	Distribution	Type of myelin damage
Multiple sclerosis	Multifocal CNS lesions of varying age	Inflammatory
Devic's disease	Optic nerve/cervical cord lesions	Inflammatory
Acute disseminated		
encephalomyelitis	Multifocal CNS lesions	Inflammatory
transverse myelitis	Focal spinal cord lesion	Inflammatory
optic neuritis	Focal optic nerve lesion	Inflammatory
other isolated lesions	Focal CNS lesions	Inflammatory
Leucodystrophies		
adreno-	Damage to CNS	Dysmyelination
Krabbe's	and/or PNS with	associated with
sudanophilic	involvement of other	sex-linked or autosomal
metachromatic	tissues in some cases	recessive enzyme
Refsum's		deficiencies
Central pontine		Non-inflammatory
myelinolysis	Pons or extrapontine	associated with hyponatraemia
Progressive multifocal		Non-inflammatory
leucoencephalopathy	Diffuse CNS lesions	due to SV40 or JC virus infection
Progressive rubella		Non-inflammatory
panencephalitis	Diffuse CNS lesions	due to persistent Rubella infection
Guillain–Barré syndrome	Peripheral nerve roots	Inflammatory
Brachial neuritis	Brachial plexus	Inflammatory
Hereditary sensorimotor		
neuropathy type 1	PNS	Non-inflammatory
other acquired neuropathies		
e.g. carcinomatous		
some diabetic	PNS	Non-inflammatory
diphtheritic		

PATHOPHYSIOLOGY

Conduction in myelinated axons is normally fast and saltatory, with the process of depolarisation and conduction differing between the nodes of Ranvier and internodal segments. The graded effect of myelin damage is best understood in the peripheral nervous system. Conduction may be completely blocked, it may be preserved but slowed through partial lesions, or the nerve may be unable to transmit fast trains of impulses. Severe central demyelination probably also leads to a failure of nerve conduction through the damaged segment. The proportion of partially demyelinated CNS fibres that are blocked increases with a rise in temperature or calcium ion concentration. Remyelination restores conduction but impaired ability to transmit fast trains of impulses may persist; continuous but very slow conduction may replace the normal saltatory pattern in partially demyelinated or remyelinated fibres.

Although many symptoms of demyelination can be

explained by conduction block, this develops slowly and the fact that symptomatic changes are often rapid indicates that other factors are important. Temporary increase in symptoms with rise in temperature (Uthoff's phenomenon) can be explained by the known effect of temperature on conduction in partially-demyelinated CNS axons. Other symptoms can be explained by abnormal spread of excitation between adjacent demyelinated nerve fibres (ephaptic transmission) or by increased sensitivity to movement as, for example, in the optic nerve (causing flashes of light on eye movement) or spinal cord, causing an electric sensation in the limbs on neck flexion (Lhermitte's symptom). Slowed conduction velocity or conduction block is often asymptomatic, but the lesions can sometimes be detected electrophysiologically or by imaging techniques (see p. 63). Symptomatic recovery could follow remyelination, dispersal of oedema, or synaptic reorganisation, but the relative importance of these and other mechanisms is poorly understood at present.

SYMPTOMS

The determination of symptoms in patients with MS is dependent more on the part that is affected than on the nature of the disease process. Visual, motor, sensory and sphincter symptoms are common because of the high prevalence of lesions affecting the optic nerve (85%), brainstem or cerebellum (70%) and spinal cord (75%).

Acute optic neuritis (see also p. 28) produces pain on ocular movement followed by a significant fall in visual acuity due to a central scotoma. The prognosis for vision after a single attack is good even in severe cases, but recovery may take several months and there is often a residual defect of colour vision, a relative afferent pupillary defect (see p. 36), and pale optic disc. Abnormal eye movements occur in 80% of patients but the commonest – nystagmus or jerky pursuit movements – are usually asymptomatic since the two eyes remain conjugate. Internuclear ophthalmoplegia due to a lesion in the medial longitudinal bundle produces dysconjugate movements (see p. 36), causes diplopia, and may be associated with other symptoms of brainstem disturbance such as vertigo.

Focal tingling or numbness occurs at some stage in most patients. Electric sensations in the spine or limbs on neck flexion (Lhermitte's symptom) and a sense of constriction or burning are particularly characteristic of MS. Proprioceptive loss leads to difficulty in using a limb and may be more disabling than weakness. Other painful symptoms include trigeminal neuralgia which, unlike the idiopathic form (see p. 247), is usually associated with facial numbness and sensory loss on examination. Frequent paroxysmal unpleasant sensory symptoms and tonic spasms, which may mimic focal epilepsy in their duration and distribution, occur in 5% of patients, probably due to ephaptic transmission.

Eighty per cent of patients experience weakness or clumsiness due to lesions in the corticospinal and cerebellar pathways; depressed reflexes or muscle-wasting indicating lower neurone involvement are rare. Whereas sensory symptoms may occur without signs, the reverse is true of motor involvement and it is common to find corticospinal signs (e.g. extensor plantar and absent abdominal reflexes) in patients without motor symptoms.

Sphincter disturbance occurs in 75% of patients, particularly urinary urgency with frequency due to a small spastic bladder; in males, impotence is equally common.

Lesions of cerebral hemisphere white matter are often found at autopsy but these usually cause few clinical symptoms early in the disease; some patients show a change in mood or personality, general fatigue and, rarely, epilepsy at some time during the illness. In long-standing disease, extensive cerebral involvement may lead to dementia.

Natural History (Fig. 9.2)

MS usually starts between the ages of 10 and 50, and is slightly more common in females than males. In 75% of patients the early course of the disease is characterised by irregular periods of disease activity (relapses) lasting from a few days to several weeks, interspersed by intervals of spontaneous remission which may last for several years. Although complete spontaneous recovery usually occurs between episodes at first, in most patients the cumulative effect of earlier lesions eventually produces a disability which appears to progress without further discrete episodes and, in some patients, MS may present insidiously with symptoms which do

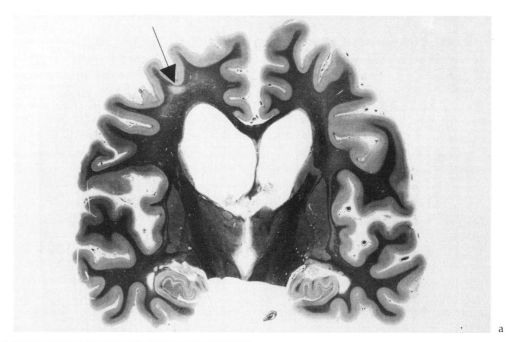

a

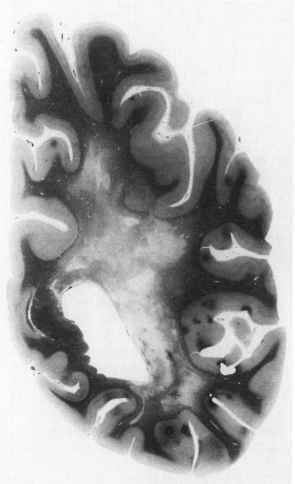

b

Fig. 9.1 (a) *Coronal section through the fronto-temporal lobes, stained for myelin showing a single subcortical plaque.*
(b) *Coronal section through the occipital lobe, stained for myelin, showing a large confluent periventricular area of demyelination.*
(c) *Transverse section of spinal cord stained for myelin showing complete demyelination of one half.*
(d) *Perivascular lymphocytic infiltration in an early MS plaque.*

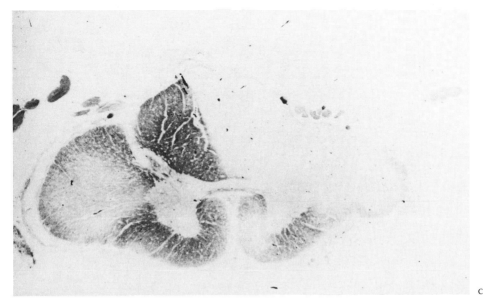

c

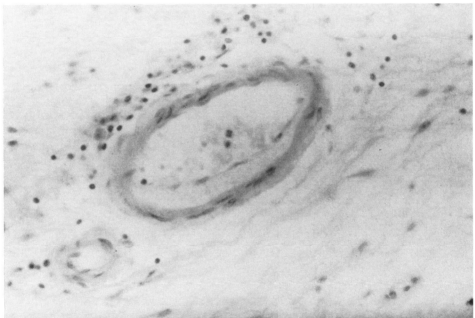

d

not remit but progress slowly from onset. Some episodes are preceded by identifiable infections and other illnesses, but in most instances no provoking factor can be discerned.

The frequency of relapse varies considerably between patients but, on average, it occurs once every 2 years per patient in the first 5 years, decreasing thereafter. Seventy-five per cent of patients will have had one or more relapses within the first 5 years, and 95% within 15 years.

In 5–10%, a pattern of frequent attacks, incomplete recovery, rapidly-accumulating disability and early death develops within one or two years of presentation, whereas approximately 25% of cases have a low frequency of relapse, complete recovery from each, and no significant disability after two or three decades.

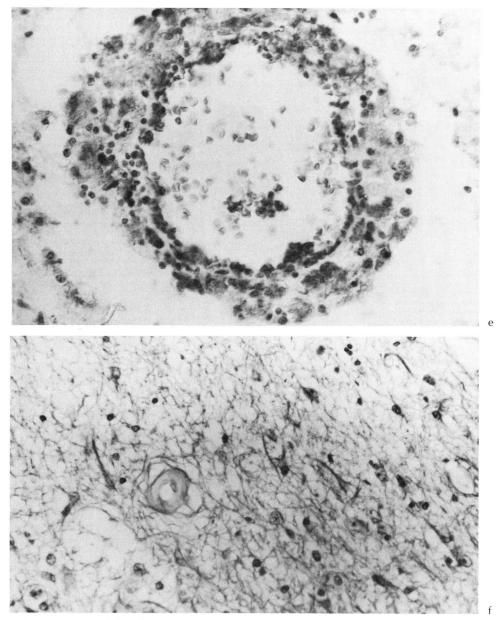

Fig. 9.1 (e) *Single vessel surrounded by lipid laden macro-phages stained for fat, indicating active myelin breakdown.*
(f) *Single vessel surrounded by area of dense gliosis in a chronic MS plaque.*

A distinction must be made between temporary disability, which depends as much on the region affected as on the severity or extent of demyelination, and fixed disability – the outcome of a complex inter-action between frequency, severity, degree of recovery and site of individual plaques. There are no reliable prognostic guides which can be applied to the indi-vidual case; factors which may indicate a benign course include a low relapse rate in the first few years, acute onset and recovery involving, in particular, visual or sensory symptoms. In many patients who have had the disease for several years the progress can be reliably predicted from the existing course of the illness. Neither a young age of onset nor severity of the initial attack necessarily carries a bad prognosis. Conversely, slowly progressive symptoms from onset or after relapse, and motor or cerebellar involvement, carry a poor prognosis. As a generalisation, one-third of patients are unrestricted, one-third significantly affected, and one-third severely disabled 15 years after presentation. The average life expectancy is at least 25 years from onset.

Immunology

Several observations suggest that an immunological process is involved in the pathogenesis of MS. Although the CNS is normally immunologically protected by the blood–brain barrier, this structure is easily damaged, allowing CNS invasion by systemic immune cells from which the Ig-secreting cells in the brain of patients with MS are derived. Myelin damage is probably carried out by macrophages, and the extent to which local antibody formation or sensitised cytotoxic lymphocytes are involved in this process is uncertain. Nevertheless, the immunological events in plaques are reflected in the CSF, which is abnormal in over 90% of patients; the total cell count is raised in 35% due to an increase in T and B lymphocytes, and cells are morphologically abnormal in most of the remainder. Total protein is raised in 10%, but 70% have an increase in IgG concentration, and in over 90% of patients electrophoresis shows abnormal immunoglobulin bands – the oligoclonal pattern (Fig. 9.3) – which are present early in the disease and remain during remission (see p. 150).

Attempts to show abnormalities in peripheral blood, which might explain why an autoimmune process develops in the CNS of patients with MS, have provided some evidence for periodic reductions in nonspecific suppressor cell number or function; these changes show some correlation with disease activity, but the precipitating factors or target of the presumed autoimmune attack in MS remain unknown.

The course of multiple sclerosis

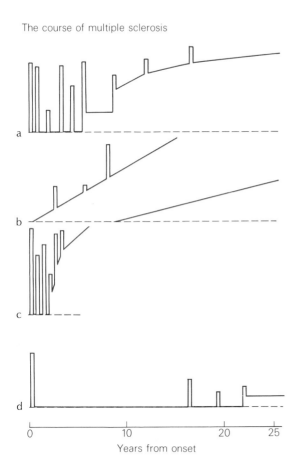

Fig. 9.2   (a) *(75%) Relapsing/remitting cases becoming progressive. Frequency of relapses decreases with time: 75% of all patients will have had one relapse within 5 years and 95% within 15 years of onset.*
(b) *(10%) Progressive from onset, with or without superimposed relapses. Many cases have a late age of onset.*
(c) *(10%) Malignant course with rapidly-accumulating deficit and short life expectancy.*
(d) *(5%) Benign cases with full recovery from each episode and/or a low frequency of relapse.*
Adapted from McAlpine D., Compston N.D., Lumsden C.D. (1955) Multiple Sclerosis. Edinburgh: E & S Livingstone.

Genetics

MS is most common in North Europeans, particularly those of Scandinavian origin, and rare in other populations – including those consisting of black and oriental races. In 8% of patients with MS, another family member is affected (Fig. 9.4). The lifetime risk to individual relatives of a patient rises from 1 in 1000 in the normal population to 1 in 100 for siblings including dizygotic twin partners and 1 in 3 for monozygotic twins.

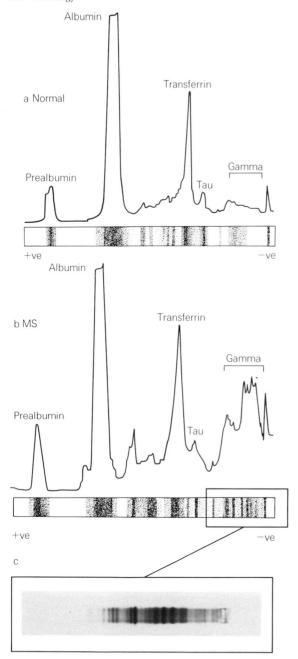

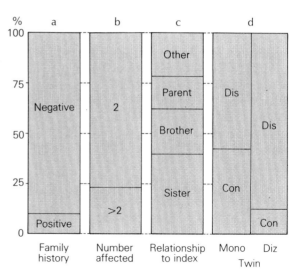

Fig. 9.4 (a) Frequency of a positive family history (multiplex) in patients with MS.
(b) Frequency of two or more affected individuals in multiplex families.
(c) Common relationships between affected individuals in multiplex families.
(d) Concordance rate for MS in monozygotic and dizygotic twin pairs, one of whom is already known to have the disease.

Fig. 9.3 CSF protein abnormalities in patients with MS.
(a) Diagram of electrophoretic separation of normal CSF proteins and densitometer scan allowing calculation of total amount of protein present.
(b) Same as A but from a patient with multiple sclerosis showing selective increase in gamma globulins.
(c) Expanded photograph of gamma region proteins immuno-fixed with anti-human IgG and stained with Coomassie blue to show at least 20 IgG bands making up the oligoclonal pattern. Adapted from Johnson M., Thompson E.J. (1981). Proteins of the Cerebrospinal Fluid. Hospital Update: November; 1155–63.

Cellular interaction involved in the immune response requires recognition by participating cells of the target antigen, in association with genetically determined HLA substances (Fig. 9.5). Gene products of the separate loci which make up the HLA system on the sixth chromosome function together in this role, but the HLA–DR products are involved primarily at the induction/intermediate stages and HLA–A, –B and –C products at the effector stage. Populations of unrelated individuals with MS from northern Europe have an increased frequency of specific antigens coded for at several HLA loci (A3, B7, Dw2, DR2 and BfS) (Fig. 9.6). The presence of any one antigen increases the risk of MS developing in an individual by up to 5 times, but the strongest association is with DR2. Associations between HLA–DR2 are found in some other groups, mostly but not all originating from northern Europe, whereas in other populations there is either no association or a different HLA gene product is implicated. In some families in which more than one case of MS has occurred, the disease segregates in association with HLA type within the family. This evidence indicates that

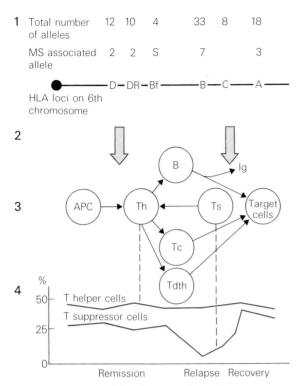

1 Total number   12 10   4   33   8   18
of alleles

MS associated   2   2   S   7   3
allele

HLA loci on 6th
chromosome
D – DR – Bf ———— B — C —— A ——

2

3 APC → Th → B → Ig
   Th → Ts → Target cells
   Tc
   Tdth

4 %
50 T helper cells
    T suppressor cells
25

0
Remission   Relapse Recovery

Fig. 9.5 *1. Diagram of the short arm of the 6th chromosome showing the 4 main HLA loci (D,B,C,A,) and the DR/Bf loci. Each is polymorphic but individuals have any two alleles encoded at each locus. In N.Europeans, MS is associated with HLA Dw2 DR2 BfS,B7 and A3.*
2. HLA antigens exert a controlling effect on cellular interactions involved in the immune response; HLA D/DR are required at the induction stage and HLA A and B antigens at the effector stage.
3. APC = Antigen presenting cells, B = B lymphocytes, Tc = T cytotoxic cells, Th = T helper cells, Ts = T suppressor cells, Tdth = T delayed type hypersensitivity cells.
4. The percentage of T suppressor cells decreases significantly in patients with active MS but T helper cells are unaltered.

genes in or near the HLA complex of the sixth chromosome increase susceptibility to the disease, exerting an effect through HLA-regulated control of the immune response. However, genetic susceptibility to MS is probably polygenic, involving other as yet unidentified genes.

Epidemiology (Fig. 9.7)

Epidemiological patterns of MS cannot be explained solely by genetic susceptibility; most individuals with

HLA–DR2 do not develop MS so that other aetiological factors must be involved. The most striking epidemiological finding is that the prevalence of the disease is high in northern Europe (latitude 43°N–65°N) and in North America (37°–52°N), decreasing towards the equator. Individuals who migrate from high to low risk areas acquire a lower prevalence if they migrate before the age of 15, but retain the high risk if they migrate after that age, suggesting that an environmental factor operates in childhood. Epidemics of the disease seem to have occurred in Iceland and the Faroe Islands. The nature of the environmental agent implicated by these epidemiological studies is unknown; there is a significant but non-specific increase in measles antibody titre in serum and CSF from patients with MS. Occasionally viruses have been seen and cultured from MS tissue but, despite the use of very sensitive methods, no single conventional virus can regularly be recovered.

Isolated Demyelinating Lesions

An isolated episode of demyelination may be the first event in a relapsing illness or in a monophasic post-infectious illness without recurrence. Some symptoms and signs are unusual as early manifestations of MS and their presence makes another diagnosis more likely, but it is rarely possible to make this distinction on purely clinical grounds. This problem is well illustrated in patients who have had a single episode of optic neuritis. Twenty-five per cent of patients with MS in the UK present with optic neuritis, 50% have an attack at some stage, over 60% with no symptoms of visual loss have abnormal visual-evoked potentials (VEPs, see p. 63) and at autopsy virtually all patients show lesions of the visual pathways. Fifty per cent of patients with optic neuritis who subsequently develop MS have CSF changes typical of MS at the time of first presentation and most of the rest develop oligoclonal bands before symptoms of more widespread demyelination are evident. The frequency of HLA–B7/DR2 in patients with optic neuritis is intermediate between controls and patients with MS, and there is a higher risk of MS developing in patients with optic neuritis if they have DR2, but the absence of this antigen and presence of normal CSF do not preclude the subsequent development of MS nor do their presence make the eventual diagnosis certain. Actuarial analysis of follow-up studies

c	Decreased	W7		7	F^C	12		2
a	6th Chromosome	D ———	DC/DR/SB	—Bf/C2 C4 ——	B ——	C ——	A———
b	Increased	W^2	2^A	S	7		3
			3^B		8		

Fig. 9.6 *Diagram of the separate multi-allelic loci which make up the HLA complex on the 6th chromosome. Certain alleles tend to occur together more often than would be expected from their individual frequencies in the normal population (linkage disequilibrium).*
(a) The strongest association is with DR2 and its linked alleles Dw2, BfS, B7 and A3.
(b) A subsidiary association is found with DR3 and its linked allele B8, suggesting genetic heterogeneity within a single population.
(c) Some HLA gene products have a reduced frequency in patients with MS. There is provisional evidence that the presence of BfF influences the rate of progression of disease and the tendency for individuals who have had an isolated episode of demyelination to develop recurrent or more widespread episodes.

Epidemiology of multiple sclerosis

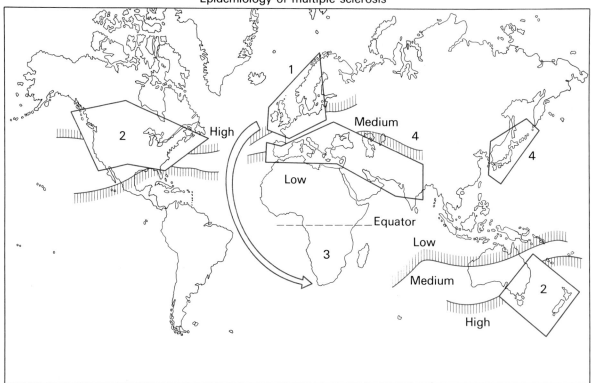

Fig. 9.7 *Hatched bars show borders between high, medium and low prevalence zones (where known).*
1. Associations with HLA A3, B7, Dw2 and DR2 in populations of northern European patients with multiple sclerosis.
2. Same associations in northern European patients who have migrated to other high or medium risk zones.
3. Low prevalence in northern Europeans migrating to low risk zone aged less than 15 years; higher prevalence in same genetic group migrating aged more than 15 years implicating an environmental risk factor. No HLA studies. Prevalence studies in migrants from other high to low, or low to high, risk zones are less detailed but agree with South African prevalence rates.
4. Mediterranean, Near Eastern, Indian and Japanese patients with multiple sclerosis show a variety of other HLA associations; this may reflect the importance of different aetiological agents in these regions.

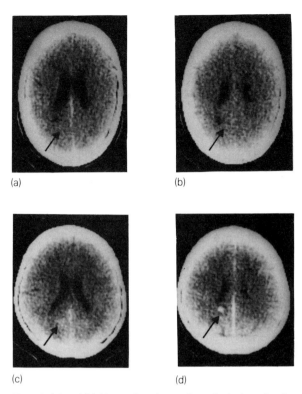

(a)   (b)

(c)   (d)

Fig. 9.8 (a) *and* (b); *Non-enhancing periventricular low-density lesions in patients with MS.*
(c) *and* (d) *Contrast-enhancing lesion in same region from same patient, scanned on a different occasion.*

suggests that approximately 75% of patients who have had an attack of isolated optic neuritis will eventually develop MS.

If it can be shown that multiple lesions have in fact occurred in patients with apparently isolated episodes, the diagnosis of MS becomes more certain. There may be a history in such patients of earlier unrecognised episodes or it may be possible to demonstrate multiple lesions which are clinically undetectable; autopsies in patients with MS usually show more extensive damage than the clinical history would suggest. CT scanning shows areas of low attenuation which may enhance after contrast injection (Fig. 9.8) and which correlate with histological lesions (Fig. 9.8). Magnetic resonance imaging seems likely to be a more sensitive method of detection. Electrophysiological tests can demonstrate latent abnormalities in sensory pathways. Evoked potentials (see Chapter 3) are recorded over the appropriate cortical area during repetitive visual, auditory and other sensory stimuli (see p. 64). In demyelination the amplitude of the evoked response may be normal but the latency is delayed. Visual evoked potentials are abnormal in more than 95% of patients who have had optic neuritis, but abnormality is also found in 90% of patients with clinically definite MS in whom there is no clinical evidence of optic nerve involvement. This technique is thus very useful for detecting multiple lesions in patients with relapsing or progressive spinal-cord and brainstem lesions. A high frequency of abnormal auditory and sensory evoked potentials is also found in MS patients with and without clinical involvement of these pathways. If, in a patient with MS involving the spinal cord, there is no clinical or electrophysiological evidence of a lesion above the foramen magnum, myelography and other investigations may be necessary to exclude other causes (especially compression).

Management and Treatment

The implications of having MS should be discussed with the patient as soon as the diagnosis is clinically definite. This usually involves waiting until at least two episodes have occurred, but special situations or a direct question from the patient may provoke an earlier discussion. Under these circumstances it is reasonable to emphasise the benign course of the disease in many patients. Many young women with MS are anxious about pregnancy. The risk of a child's being affected is higher than if the mother did not have MS but is still only 5% or less. There is a slightly increased risk to the mother of relapse during the puerperium and this may affect her ability to look after a child. Nevertheless, the diagnosis should not necessarily affect the decision to have a family, and only in exceptional circumstances are there grounds for termination of pregnancy in a patient with the disease. Patients should be encouraged to lead as normal a life as their symptoms allow, incidental infections should be treated early, and vaccinations avoided. Injections of ACTH and probably oral corticosteroids both increase the rate of recovery in acute attacks of demyelination, but neither the degree of recovery nor the overall course of the disease is influenced by short- or long-term treatments of this kind.

Some persistent symptoms can be treated. Paroxysmal painful symptoms often respond to carbamazepine or phenytoin, as may burning dysaesthesiae. Spasticity can be improved with physiotherapy, ice packs, baclofen, diazepam or dantrolene sodium; despite reducing spasticity and cramps, these drugs increase weakness and their use may reduce mobility, particularly in patients who depend on extensor tone to stand. Urinary symptoms are aggravated by infection and require treatment with antibiotics; where there is no infection, anticholinergic drugs (which inhibit detrusor contractions) reduce the urge to micturate at small bladder volumes and relax the internal sphincter, relieving urgency, frequency and retention. Alpha-blocking drugs such as phenoxybenzamine are sometimes helpful but the use of such agents should be preceded by formal urodynamic studies. Patients with MS and a fixed disability require help from physiotherapists, occupational therapists and social workers both in hospital and at home to make best use of residual neurological function (see Chapter 19).

In many patients with relapsing/remitting disease there is evidence that immunological processes continue and tissue damage accumulates during periods of apparent clinical inactivity. This evidence reinforces the need to identify potentially severe cases early in the disease, when they are leading a relatively normal life, and to find a treatment that will arrest the course of the illness at this stage. Because of very incomplete understanding of the immunological basis of MS it is not yet certain whether stimulatory or suppressive immunological treatment should be given. The results of either are difficult to assess in a disease with such a widely varying natural history. Existing trials suggest that immunological treatment can reduce the rate of disability and frequency of relapse even in severely affected patients, but in milder cases the possible benefits must be measured against potentially serious side-effects. Many trials are in progress and, at present, immunosuppression is most commonly used in patients with frequent relapses and a rapidly-accumulating deficit, but the indications and choice of immunological treatment may change with increasing experience.

10

Extrapyramidal Disease and Involuntary Movements

The basal ganglia (caudate, lentiform, thalamic and subthalamic nuclei, and substantia nigra see p. 19) are concerned with the control of movement and posture, and with patterns of learned movement. Patients with basal ganglia disorders, of which Parkinson's disease is by far the commonest type, show slowness and clumsiness of movement together with loss of associated or synergistic movements of other parts of the body. They frequently have involuntary movements and may show abnormalities of posture and equilibrium.

PARKINSON'S DISEASE

The 60–80 000 people afflicted with Parkinson's disease in England and Wales make up perhaps 1% of the population over 50 years old. Males and females are equally affected, but light-skinned races are affected more than Negroes. The majority of cases nowadays are due to a system degeneration of catecholamine-containing, mainly pigmented, brainstem neurones, particularly in the substantia nigra, locus coeruleus and dorsal motor nucleus of the vagus (Fig. 10.1). Intraneuronal inclusions (Lewy bodies) are typical of the disease and neurofibrillary tangles and plaques similar to those seen in Alzheimer's disease may be found.

There are several less common conditions in which features of Parkinsonism occur:

a. During and after the 1917–27 pandemic of encephalitis lethargica, extrapyramidal features developed in up to a quarter of the patients. A widespread neurofibrillary degeneration was found in these cases, affecting the putamen, thalamus, hypothalamus and brainstem nuclei.

b. Following the use of dopamine receptor-blocking drugs (phenothiazines, butyrophenones) (see p. 162).

c. Following repeated episodes of head trauma (boxing), and chronic manganese poisoning, although the overall clinical features differ from Parkinsons' disease.

d. In other degenerative diseases such as multi-system atrophy (Shy–Drager syndrome), progressive supranuclear palsy, olivopontocerebellar atrophy and widespread brain damage of many kinds (see pp. 193 and 194).

Biochemistry

Dopamine receptors are extensively distributed in the brain (Table 10.1). There are two types of dopamine receptor in the corpus striatum: D1 (adenylate cyclase-dependent) and D2 (independent). Many features of Parkinsonism can be related to either blockade of dopamine receptors or degeneration of dopaminergic neurones. Dietary phenylalanine and tyrosine are converted via a rate-limiting enzyme – tyrosine hydroxylase – to L-dihydrophenylalanine (levodopa) which is then decarboxylated by dopa decarboxylase to dopamine (Fig. 10.2). Levodopa crosses the blood–brain barrier whereas dopamine does not. In attempting to restore depleted brain dopamine, therefore, levodopa is often given with a peripheral dopa decarboxylase inhibitor (e.g. benserazide or 1-α-methyldopa hydrazine) which reduces systemic dopamine formation – and hence some side-effects – but allows conversion in the CNS. Dopamine is dispersed from the central synaptic clefts by active reuptake into nerve terminals; it is also metabolised intraneuronally via monoamine oxidase B, and extraneuronally by catechol-O-methyl transferase (COMT).

155

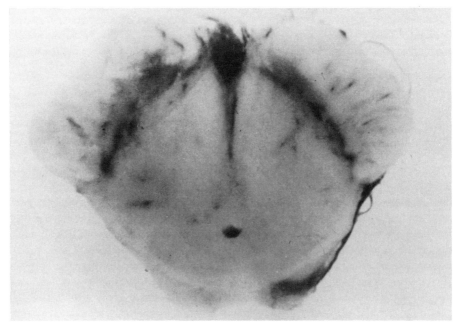

a

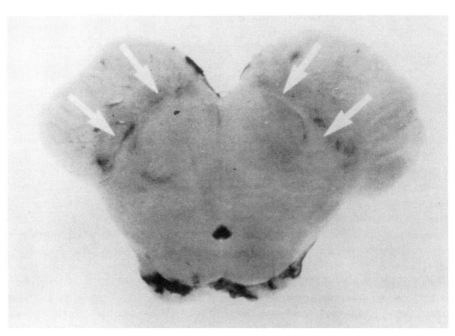

b

Fig. 10.1 *Sections through normal midbrain (a) and midbrain from a patient who had Parkinson's disease. The substantia nigra in (b) is barely evident (arrowed) due to the reduced density of pigmented nigrostriatal neurones.*

Table 10.1

Dopamine Receptor Stimulation and Blockade

Dopamine receptor site	Stimulation	Blockade
	Levodopa Dopamine agonists (e.g. bromocriptine)	Dopamine antagonists (e.g. haloperidol, phenothiazies)
Medulla	Emetic	Antiemetic
Basal ganglia	Antiparkinsonian Dyskinesia	Akathisia Parkinsonism Acute dystonia Tardive dyskinesia
Cortex (?)	Delirium, hallucinosis	Antipsychotic
Hypothalamus	Cause growth-hormone release via peptide-link	Inhibit growth hormone release
	Inhibit growth hormone (acromegalics only)	Infertility
	Inhibit prolactin release	Hyperprolactinaemia (→galactorrhoea)
Cardiac, vascular receptors	Arrhythmias Dopamine dilates renal mesenteric arterial beds Cardiac inotropic agent Pressor agent	

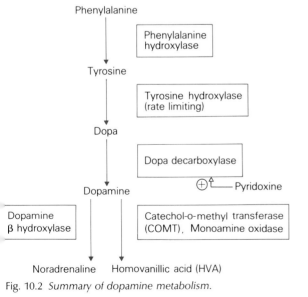

Fig. 10.2 *Summary of dopamine metabolism.*

Clinical Features

Idiopathic Parkinsons's disease (PD) commonly develops in the 6th–7th decades. The commonest initial symptom is a resting tremor affecting the hands first. The typical, 'pill rolling' tremor (4–8 Hz) may be unilateral; it characteristically lessens with the initiation of movement but is worsened by anxiety or adrenergic stimulation. A quarter of patients never have a significant tremor. Rigidity (see p. 10 and Table 2.4) results in a flexed posture and this may be particularly striking in the neck muscles so that, when lying supine, the head is held clear of the bed. Bradykinesia, with loss, fatigue or slowness of movements is characteristic. The patient walks with a shuffling gait, there is loss of arm swing, and an inability to make rapid corrective postural adjustments causes falls and unsteadiness when turning. Turning over in bed is also difficult. The face is relatively immobile and expressionless, and the speech softly slurring. Swallowing is sometimes impaired. There may be a tendency to stare, and voluntary ocular upgaze and convergence can be impaired. The patient may complain of weakness in the limbs but this is due to the reduced speed of initiation of voluntary movement, as muscle power is normal. Fine delicate finger movements in particular are impaired, and the patient's writing becomes small.

If untreated, some patients may become dependent and immobile, unable to leave the bed or chair. In other patients the condition remains mild, perhaps only affecting one limb for several years. Depression is not uncommon in PD and dementia may occur in the later stages, although it is important to distinguish this from the false impression of mental slowness caused by bradykinesia or the side-effects of anti-Parkinsonism drugs. In most early cases the intellect is well preserved.

Differential Diagnosis

Post-encephalitic Parkinsonism is suggested by a relevant history and, sometimes, by onset in youth. Particular features of this (now uncommon) condition are oculogyric crises (episodes of upward deviation of the eyes) sometimes accompanied by prominent mental and behavioural changes. Parkinsonism is a feature of multisystem atrophy (Shy–Drager syndrome) where autonomic failure – notably sexual and bladder dysfunction, postural hypotension and loss of sweating – may also be associated with cerebellar and pyramidal signs (see p. 194). In the condition of progressive supranuclear palsy (Steele–Richardson–Olzsewski syndrome) a mask-like face, dysarthria, and dysphagia are associated with early loss of conjugate downward gaze, axial rigidity often causing retraction of the neck, and bradykinesia (see p. 193). Parkinsonism due to medication is similar to idiopathic PD.

Treatment (Fig. 10.3)

Anticholinergic drugs alone such as benzhexol, benztropine, or orphenadrine depress striatal cholinergic activity. Side-effects include a dry mouth, retention of urine and blurred vision and, particularly in a mentally

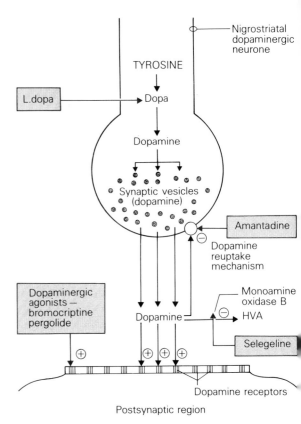

Fig. 10.3 *Sites of action of dopaminergic drugs used in Parkinsonism.*

impaired patient, confusion and hallucinations. Beta-blocking drugs and minor tranquillisers are of value in ameliorating tremor. Amantadine inhibits dopamine reuptake and has a minor effect on bradykinesia and rigidity (Fig. 10.3).

Levodopa with a dopa decarboxylase inhibitor (see above) forms the main line of treatment. Central decarboxylation may occur in blood vessels as well as in remaining dopaminergic neurones, and levodopa treatment also results in increased brain concentrations of noradrenaline as well as dopamine. The initial improvement in bradykinesia with treatment is impressive in 75% of patients, but small doses are essential initially and should be increased cautiously. Notable early side-effects are nausea, vomiting and postural hypotension. Later, dyskinesias and psychological disturbances become important problems (see p. 159).

After about 2–5 years a substantial proportion of

patients develop side-effects necessitating drug reduction or withdrawal and about half may experience sudden marked swings in mobility ('on-off' phenomena) or dyskinesias. It should also be remembered that Parkinson's disease causes progressive disability so that at 5 years only about one-third of patients have maintained their original improvement. Psychiatric complications become increasingly prominent with time, due to either the disease or the drugs, or both. Overall, however, levodopa extends the life expectancy of patients and many side-effects, in particular the 'on-off' phenomena and dyskinesias, may be countered by giving small doses very frequently (e.g. 2–3-hourly) and by reducing the total daily dosage.

The effect of a single dose of levodopa may be prolonged for perhaps 10–30 minutes by the simultaneous use of a monoamine oxidase B inhibitor, e.g. selegeline. Unlike monoamine oxidase A inhibitors, dietary restriction of cheese, wine, etc. is unnecessary, but the dosage of levodopa should initially be reduced by 25%. The place of this drug in treatment remains uncertain.

Dopamine agonists with long half-lives, such as bromocriptine (or possibly pergolide), may have a useful effect as an alternative to or in addition to levodopa if, despite frequent oral doses of the latter, dose-related fluctuations in response are troublesome. Postural hypotension, involuntary movements, confusion and hallucinations may also occur with these drugs.

INVOLUNTARY MOVEMENTS

These are summarised in Table 10.2.

Tremor (see Table 10.3)

Tremors may be categorised into those present in a relaxed rested limb (rest tremor), those evoked by movements (intention tremor), and those most prominent on maintaining a posture (postural tremor). *Rest* tremor is virtually always due to basal ganglia disease, notably Parkinsonism. *Intention* tremor is caused by damage to the cerebellum or its connections and is thus usually associated with other signs of cerebellar

disease (see p. 18). *Postural* tremor may be an exaggeration of normal physiological tremor due to anxiety, thyrotoxicosis, sympathomimetic drugs, alcohol or certain types of heavy metal poisoning (e.g. mercury), but it may also be a feature of structural disease, e.g. Wilson's disease (see p. 162), neurosyphilis, Parkinson's disease (in addition to rest tremor), or chronic neuropathies. If the underlying disease cannot be treated, many tremors are helped by reducing anxiety and/or sympathetic drive. A particularly common variety of predominantly postural tremor of unknown cause is known as benign essential tremor.

Essential tremor

This condition may start at any age; it is often familial and behaves as an autosomal dominant. The tremor is obvious on maintaining a posture and persists on movement, but disappears when the affected limb is completely at rest. Features of cerebellar disease are absent. The tremor affects handwriting and ability to pick up objects steadily but tends not to affect the legs. Frequently, there is a tremor of the head (titubation) or jaw, and the voice may sound tremulous. Alcohol temporarily alleviates this tremor. If treatment is required, the benzodiazepines (e.g. diazepam, 2–15 mg daily) or β-blocking agents (e.g. propranolol 60–120 mg daily in divided doses) are the drugs of first choice, but it may also be worth trying the affect of primidone, starting cautiously at a very low dose (e.g. 62.5–125 mg daily). Thalamic damage, e.g. following stroke, may abolish the tremor on the contralateral side.

Chorea

Choreic movements are brief, jerky, and unpredictable in site and timing, and affect muscles both at rest and during movement. Gait and posture may be interrupted by abnormal movements, as may the tongue movements, speech, swallowing, and respiration. These jerks may be associated with more complex and apparently voluntary movements so that the patient may appear 'fidgety' to the untrained observer. The limbs are hypotonic and the reflexes may be pendular (see p. 11).

Chorea may be precipitated by many different drugs, and is a recognised side-effect of treatment with

Table 10.2

Characteristics of Abnormal Movements (Dyskinesias)

Tremor	Rhythmic, sinusoidal movement
Chorea	Unpredictable, brief, jerky movements affecting any part of the body
Dystonia (athetosis)	Abnormal posture with involuntary movement
Myoclonus	Brief shock-like movement involving single or many muscle groups
Tics	Repetitive, sterotyped movement involving single (often facial) or many muscle groups

Table 10.3

Tremor Characteristics

	Character	Aggravated by	Relieved by*	Major sites	Associated features
Benign essential tremor	6–8 Hz variable amplitude	posture, movement	rest, alcohol	arms, head, voice	no rigidity, cerebellar signs not present, familial
Cerebellar tremor	6–8 Hz variable amplitude	posture, movement, terminal accentuation	rest	limbs, trunk, head	dysmetria, ataxia, nystagmus
Parkinsonian tremor	4–8 Hz variable amplitude	resting, walking, use of other limbs	some voluntary control	hands, legs, may be unilateral	bradykinesia, rigidity
Physiological tremor	10–12 Hz low amplitude	anxiety, posture, movement	relaxation, anxiolytic drugs	hands	hyperthyroidism, tachycardia, sweating, no incoordination or rigidity

* most tremors are ameliorated by reduction of anxiety and/or adrenergic blockage with, e.g., β-blockers.

levodopa and neuroleptics (often affecting the orofacial musculature). Chorea may also occur in association with rheumatic fever (Sydenham's chorea), pregnancy (chorea gravidarum) or the contraceptive pill. It may occur with vascular lesions caused by polycythaemia or systemic lupus erythematosus, in Wilson's disease (see p. 162), or as an autosomal dominant condition (Huntington's chorea). It may also rarely be associated with neuropathy and acanthocytosis in the peripheral blood (but – unlike Huntington's chorea – there is no dementia). Acute hemichorea (hemiballismus) follows a vascular lesion in the region of the subthalamic nucleus. In this condition the movements are of large amplitude and may prove quite exhausting to the patient.

Huntington's Chorea

There are about 4000 patients with this autosomal dominant condition in Great Britain. It may be commoner in parts of the USA, where it was taken by East Anglian migrants who landed in Salem, Massachusetts in 1632. Some patients are said to have the blue eyes and prematurely grey hair of the original stock. Symptoms usually commence between 30 and 50 years. The features of the condition are increasing dementia and personality change, with depression, paranoia and a suicidal tendency, together with progressive choreic movements. A juvenile onset (< 20 years) also occurs, presenting with rigidity, ataxia, akinesia and epilepsy rather than chorea and, in this case, the affected parent is more often the father. The condition should be distinguished from the chorea–acanthocytosis syndrome referred to above.

A progressive loss of neurones in the forebrain and corpus striatum (particularly the caudate nucleus) is found, and there appears to be a decrease in choline acetyl-transferase with a relative increase in dopamine content of the nigrostriatal and mesolimbic systems. Gamma aminobutyric acid (GABA) and glutamic acid decarboxylase are decreased in the caudate nucleus and putamen.

Treatment

Dopamine receptor antagonists such as phenothiazines and butyrophenones reduce chorea, but they may cause Parkinsonian features and, paradoxically, choreiform movement as a long-term side-effect (see p. 162). Tetrabenazine depletes the central neurones of amines, and this is effective but may cause severe depression. These drugs do not influence the underlying cause of any of the above diseases. Genetic counselling of the patient and his family is a most important aspect of management of Huntington's disease, but at present no established predictive tests exist for the disease, which often only presents clinically after the next generation has been born. Recently, recombinant DNA techniques have allowed the identification of a DNA sequence which may be close to the gene for Huntington's disease on chromosome 4. Future developments may perhaps allow identification of gene carriers before the disease is clinically manifest – even *in utero*.

Dystonia

In this group of conditions, sustained co-contractions of agonist and antagonist muscle groups result in abnormal (sometimes painful) postures. There may be associated slow writhing movements of the affected parts (athetosis). The condition may be very localised, affecting the use of the hand during writing (writer's cramp), causing spasmodic turning of the head and neck to one side (spasmodic torticollis), of closure of the eyes (blepharospasm). On the other hand, it may be quite generalised, resulting in such gross distortions of body posture as in idiopathic torsion dystonia. These conditions are either genetically determined (idiopathic torsion dystonia) or may be symptomatic of structural brain disease following hypoxic damage (including cerebral palsy see p. 184), Wilson's disease or encephalitis lethargica, or may follow the use of neuroleptic drugs. The initial focal or segmental patterns of the disease sometimes spread to become more generalised.

If acute dystonia is drug-induced as, for example, following phenothiazine ingestion, the administration of intravenous anticholinergic drugs (e.g. benztropine) will rapidly reverse the situation. Otherwise the dystonias are difficult to treat although a wide range of centrally-active drugs, such as anticholinergic agents, dopamine agonists or antagonists, or benzodiazepines, are often tried.

Dystonia musculorum deformans (torsion spasm)

This is a condition where dystonia is the major feature. The bizarre and severe involuntary movements and postures usually start in childhood, first with spasms of one foot and ultimately spreading to the whole body. Initially, the movements are intermittent but later they are continuous except during sleep; they are frequently diagnosed as being 'hysterical' at first. There are two patterns of inheritance; the autosomal recessive variety is often severe and tends to be commoner in Ashkenazi Jews, whilst the dominant form is later in onset. The condition may cause dysarthria, dysphagia, blepharospasm, torticollis, a bizarre 'dromedary' gait and mild choreoathetosis or tremor of the limbs. Higher cerebral function is normal and there is no sensory abnormality. In contrast to Wilson's disease, no brain lesion has yet been documented in this condition.

Spasmodic torticollis and writer's cramp

These are examples of focal dystonia and are not usually hereditary. Mild or severe head turning, uncontrollable by the patient except for brief periods, may be accompanied by fragments of dystonia elsewhere, e.g. the trunk, arms or face, with or without tremor. The active muscles (e.g. sternomastoid) may become hypertrophied. This condition overlaps with writer's cramp and other 'occupational' cramps such as those occurring in musicians, telephone exchange operators or darts players. In these conditions painful cramps and inability to use a limb normally occur when specific tasks are attempted, but may later affect function more widely. The evidence suggests that these are not 'psychiatric' disorders but that they are organically determined, although the neural basis remains elusive.

Wilson's disease

Wilson's disease is a rare autosomal recessive disease of great diagnostic significance, since it is treatable. It is a disorder of copper metabolism which leads to increased copper deposition in certain tissues. In the CNS, there are degenerative changes in the lentiform nucleus (notably the putamen) and caudate nucleus. In the liver, a multilobular cirrhosis occurs and, in the cornea, a deposit of copper (the Kayser-Fleischer ring) occurs near the limbus. Renal function is impaired, with aminoaciduria and renal tubular acidosis. The plasma caeruloplasmin and copper concentrations are reduced, the urinary copper excretion is greater than normal and the hepatic copper content is raised.

Clinical features

The condition presents in children or young adults. The neurological features are a flapping tremor, choreiform movements of the face and hands, and dystonic movements causing abnormal limb and trunk postures, rigidity, and contractures. School performance may decline and epilepsy or dementia may occur. Emotional control is impaired. Rapid accurate diagnosis is essential – with differentiation from athetoid cerebral palsy, familial degenerative basal ganglia disease (e.g. torsion dystonia), and drug-induced disorders. The condition can also present as a hepatic disorder, as a renal problem, or as a wholly psychiatric disturbance.

Treatment

The manifestations of the disease can be largely reversed by treatment with d-penicillamine, which chelates copper and increases its urinary excretion. Side-effects can occur, notably disturbance of taste, blood dyscrasias, and nephrotic syndrome. Without treatment the disease is fatal; with treatment, even gross CT scan abnormalities can be reversed. Alterna-tive drug treatment is available if d-penicillamine cannot be tolerated.

Tics

These are sudden, rapid, stereotyped and purposeless jerking movements. Many tics are perhaps psychologically determined but exactly similar movements can be caused by organic conditions, notably encephalitis lethargica, as well as by psychotropic drugs. Tics are common in children but often resolve spontaneously. A bizarre syndrome of multiple motor and vocal tics, the latter including grunts, repetitions (echolalia) or obscenities (coprolalia), may start in childhood or adolescence – Gilles de la Tourette syndrome. The condition responds well to treatment with neuroleptics (often haloperidol), but these may impair school performance as well as stunting growth.

Drug-induced Movement and Extrapyramidal Disorders

Neuroleptic medication (e.g. phenothiazines, butyro-phenones, thioxanthenes), which block central dopamine receptors, cause a range of disorders:

a. Acute dystonic reactions such as protrusion of the tongue, oculogyric crises or retrocollis are *sensitivity-related*; they occur in 2–5% of patients after the initial one or two doses. The dystonia is abolished by intravenous benztropine or by diazepam.

b. All neuroleptics may cause *dose-related* Parkinsonian features; these usually start within 4–12 weeks of commencing the drugs. Drug-induced Parkinsonism can take many months or even years to disappear after drug withdrawal. Anticholinergic agents alleviate these symptoms in part but may predispose to tardive dyskinesia and should not be given as a routine accompaniment.

c. Motor restlessness (akathisia) is the commonest side-effect of phenothiazines, and this may also be relieved by anticholinergic agents.

d. Orofacial, lingual, mandibular and other choreiform movements are an increasingly recognised long-term complication of neuroleptic therapy and, unlike the other side-effects mentioned, may be irreversible despite drug withdrawal (tardive dyskinesia). The movements are lessened by increasing neuroleptic medication but this benefit is short-lived and, on the whole, attempts should be made to withdraw such medication. Similar movements do sometimes occur in the elderly without any prior neuroleptic drug history.

Myoclonus (see also Chapter 7)

Spontaneous jerking movements of one or more muscle groups (myoclonic jerks) are normal phenomena on falling asleep or waking. Such myoclonic jerks are prominent in patients with sleep *epilepsy*, when they may persist for up to an hour or so after waking. The combination of increasingly severe epilepsy and myoclonus with mental impairment starting in childhood or adolescence may be caused by a number of rare disorders including Lafora body disease, lipid storage disease (e.g. Tay–Sachs disease, see p. 218), or in association with a cerebellar degeneration.

Myoclonus can also occur on a genetic basis, independent of epilepsy (essential myoclonus). Generalised myoclonic jerks are common following anoxic brain damage or in major *metabolic* disturbances e.g. renal, hepatic or respiratory failure, or with drug/alcohol withdrawal. When associated with subacute *dementia*, myoclonus may suggest Creutzfeldt–Jacob disease (see p. 238) in adult life, or subacute sclerosing panencephalopathy (see p. 237) associated with a high titre of measles antibody in childhood. Segmental forms of myoclonus occasionally occur with *focal disease* of the spinal cord or brainstem. The treatment is that of the underlying conditions but the benzodizapines (clonazepam has been the drug most investigated) are sometimes beneficial, as are drugs which increase 5-hydroxytryptamine concentrations in the brain.

11

Diseases of the Spinal Cord

The spinal cord extends from its junction with the medulla oblongata, opposite the odontoid peg at C1 level, to the conus medullaris, which in the adult lies opposite the body of L1 vertebra (Fig. 2.2). It reaches this position by the fifth year of life, the rapidly-elongating vertebral column having outstripped the development of the cord. Developmental anomalies (see Chapter 12) at the lower end of the spinal canal may cause increasing damage to the cauda equina during the first five years of life.

BLOOD SUPPLY OF THE SPINAL CORD

At segmental level (Fig. 11.1), a fairly constant pattern of supply is found. An arterial plexus on the posterior cord

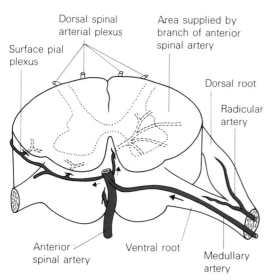

Fig. 11.1 *Segmental blood supply of the spinal cord.*

nourishes the posterior columns and posterior horns and a single anterior spinal artery lying in the anterior fissure supplies the core of the cord and the anterior horns. The peripheral rim of the cord is supplied by short branches from circumferential vessels. This vascular network is fed by 7–10 spinal medullary arteries which are derived from: the vertebral arteries; the thyro-cervical trunk; a branch from one of the intercostal vessels; a major vessel from a lower intercostal or upper lumbar artery, usually on the left-hand side (known as the arteria magna); and a variable vessel entering on one of the upper lumbar nerve roots to supply the terminal cord and the cauda equina. At many levels small radicular arteries supply the nerve roots, but these vessels do not contribute to the supply of the cord.

ANATOMICAL FEATURES OF THE SPINAL CORD

The anatomy of the spinal cord is described in Chapter 2. For diagnostic purposes, the following are the important features (Fig. 11.2).

Motor pathways

The motor pathways may be damaged at corticospinal-tract level (upper motor neurone lesion), or at anterior horn-cell and anterior-root level (lower motor neurone lesion).

The upper motor neurone lesion, whatever the cause, will produce varying degrees of spasticity below the level of damage. Weakness (mainly shoulder abduction, elbow, wrist and finger extension in the arm

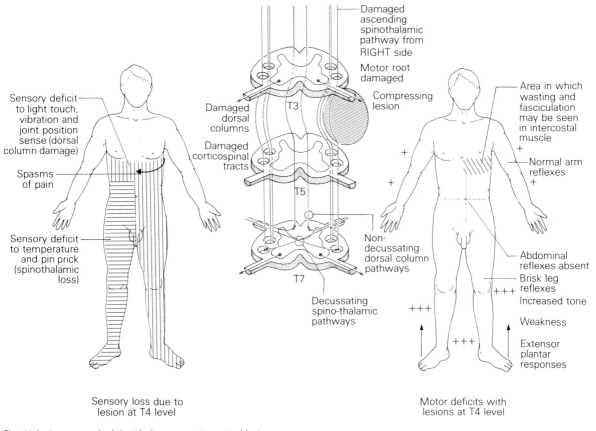

Fig. 11.2 *Anatomy of a left-sided compressive spinal lesion at T4. The corresponding motor and sensory features are shown.*

and the flexor groups in the leg), is accompanied by reflex enhancement, increased tone (spasticity, see p. 17), and extensor plantar responses; the abdominal reflexes are variably absent or depressed if the lesion is above T8 level.

The lower motor-neurone lesion causes a flaccid muscle weakness, wasting and fasciculation of the affected muscle groups and loss of the segmental tendon reflex. Using the combination of upper and lower motor-neurone signs, localisation of the level and extent of cord damage is often possible.

Sensory pathways

Sensory pathway damage falls into two major groupings; posterior column function (joint position sense, accurately localised light touch and two-point discri-

mination), and spinothalamic sensation (pain and temperature). The posterior columns contain fibres carrying sensation from the *same* side of the body, and the relay to the opposite side of the brain occurring at medullary level. In contrast, spinothalamic sensation is relayed across the cord within two or three segments of entry and ascends in the cord on the opposite side (see p. 21). Combining sensory abnormalities with the motor findings usually allows accurate localisation of spinal cord damage.

Autonomic pathways (see also p. 54)

The supra-segmental control of sweating, blood vessels and bladder function is conveyed in pathways close to the corticospinal tracts; alterations in bladder function in particular tend to parallel motor pathway involvement in many conditions. Impaired inhibitory control of the bladder produces the earliest symptoms of spinal cord involvement of this type, i.e. urgency of micturition. Awareness of bladder filling is almost immediately followed by uncontrolled voiding, especially if there is delay in reaching a toilet. This is known as a spastic bladder. If caused by total cord transection, with loss of sensation, the patient may be aware of bladder filling because of reflex autonomic activities, such as sweating, pallor, tachycardia and rise in blood pressure.

By contrast, damage to the cauda equina produces a bladder that fills passively, with ineffectual spontaneous contractions producing slight continuous dribbling incontinence. A similar situation may exist when severe posterior column damage prevents recognition of bladder filling. Both situations lead to back pressure, high residual urine volumes, and recurrent urinary tract infections.

COMPRESSIVE DISEASE OF THE SPINAL CORD AND ROOTS

Spinal cord compression is one of the most urgent clinical situations; its recognition requires skill and necessitates prompt action. Some major causes of spinal cord compression are indicated in Table 11.1. The clinical features tend to be similar whatever the cause. Acute spinal cord compression is quite unmistakable with sudden paralysis and loss of sensation below the level of the lesion. In this situation the cause is usually obvious, e.g. spinal fracture (see p. 92). Gradual development of spinal cord compression is

---

Table 11.1

Causes of Spinal Cord Compression

Neoplasms	(See Table 11.2)
Disc lesions	Acute traumatic, chronic degenerative
Inflammatory	Epidural abscess, spinal granuloma, Tuberculosis
Vertebral Tumours	Metastatic carcinoma, chordoma, myeloma, aneurysmal bone cyst, vertebral angioma
Cysts	Epithelial, endothelial, parasitic
Haematoma	

---

usually dominated by progressive motor disabilities. This is thought to be due to impaired venous drainage of the spinal cord which specifically damages the central part, notably the corticospinal tracts. The symptoms include stiff legs, clumsy walking, inability to run, involuntary spasms in the legs in bed and spontaneous clonus when stepping downwards. These symptoms may evolve over days or years, depending on the pathology. Sometimes they are worsened by exercise.

Sensory symptoms tend to appear later and consist of tingling and numbness in the feet, evolving gradually over hours or days and ascending up to or below the level of the compressive lesion. Once sensory symptoms appear, a diagnosis must be rapidly established. Bladder dysfunction is a late feature of cord compression and may quickly become irreversible.

Progressive spinal cord compression therefore requires urgent investigation and treatment. Spinal x-ray and myelography via the lumbar or cervical route are the definitive investigations but should be carried out in the knowledge that neurosurgery may be necessary immediately or shortly afterwards. Myelography may, by virtue of setting up pressure gradients across masses which obstruct the spinal canal, precipitate further clinical deterioration and should therefore be performed in or near to a neurosurgical facility. Patients who have cord compression demonstrated at myelography must be closely observed in the hours after the investigation.

Tumours (Table 11.2)

Spinal tumours can be classified by their position in relation to the cord and covering membranes. Extradural tumours lie in the canal outside the dura in the extradural fat; they are usually malignant, either due to extension of metastatic malignant disease from adjacent vertebrae or due to remote spread, particularly by malignant lymphomas.

Intradural extramedullary tumours lie inside the dura against the spinal cord. Commonly these tumours are derived from the meninges (meningiomas) or the nerve roots (neurinomas or neurofibromas). Meningiomas are more common in women and tend to occur in the thoracic region. Neurofibromas may be single or multiple (see also neurofibromatosis, p. 181) and may extend through the intervertebral foramen, enlarging it

Table 11.2

Spinal Cord Neoplasms

	Adults
Extradural	metastatic disease, from lung, breast, prostate, lymphoma, thyroid, melanoma
Extramedullary	neurofibroma, meningioma, ependymoma (sacral) sarcoma, vascular tumours, A-V malformation
Intramedullary	ependymoma, astrocytoma, epidermoid, haemangioblastoma, oligodendroglioma, lipoma, A-V malformations
	Children
Extradural	ganglioneuroma, neuroblastoma, metastases, neurofibrosarcoma
Extramedullary	metastatic (from cerebellar medulloblastoma), dermoid, arachnoid cyst, ependymoma (sacral)
Intramedullary	astrocytoma, ependymoma, teratoma

and sometimes causing an associated paraspinal mass. Intramedullary tumours arise in the spinal cord itself and are usually gliomas of varying degrees of malignancy or ependymomas derived from the lining cells of the central canal, often extending up and down the cord over many segments.

Extradural and intradural extramedullary tumours produce a picture of cord compression gradually over weeks to months, often with local pain (extradural lesions) or referred root pain (intradural lesions). Intramedullary tumours typically have a very slowly progressive course, in some instances extending over two to three years, before definite physical findings appear. They produce low-grade backache in the region of the tumour as the presenting symptom, the ultimate neurological picture being similar to syringomyelia, as discussed below. The characteristic finding is a segmental pattern of sensory deficit (Fig. 11.2).

DEGENERATIVE VERTEBRAL COLUMN DISEASE

Degenerative changes, particularly in the highly mobile cervical and lumbar regions, are important causes of damage to the spinal cord and spinal roots.

Cervical Region

At cervical level, degenerative prolapsing intervertebral discs provoke bony overgrowth of adjacent vertebral margins; this composite lesion compromises both the canal's sagittal diameter and the exit foraminae (Fig. 11.3). How severely these normal ageing processes affect the neural structures depends on the pre-existing sagittal diameter of the canal, the thickness of the ligamenta flava posteriorly, and the overgrowth of the soft tissues around the apophyseal joints laterally. These lesions may not only compress the spinal cord and nerve roots in the neutral position but there is considerable dynamic variation in their compressive effects during neck extension and flexion. Sudden hyperextension of the neck in a whip-lash injury or a fall onto the chin, may cause irreversible damage in a previously asymptomatic patient. In addition, degenerative disease probably influences cord function by an effect on blood supply and venous drainage.

Degenerative cervical spinal (column) disease most commonly affects discs at C5/6, 6/7 and 4/5, in that order. Patients with rheumatoid arthritis may develop damage at other levels and degeneration of the cruciate ligaments or resorption of the odontoid peg produce sliding atlanto-axial dislocation, with the

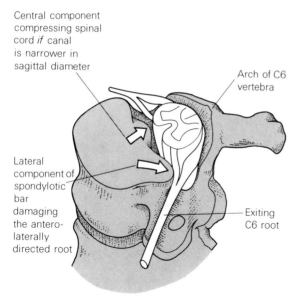

Central component compressing spinal cord *if* canal is narrower in sagittal diameter

Arch of C6 vertebra

Lateral component of spondylotic bar damaging the antero-laterally directed root

Exiting C6 root

Fig. 11.3 *The anatomical factors causing cord and root compression in degenerative disease of the cervical spine.*

potential for fatal cord transection at C1/2 level on minimal trauma.

The C5, C6 and C7 roots are those most often affected by degenerative disease. Pain is commonly felt in the myotome supplied by that root, with sensory symptoms being more prominent in the dermatome. A C5 root lesion causes pain around the shoulder spreading into the upper arm: there may be weakness and wasting of deltoid, the spinati and elbow flexion, variable reduction of the brachioradialis and biceps reflexes, and sensory loss in the C5 dermatome (see Fig. 2.12). A C6 lesion causes pain spreading down the arm, sometimes with sensory disturbance in the thumb and index finger: weakness is most noticeable in the radial wrist extensor. A C7 lesion quite frequently causes pain around the scapula and this rather than pain in the neck or arm may be the main presenting feature: weakness mainly affects elbow and finger extension (wrist extension less so) but brachioradialis is not affected (a distinguishing feature from a high radial nerve lesion), and there may be sensory disturbance on the back of the hand, middle and ring fingers.

Treatment

Much of the radicular pain and muscle spasm asso-

ciated with root irritation or compression may settle if the neck is rested by the use of a well-fitting surgical collar. The latter must prevent major neck movements and be worn the whole day but can be substituted by a soft collar at night for comfort. Analgesics also help in the acute phase. Progressive radicular signs despite rest are an indication for myelography, to confirm the diagnosis and as a necessary preliminary to surgical decompression.

When there are signs of cord compression with evidence of a cervical lesion, management will be influenced by several factors including the age and fitness of the patient, tempo and severity of lower limb involvement, and the presence of bladder dysfunction. Myelography is necessary to confirm the diagnosis. In some patients useful improvement in symptoms and signs occurs with simple immobilisation of the neck using a collar, and this management can be quite appropriate in the elderly patient. In a younger person, once the precise level of the lesion is defined radiologically an anterior decompression of the cord, with removal of degenerate material and bone grafting (Cloward's procedure), is a currently favoured procedure. Cord compression at multiple levels may also be treated with a decompressive laminectomy. Surgery can usually be expected to arrest progression of signs and symptoms and, less commonly, to lead to major improvements.

Lumbosacral Region

Root lesions

In the lumbosacral region similar pathological processes to those in the neck may occur, impinging either on the nerve roots as they pass downwards and laterally to the intervertebral foramina or on the main cauda equina when the central part of the canal is most affected. The L5 and S1 roots are most susceptible to lateral prolapses of the L4/5 and L5/S1 discs respectively. Commonly, this presents with local back pain as well as referred pain, motor or sensory symptoms. With an L5 lesion, pain tends to be felt in the buttock and lower leg; weakness affects extensor hallucis longus, extensor digitorum brevis, peronei and hip abductors in particular, with sensory disturbance in an L5 dermatomal pattern (see Chapter 2, Fig. 2.12), but there may be no reflex change. An S1 lesion causes pain mainly in the back of the leg from buttock to ankle and may cause weakness and wasting of gastrocnemius/soleus (best observed with the patient standing) and a depressed ankle reflex. Less commonly, the higher roots are affected. Passive traction on the lower lumbosacral roots (supine straight leg raising) or upper roots (femoral stretch test – lying prone) is limited by pain and reflex muscle spasm. There is local back tenderness, paraspinal muscle spasm, and frequently a pelvic tilt or limp is apparent on walking.

When investigating lumbosacral root pain it is important to note that the roots take their origin at the L1 vertebral level. Plain x-rays and radiculography must therefore fully encompass this region so that the rare case of a neurofibroma or ependymoma presenting with low back pain or radicular pain is not missed. In addition, involvement of roots or plexuses in the retroperitoneal space or pelvis needs to be considered and excluded by appropriate investigation.

Cauda equina claudication

When the diameter of the lumbar spinal canal is narrow, transient neurological symptoms and signs may appear on exercise and be relieved by a period of rest, often in the sitting position with the lumbar spine flexed. These symptoms include pain spreading from the buttocks into the legs, paraesthesiae and numbness, weakness and eventual wasting of muscles; they are attributed to 'claudication of the cauda equina', implying a disturbance of blood-flow to the nerve roots in the tight canal, and they require differentiation from claudication of the limb muscles due to vascular obstruction. The latter usually causes pain (not weakness or numbness) which is relieved by a minute or two of rest (rather than 5 to 15 minutes); it is valuable to ask the patient to exercise until symptoms appear and then to examine him when they are severe – the onset of neurological signs, the presence of obvious circulatory disturbance in the limb, and the description of the symptoms as they develop usually allow clear distinction to be made.

Central disc prolapse

An acute central disc prolapse in the lumbosacral region is a serious condition, often requiring urgent intervention. The patient complains of severe back pain with or without radiation into the legs, weakness of both legs which varies depending on the level of cauda equina compression, and retention of urine. Sensory loss may be quite minor, often only involving the lower sacral sensory dermatomes, and it is essential to examine these carefully. Plain x-rays and radiculography are usually a prerequisite to decompressive laminectomy, which needs to be performed early if irreversible sphincter disturbance is to be prevented.

Treatment

A wide variety of techniques exist which claim to mitigate symptoms of low back pain due to degenerative disease. Root symptoms are still, however, most effectively treated with bed rest followed by careful mobilisation with a lumbar support, although local injection of steroid and local anaesthetic may speed up pain relief. Symptoms and signs of root compression (other than central disc prolapse) which persist or advance despite medical measures and rest may be treated by surgical decompression of the affected nerve root. The disc is removed at formal laminectomy, or the exit foramen is unroofed at a fenestration operation. It is of note that a very laterally placed root compression may not be visible on routine radiculography and is better seen on CT scanning of the relevant level after insertion of contrast. With the claudication syndrome the canal may be narrowed at multiple levels and a more extensive laminectomy is required; dramatic relief of symptoms is often obtained.

Thoracic Region

Thoracic discs may present with either severe radicular pain (usually around the trunk) or with a progressive paraparesis. Diagnosis usually entails seeing calcification in a disc space at the relevant level and myelography. Thoracic disc prolapse is relatively rare.

Treatment

By contrast with the neck, thoracic disc compression of the cord is not usually managed conservatively. However, the more tenuous blood supply of the cord at this level, the narrower spinal canal, and the technical operating difficulties make operation more hazardous.

TRANSVERSE MYELITIS

Transverse myelitis has many possible causes (Table 11.3) but the commonest in the United Kingdom is probably multiple sclerosis (see Chapter 9).

This condition typically presents with a variably rapid onset of motor and sensory impairment below the level of the lesion, which is usually mid-dorsal; sphincter disturbance is common. These features are sometimes accompanied by very severe local pain simulating a surgical lesion and myelography is usually necessary to exclude a compressive lesion. Although very dramatic at the onset, substantial and often complete recovery occurs. Rarely, simultaneous or subsequent unilateral or bilateral retrobulbar neuritis accompanies acute transverse myelitis (Devic's syndrome).

In the older age range (35–60), demyelinating disease may present with a slowly progressive essentially motor picture often evolving over several years before medical advice is sought. Sensory features are relatively minor but eventually a moderate to severe spastic paraparesis with ataxia becomes apparent. In this situation, other causes must be excluded and evidence of lesions is sought elsewhere in the CNS by clinical examination and evoked potential studies (see p. 62) and the CSF is examined for immunoglobulins to try and confirm the diagnosis of multiple sclerosis (see p. 149). In many instances, myelography needs to be combined with CSF examination for definitive exclusion of a compressive lesion.

INFECTIVE SPINAL CORD LESIONS

Three major diseases, syphilis, poliomyelitis and tuberculosis were frequent causes of spinal cord disease in the past, only the latter remaining a relatively common disease in third world countries and in immigrants in the United Kingdom.

Syphilis (see also p. 234)

Syphilis causes three main types of spinal cord damage. A leptomeningitis affects the cervical region leading to cord compression, pain in the arms and wasting in the hand muscles. It seems quite possible that many so-called cases of this condition could have been due to unrecognised complications of cervical spondylosis. Endarteritis of the spinal cord arteries may cause acute vascular cord lesions, usually the syndrome of occlusion of the anterior spinal artery (see p. 171).

Tabes dorsalis

In this rare chronic condition there is demyelination and subsequent atrophy of the central processes of the dorsal root ganglion cells which make up the posterior columns. The loss of afferent input causes a major part of the clinical picture. Thus profound loss of joint position and kinaesthetic sensation causes an ataxic broad-based stamping gait with a positive Romberg

---

Table 11.3

Causes of Acute Transverse Myelitis

Acute infective	enterovirus, cytomegalovirus, Epstein–Barr virus, rabies, herpes zoster (see p. 223)
Following vaccination	rabies, smallpox, polio, tetanus vaccinia (acute disseminated encephalomyelitis)
Post infectious	rubella, rubeola, varicella, vaccinia, mumps, influenza, mycoplasma, Epstein–Barr virus
Demyelinating disease	multiple sclerosis, Devic's disease (see p. 143)
Vascular	shock, aortic dissection, thoracic surgery
Radiation myelopathy	

test (the original use of this sign); the tendon reflexes, especially knee and ankle jerks, are absent, and the plantar responses flexor. Severe spontaneous lancinating pains occur at various points in the lower limbs and patches of analgesia occur, particularly on the trunk and down the inner aspects of the arms. Loss of deep pain sense results in trophic changes in the limbs, causing perforating ulcers, and promotes florid degenerative changes and painless hypermobility of joints (Charcot's joints). Sphincter disturbance is common and loss of sensation results in painless retention of urine in a dilated atonic bladder, eventually causing secondary obstructive nephropathy. Other autonomic features include painful paroxysmal attacks ('crises') affecting various viscera, including the larynx, stomach, bladder and rectum. Optic atrophy, Argyll Robertson pupils (see p. 38) and ptosis are further manifestations of the condition. Treatment of syphilis is considered on p. 235.

Tuberculosis (See also p. 226)

This condition typically causes destruction of the intervertebral discs as well as the vertebral bodies, commonly in the cervical and upper thoracic region. Infection may spread into the extradural space to involve the cord and its blood supply or there may be compression secondary to vertebral collapse. Occasionally there is an associated paraspinal cold abscess. Management is with the use of antituberculous drugs together with judicious surgery to decompress the spinal cord if necessary. Immobilisation and stabilisation of the spine are important and specialised aspects of treatment in many cases.

Poliomyelitis (See p. 231)

Acute Bacterial Infections (See also p. 230)

Bacterial infections, particularly septicaemia due to staphylococcal or streptococcal infections, are the usual cause of epidural abscess. This produces acute pain and spinal cord compression and the diagnosis is usually made at operation. Little evidence of systemic infection is apparent in most instances. Surgical evacu-ation of pus and prolonged antibiotic therapy is the treatment of choice.

METABOLIC DISORDERS AFFECTING THE SPINAL CORD

The classical metabolic disorder of the spinal cord is subacute combined degeneration of the cord. This is usually due to vitamin B_{12} deficiency but can also be caused by folate deficiency.

The posterior columns and corticospinal tracts are specifically damaged, but the clinical picture is complicated by the early development of coexistent peripheral nerve damage. The patient usually complains of paraesthesiae, unsteadiness and weakness, and is found to have spastic legs, reflex loss (usually ankle jerks), extensor plantar responses and impaired posterior column functions. The marked loss of postural sense may be severe enough to prevent walking. A poorly-explained sphincter disturbance similar to that in tabes dorsalis occasionally produces a dilated hypotonic bladder with loss of sense of bladder fullness.

Treatment

Hydroxycobalamin therapy improves peripheral nerve damage but the improvement in spinal cord function is often disappointing. The condition is generally treated with large doses of vitamin B_{12}, e.g. 1000 μg daily for three weeks, followed by weekly injections for three months and 1000 μg monthly thereafter.

VASCULAR LESIONS OF THE CORD

Surgical damage to the main spinal medullary arteries is an important cause of spinal cord disease. Operations on the lateral neck, mid-thoracic approaches to the posterior mediastinal structures, to the renal bed and to the posterior abdominal wall, all carry the risk of ligation or coagulation of an apparently-insignificant vessel entering the canal with a nerve root to supply the cord. The territory supplied by the anterior spinal artery is maximally affected, with sparing of the posterior columns and the periphery of the cord (Fig. 11.1). This results in acute paraparesis or paraplegia and sphincter disturbance with sparing of posture sense and light touch; pain and temperature sensation are often impaired from just below the level of the lesion, but may be intact in the perineum (sacral sparing) due to the preservation of the spinothalamic tracts on the periphery of the cord. In many instances, however, the picture is one of total cord transection at the upper limit of the feeder vessel, C2 in the cervical region and T4 in the thoracic region.

Cord infarction may also occur with any thrombotic or embolic vascular disease (subacute bacterial endocarditis, atrial fibrillation, thrombotic thrombocytopenic purpura, sickle cell anaemia, decompression sickness and prolonged hypotensive shock). Feeder vessel occlusion may complicate diabetes mellitus, polyarteritis nodosa, meningovascular syphilis and dissecting aneurysm of the aorta.

Haemangioblastoma usually presents as an intramedullary lesion of the cord and often has a substantial cystic component. Arteriovenous malformations (AVMs) of the dura or cord present with a wide variety of features, including subarachnoid haemorrhage, acute cord dysfunction due to haemorrhage, slowly progressive neurological signs such as paraparesis with bladder disturbance, or typical signs of an intrinsic cord lesion: neurological symptoms are sometimes prominently related to exercise. AVMs are usually diagnosed on myelography but spinal angiography may be required as a preoperative investigation to identify the main feeding vessel to be occluded.

SYRINGOMYELIA AND SYRINGOBULBIA

These conditions consist of fluid-filled cavities within the spinal cord or brainstem. The dilatation of the spinal cord may lead to widening of the cervical canal, seen on plain x-ray, and may be associated with bony anomalies at the atlantoaxial or atlanto-occipital junction, spina bifida or hydrocephalus. Frequently there is obstruction to the normal circulation of CSF at the foramen magnum associated with these bony anomalies, cerebellar tonsillar prolapse into the cervical canal (Chiari malformation), or arachnoid adhesions (Fig. 11.4). A history of birth injury is fairly frequent but clinical presentation is not usually until the third or fourth decade. Syrinxes also occur in later life as a complication of major spinal cord trauma or as a cavitation above or below an intramedullary tumour.

The condition often has a very chronic course, punctuated by periods of deterioration. Expansion of the syrinx causes pressure on crossing spinothalamic fibres resulting initially in severe pains, worsened by cough or physical exertion, and later a dissociated sensory loss (see p. 23) which spreads in a segmental distribution up and down from the original site of the lesion. This results in anaesthetic segments (commonly hands and forearms) scarred by unnoticed burns, severe skin ulceration, and joint damage. If the syrinx disrupts the monosynaptic reflex arcs, tendon jerks are lost, and lower motor neurone features with wasting of the hands and forearm are typical. A spastic paraparesis indicates corticospinal tract involvement. Scoliosis is frequently associated. Involvement of the brainstem may cause atrophy and fasciculation of the tongue, dysarthria and dysphagia, ataxia, nystagmus, and hearing loss. A dissociated sensory loss may extend onto the face (see p. 39). The presence of a Chiari malformation is suspected clinically from the presence of a characteristic 'down-beating' nystagmus particularly on lateral gaze.

Treatment

Plain radiographs of neck and skull looking for bony anomalies are usually followed by CT scan of the head to exclude hydrocephalus. The definitive investigation is myelography to look for cord expansion, with CT scanning if available to demonstrate the intramedullary cavity: the position of the cerebellar tonsils is also shown at myelography. The most common operation is a foramen magnum decompression with removal of the laminae of C1 and C2 and the posterior part of the foramen magnum itself. The fluid from the syrinx may be shunted into the subarachnoid space (syringostomy). In a modest number of patients there is improvement after operation, but, in a greater number, cessation of deterioration is the best attainable result.

RADIATION DAMAGE

The use of radiotherapy to treat lesions in or adjacent to the vertebral column, and as palliative treatment for

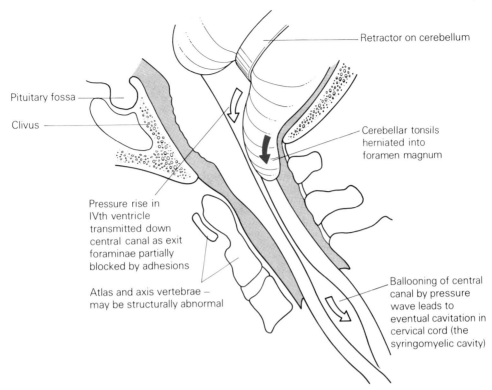

Retractor on cerebellum

Pituitary fossa

Clivus

Cerebellar tonsils
herniated into
foramen magnum

Pressure rise in
IVth ventricle
transmitted down
central canal as exit
foraminae partially
blocked by adhesions

Atlas and axis vertebrae –
may be structurally abnormal

Ballooning of central
canal by pressure
wave leads to
eventual cavitation in
cervical cord (the
syringomyelic cavity)

Fig. 11.4 *Illustration of possible hydrodynamic mechanism for the formation of a syrinx.*

carcinoma of the oesophagus and bronchus, carries a risk of damaging the spinal cord. The dosage which causes cord damage depends on total dose, the fractionation of the total dosage (i.e. dose per treatment and total length of treatment), and the site: areas of the spinal cord with a more tenuous blood supply, e.g. upper thoracic, seem most susceptible. Radiation myelitis occurs either a few weeks after irradiation (possibly due to acute effects on the blood vessels of the cord) or nine to fifteen months later, when progressive spinothalamic loss and mild spastic paraparesis develops over a few weeks and then arrests. Myelography may be required to differentiate this picture from cord compression, caused by direct extension or metastatic spread of the underlying malignancy into the spinal canal. Further 'blind' irradiation at the suspected level of the lesion is unwise under these circumstances. (See also p. 221.)

MANAGEMENT OF PARAPLEGIA

Acute Stages

In acute paraplegia, the urgency of establishing the diagnosis and initiating any effective treatment should be coupled with early steps to avoid long-term complications, especially if the condition is irreversible. This requires special attention to bladder management, skin care to avoid ulcers and passive physiotherapy to avoid contractures.

Intermittent catheterisation every four to six hours to prevent bladder stretching lessens the risk of infection and increases the likelihood of the patient developing a reflex autonomic bladder. This technique is more successful than permanent catheterisation.

Sensory loss predisposes to the development of

pressure sores. From the outset, the use of a ripple bed or nursing on bolsters, with strict two-hourly turning, is essential to prevent pressure on the sacrum, iliac crests, greater trochanters, knees, heels and malleoli. Avoidance of skin maceration by sweat, urine or faecal soiling is also important.

Passive movements of the joints of paralysed limbs through a full range, at least twice a day, is essential to prevent contractures. Foot position is important and a foot board to hold the ankles in a normal position is essential to prevent Achilles tendon shortening, which may develop very rapidly unless this simple precaution is taken.

Chronic Stages

When paraplegia has become a permanent state the problems remain the same.

A reflex emptying bladder is preferable to permanent catheterisation, as the latter can lead to chronic urinary tract infection, urinary calculi and eventually renal failure. Even in established paraplegia, an intermittent catherisation programme may reestablish reflex bladder control when the patient has initially been put on permanent drainage.

With the return of reflex motor activity, extensor spasms in the legs may cause problems in bed and in using a wheelchair. Conversely, the development of flexor spasms often indicates a urinary tract infection, faecal impaction or an infected pressure area. In both instances, passive movements supplemented by diazepam, baclofen or dantrolene sodium, may be of benefit but the cause of a change to flexor spasms should be sought urgently and treated.

The risk of pressure sores is ever-present unless meticulous attention is given to cleanliness and the avoidance of maintaining any position for longer than two hours. Once chronic pressure sores develop they may require plastic surgical repair since, if untreated, they destroy the general health of the patient, leading to anaemia, hypoalbuminaemia and chronic low-grade fever. Further complications of this type, combined with renal impairment due to poor bladder management, ultimately shorten the paraplegic patient's life.

The specialised nature of care of the paraplegic or qaudriplegic patient, particularly following injury, has led (in the United Kingdom) to the early referral of many of these patients to spinal injuries units.

12

Congenital Diseases of the Central Nervous System

Congenital diseases are those existing or dating from birth or from fetal development (Table 12.1). Most are recognisable at birth but some may have onset delayed until childhood or adolescence. The group of heredofamilial diseases coming on in adult life are usually classified separately.

There are two basic causes of congenital disease:

a. Abnormalities in the genetic material which include conditions with clear inheritance or a demonstrable chromosome anomaly. Examples are neurofibromatosis with a dominant inheritance, and Down's syndrome with trisomy 21.

b. Noxious agents acting on the fetus at critical periods, usually in the first trimester of pregnancy when embryological development of the CNS is most active. Such agents include infections, chemicals, vitamin deficiency, drugs, radiation and anoxia. Examples are rubella infection in the first trimester causing congenital rubella syndrome, possibly folate deficiency soon after conception causing anencephaly, and birth hypoxia causing cerebral diplegia.

The cause of most congenital disease is not known – either whether it is genetic or not or which noxious agent might have acted. A further problem is that siblings not only share genetic material but also have the same environment *in utero*. Noxious agents are often not recognised by the pregnant mother. The timing of a noxious agent is critical, as its effects at two gestational ages will be different. Different agents can cause the same clinical syndrome in the neonate.

DEVELOPMENT OF THE CENTRAL NERVOUS SYSTEM

The central nervous system develops from the neural plate, which is a thickened area of ectoderm in the mid-dorsal line. In the third week of gestation the edges of the plate enlarge, forming the neural folds which fuse to form the neural tube (Fig. 12.1). The fusion starts in the cervical region and extends cranially and caudally, completely closing by the fourth week. At the edge of the neural plate are the cells of the neural crest which

Table 12.1

Congenital CNS Disease

Agents		Clinical syndrome (examples)
Chromosome abnormality	Trisomy 21	Down's syndrome
Inherited conditions	Dominant	Neurofibromatosis Tuberose sclerosis
	Recessive	Dandy–Walker syndrome Agenesis of corpus callosum
	Sex-linked	Aqueduct stenosis
Infections		Congenital rubella Cytomegalic inclusion disease Congenital neurosyphilis
Possible vitamin deficiency		Anencephaly
Drugs	Ethyl alcohol Anticonvulsants Thalidomide	Various malformations
Chemicals	Bilirubin	Kernicterus
Anoxia		Spastic diplegia
Irradiation		Cerebellar hypoplasia

Neural plate

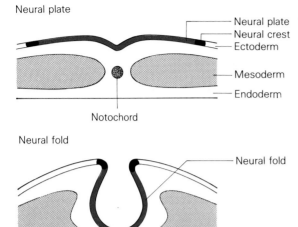

Neural plate
Neural crest
Ectoderm

Mesoderm

Endoderm

Notochord

Neural fold

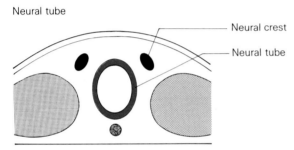

Neural fold

Neural tube

Neural crest

Neural tube

Fig. 12.1 *Development of the nervous system.*

migrate to form the sensory and autonomic ganglia, Schwann cells, and pigment cells. The differentiation into the spinal cord and brain is obvious by the third week.

Spinal Cord

Three layers develop round the central canal. The inner is the ependyma, which persists as an epithelial layer. The mantle layer proliferates to form the dorsal and ventral horns. The outer marginal layer develops into the white matter.

The spinal tracts first appear in the second month, the long association tracts develop in the third month, and the corticospinal tracts in the fifth month. Myelination starts in the fifth month; the phylogenetically older tracts myelinate first and the corticospinal tracts do not

myelinate until the second postnatal year. Myelination is not complete until adult life.

The mesoderm around the neural tube forms the vertebral bodies and arches, the meninges and blood vessels.

Brain

By the time the neural tube has closed, the three primitive vesicles of the brain are apparent. In the fourth and fifth weeks, development of the brain is rapid and, by the sixth week, the definitive structures can be recognised (Fig. 12.2). The telencephalon gives rise to the cerebral cortex, striate bodies and rhinencephalon. The diencephalon forms the thalamus, hypothalamus and optic chiasm. The mesencephalon develops into the midbrain. The metencephalon forms the cerebellum and pons and the myelencephalon the medulla oblongata. The ventricular system, which has been formed by this stage, communicates with the central canal of the spinal cord.

The brain continues to develop but at a slower rate and the grey matter, central nuclei and tracts form. The cerebral hemispheres show the greatest growth, with differentiation into the cerebral cortex, white matter and commissures including the corpus callosum. Initially the cerebral hemispheres are smooth but in the sixth month gyri and sulci develop, the phylogenetically older ones developing first. Development of the cortex and myelination of the spinothalamic and pyramidal tracts continues for many years after birth.

The mesoderm grows around the developing brain to form the skull and meninges.

The CNS is susceptible to damage at all stages up to and beyond parturition. Maximal disruption is liable to be in the early stages of development where major defects will result, e.g. anencephaly.

DYSRAPHISM

Failure of the normal folding and fusion of the neural plate, failure of closure of the overlying skin, and failure of development of the bony structures results in dysraphism (Fig. 12.3).

Anencephaly is an absent brain and cranial vault and

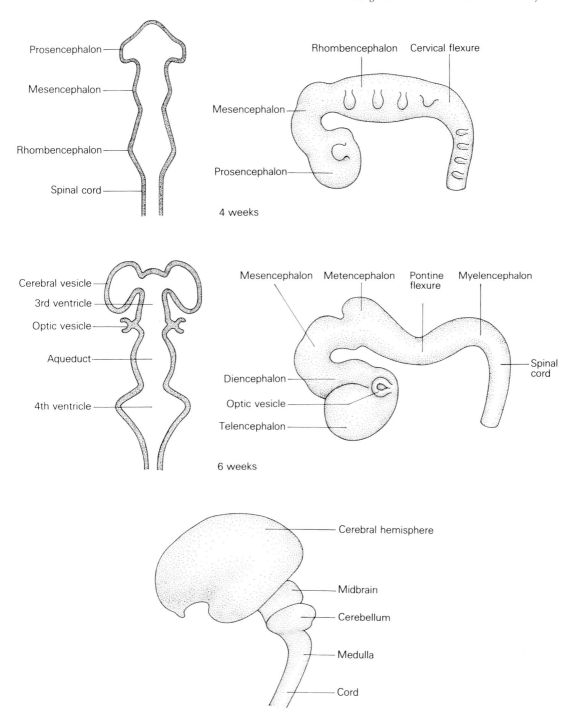

Fig. 12.2 *Development of the brain*

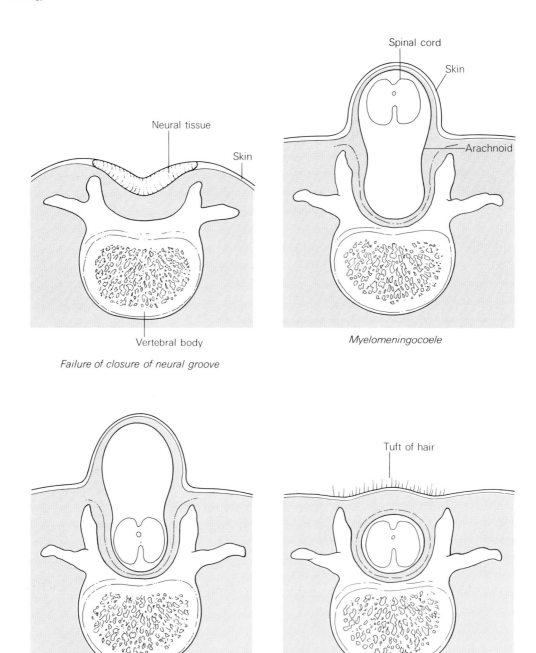

Failure of closure of neural groove

Myelomeningocoele

Meningocoele

Spina bifida occulta

Fig. 12.3 *Spinal dysraphisms.*

and ventricular drainage has to be undertaken. Minor spinal meningocoeles present no surgical difficulties. Infection of the CNS can result from organisms gaining entry through a defect: occasionally a sinus tract leads from a small dimple on the skin to the meninges. In cases of bacterial meningitis, in particular recurrent meningitis, a careful search should be made for such tracts.

The diagnosis of a neural tube defect can often be made antenatally. Serum alphafetoprotein estimations are done routinely in many pregnant women; they are persistently raised in neural tube defects (there are other causes of raised levels which have to be excluded). Ultrasound examinations of the fetus after the fourteenth week of gestation should demonstrate the major defects. If doubt exists, the amniotic fluid should be analysed for a high alphafetoprotein level.

Aetiology

The cause of neural tube defects is not known but there are a number of interesting observations. There is a definite increased risk for subsequent pregnancies; after one affected child the risk is 4%, after two affected children it is 8%. For anencephaly there is a strong geographical distribution, with the highest incidence in the west of Europe and the lowest in the east. The British Isles has a very high incidence. There appears to be no seasonal variation but there is a year-to-year variation. At times the incidence reaches almost epidemic proportions (Dublin 1935–39 and 1960–65). There is preliminary evidence that folate and/or other vitamin deficiencies in early pregnancy may be relevant.

ENCEPHALOCRANIAL DISPROPORTION

Craniostenosis

This results from premature fusion of the cranial sutures. When the sagittal and coronal sutures fuse, the head grows vertically producing a tower skull (turrecephaly, oxycephaly). Fusion of the sagittal suture produces a long narrow head (scaphocephaly), and fusion of the coronal suture produces a wide short head (brachycephaly). When severe craniostenosis interferes

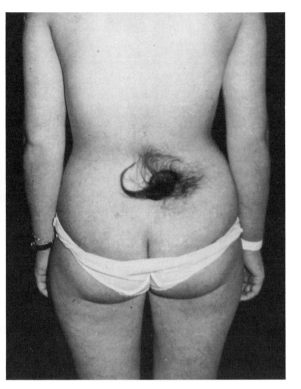

Fig. 12.4 *Tuft of hair overlying spina bifida occulta.*

is incompatible with life. Extrusions of brain and meninges through midline defects in the skull, usually in the frontal and occipital regions, are termed *meningoencephalocoeles* and they vary from minor protrusions to massive abnormalities. *Meningocoeles* are protrusions of a meningeal sac but not brain tissue. Spinal abnormalities also vary in severity and are most frequent in the lumbo-sacral region.

Meningomyelocoeles consist of neural elements of the spinal cord contained within a sac: in severe cases the legs and sphincters are paralysed. *Meningocoeles* also occur, and both latter conditions may lead to hydrocephalus. *Spina bifida occulta* is the mildest variety of dysraphism and is a failure of bony fusion only. There is no external sac, but a tuft of hair (Fig. 12.4) or a dimple may overlie the lesion and 5% of the population have a bony abnormality in the lumbo-sacral region.

Multiple defects often exist and the treatment of severe abnormalities in neonatal life is open to many ethical considerations. Sometimes extensive surgery with brain development, surgical treatment is necessary.

Microcephaly

This is an abnormally small head associated with an abnormally small brain.

Hydrocephalus (see p. 80)

In congenital hydrocephalus the head usually expands because the cranial sutures have not fused: accurate measurements of head circumference will show a disproportionate increase in size compared to the body growth curve. The appearance is of a broad forehead, bulging fontanelles, eyelid retraction, prominent scalp veins and a 'crack pot' percussion note. Plain skull x-ray will show the enlargement, but CT scanning is usually required for accurate diagnosis. Ultrasound may also help in diagnosis, and ventriculography is occasionally required. The cause of the hydrocephalus can be congenital anomaly, intracranial haemorrhage, infections, neoplasms or trauma. Treatment depends on the cause, but often the ventricles have to be shunted.

Aqueduct Stenosis

The aqueduct of Sylvius can become blocked either by a congenital defect (often associated with other defects) or as a result of haemorrhage or infection. In severe cases, congenital hydrocephalus results. In mild cases, presentation can be delayed until adult life. The lateral skull x-ray shows a shallow posterior fossa and the CT scan shows dilated lateral and third ventricles but normal fourth ventricle.

Chiari Malformation (see also p. 172)

This is the downward displacement of a tongue of cerebellum and the medulla oblongata into the spinal canal, and there are often other congenital defects. The infantile variety (type II) has an associated meningocoele and presents in early life with hydrocephalus and lower cranial nerve palsies. The adult variety (type I) has no meningocoele and presents in adolescence or adult life with syringomyelia, progressive cerebellar ataxia, hydrocephalus or lower cranial nerve palsies. The diagnosis is often difficult to establish and requires myelography. Where there is an advancing neurological deficit decompression of the foramen magnum and removal of the high cervical laminae can be successful in arresting the symptoms.

Dandy Walker Syndrome

An outflow obstruction to the fourth ventricle results in enormous dilatation. It is associated with an occipital meningocoele, agenesis of the cerebellar vermis, and hydrocephalus.

Basilar Impression

This is an abnormal invagination of the cervical spine into the base of the skull. The diagnosis is made from the lateral skull x-ray where the tip of the odontoid peg protrudes above a line drawn from the back of the hard palate to the posterior margin of the foramen magnum. There are often associated defects such as atlanto-occipital fusion, atlanto-axial subluxation, Klippel–Feil and Arnold–Chiari malformations. On clinical inspection the neck is short with a low posterior hair line. With severe deformity there may be involvement of cerebellar pathways, lower cranial nerves, corticospinal tracts and dorsal columns. In advanced cases surgical decompression may be indicated. Occasionally basilar impression results from metabolic bone disease (osteogenesis imperfecta).

Platybasia refers to flattening of the base of the skull which, in itself, is asymptomatic.

MYELOSPINAL ANOMALIES

Klippel–Feil Syndrome

This results in a fusion of one or more cervical vertebrae. It is often asymptomatic and incidentally found on x-ray. If severe it can cause shortening of the neck, with limited movements. Other anomalies often coexist. A compressive cervical myelopathy can result later in life from spondylosis at the mobile joints above and below the fusion. An interesting association is synkinetic 'mirror movements' in the arms.

Tethered Cord

This condition can result from a number of congenital anomalies associated with spina bifida. In myeloschisis, the spinal cord is attached to the sacrum by a thickened filum terminale. In diastematomyelia there is a bony spicule or fibrous band in the lower thoracic or upper lumbar canal which passes through the cord (which may be reduplicated – biplomyelia). Congenital lipomas, dermoids, teratomas and cysts can also be present. Presentation is varied, occurring at any age and in many clinical forms. Not uncommonly, a progressive spastic paraparesis develops during the adolescent growth spurt due to progressive traction on the cord. Sudden cauda equina syndromes can follow unusual exercises or trauma due to stretching and damage to nerve roots. Progressive cauda equina syndromes can be due to chronic compression or traction. Plain x-rays are helpful but usually myelography is needed to reveal the defect. Surgery can given excellent results.

A marked scoliosis or kyphosis from whatever cause can result in damage to the spinal cord and nerve roots.

CEREBRAL ANOMALIES

The brain itself is subject to many malformations. *Agenesis of the corpus callosum* results in deficient commissures. *Porencephaly* is characterised by large cortical cysts, usually communicating with the ventricles. Abnormal cortical gyri can occur in *microgyria* and *pachygyria*.

COMBINED MALFORMATIONS

There are many syndromes with anomalies of the brain, skull and spine together with skeletal and visceral malformations. Examples are: *Down's syndrome* with a typical facial appearance and multiple somatic defects, *Apert's syndrome* with a flat skull and syndactyly, and *Greig's syndrome* with hypertelorism.

Phakomatoses (Table 12.2)

These are inherited conditions where ectodermally-derived organs have a tendency to form benign tumours and hamartomas.

Neurofibromatosis (Von Recklinghausen's disease)

This is an autosomal dominant condition with a prevalence of about 40 per 100 000: one new case occurs in every 3000 live births. It is characterised by malformations and benign tumours of skin, nervous tissue, bone, endocrine glands and other organs. The typical skin appearance is of numerous ($\geqslant 5$) brown patches (café-au-lait naevi) and cutaneous tumours (Fig. 12.5). The peripheral nerves are studded with firm neurofibromas, composed of fibroblasts and Schwann cells. The cranial nerves, notably the acoustic nerve, and spinal nerve roots (Fig. 12.6) can also harbour these tumours, which may require surgery. Other recognised features are an increased incidence of meningiomas, gliomas of the optic nerve and brain, malignant change of the neurofibromas, massive cutaneous overgowth (plexiform neuroma), bony abnormalities resulting in skull defects and scoliosis, iris lesions and endocrine adenomas such as phaeochromocytomas.

Tuberose sclerosis (epiloia)

This is an autosomal dominant condition with a prevalence of about 5 per 100 000. Its features are adenoma sebaceum, epilepsy, mental retardation and abnormalities of other organs. The adenoma sebaceum are reddish nodules (angiofibromas) which develop in childhood on the face especially the cheeks and nasolabial folds (Fig. 12.7). In infancy one of the first changes is hypomelanotic macules, which are best seen under ultraviolet light (Wood's lamp). The brain exhibits tubers which are firm white areas containing astrocytes which distort and broaden the cortical gyri. The ependyma of the lateral ventricles is encrusted with astrocytic masses (candle-guttering), which calcify to give a characteristic x-ray appearance. The cerebral

Table 12.2

The Phakomatoses

	Nervous system	Skin	Eyes	Viscera	Bone
Neurofibromatosis (von Recklinghausen)	Cranial schwannomas Spinal schwannomas Peripheral neurofibromas Optic nerve glioma Gliomas Meningiomas Hamartomas	Café-au-lait patches Cutaneous neurofibromas	Eyelid neurofibromas Orbital wall defects Iris lesions	Neurofibromas Endocrine adenoma malformations	Bone cysts Scoliosis Fibrous dysplas
Tuberose sclerosis (Bourneville)	Mental retardation Epilepsy Cortical tubers Subependymal nodules Gliomas	Adenoma sebaceum Subungual fibromas Shagreen patches Amelanotic naevi	Retinal phakomas	Hamartomas Rhabdomyomas Renal tumurs Endocrine tumours	Bone cysts
Encephalo-facial angiomatosis (Sturge–Weber)	Meningeal angiomatosis Cortical malformation Calcification	Port-wine facial naevus Other naevi	Buphthalmos Glaucoma Retinal angioma Exophthalmos	Angioma	Atrophic hemiplegi
Retino-cerebellar angiomatosis (von Hippel–Lindau)	Cerebellar haemangioblastoma (cerebral and spinal)		Retinal haemangioblastoma	Haemangioblastoma Hypernephroma Phaeochromocytoma Polycythaemia	Cysts
Ataxia telangiectasia (Louis Bar)	Cerebellar degeneration Spinal cord degeneration Peripheral nerve degeneration Gliomas	Cutaneous telangiectasia	Conjunctival telangiectasia	Thymic hypoplasia IgA/IgE deficiency Lung abscesses Lymphomas	Growth retardatio
Familial telangiectasia (Osler–Weber–Rendu)	Arteriovenous fistulas Brain abscesses	Cutaneous telangiectasia Mucous membrane telangiectasia		Gastrointestinal, pulmonary and genito-urinary telangiectasis Gastrointestinal haemorrhage Pulmonary fistulae Polycythaemia	

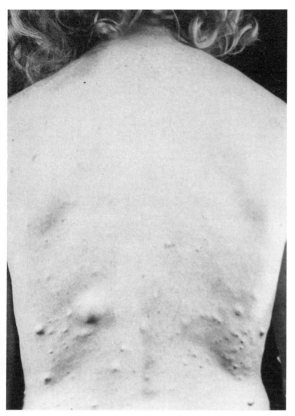

Fig. 12.5 *Multiple cutaneous and subcutaneous tumours in neurofibromatosis.*

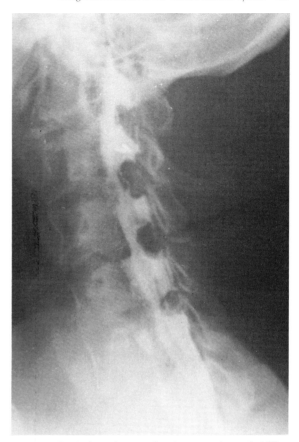

Fig. 12.6 *Cervical myelogram showing several rounded filling defects – schwannomas in neurofibromatosis.*

cortex exhibits disorganisation of the normal neuronal architecture and is subject to malignant transformation. Phakomas are discrete white gliomatous tumours of the retina. There is no treatment other than control of seizures.

Encephalo-facial angiomatosis (Sturge–Weber syndrome)

In this condition there is an extensive port-wine naevus on one side of the face with an angioma of the leptomeninges on the same side, usually in the parieto-occipital region. The underlying cortex is abnormal and calcified, giving rise to the typical 'tramline calcification' on skull x-ray. In severe cases there is a motor, sensory or visual defect on the contralateral side and epilepsy is common. The cause is unknown and familial occurrence is exceptional.

Retinocerebellar angiomatosis (Von Hippel–Lindau syndrome)

This is a familial condition with multiple haemangio-blastomas of the retina and cerebellum and, less commonly, of the spinal cord and cerebrum. Visceral tumours and cysts of the pancreas and kidney are associated.

Ataxia Telangiectasia (Louis Bar syndrome): see p. 197 and Table 12.2.

Familial telangiectasia (Osler–Rendu–Weber syndrome)

This is a dominant condition with multiple vascular anomalies of skin, mucous membrane, gastrointestinal

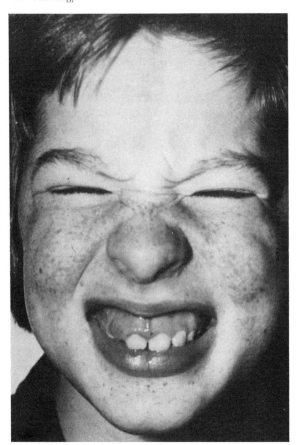

Fig. 12.7 *Adenoma sebaceum in a child with tuberose sclerosis: note gum hypertrophy secondary to phenytoin treatment for epilepsy.*

tract, and occasionally the nervous system. The small red angiomas can be found on the face and mucous membranes in adolescent and adult life. The usual presentation is with repeated gastrointestinal haemorrhage. The central nervous system can be affected by angiomas, which can bleed. Pulmonary fistulas can develop and predispose to brain abscess.

There are numerous other phakomatoses and reference should be made to specialist texts.

CEREBRAL PALSY

The cerebral palsies of childhood are predominantly motor syndromes, not diseases, caused by a variety of pathologies. There is an abnormality of movement, posture and tone which is usually not progressive but is commonly associated with sensory abnormalities, cognitive deficits and epilepsy. The prevalence is about 1 per 1000 live births and is greater in the lower socio-economic groups. There are three basic types of disorder; spasticity, choreoathetosis and ataxia.

Spastic cerebral palsy

In *spastic diplegia* (Little's disease) both legs are spastic, weak and clumsy, and are held usually in extension and adduction. The gait is the typical 'scissor gait' due to severe spasticity. The arms, face and bulbar muscles are involved to a lesser extent. Motor development is delayed and there is often mental retardation. The condition is associated with prematurity or with birth asphyxia.

Infantile hemiplegia may be noted at birth or develop, often abruptly, in the first six months of life. The arm and leg show spastic weakness. Epilepsy is common but mental retardation is not. The pathology may be infarction from arterial or venous occlusion or, more commonly, intracerebral haemorrhage associated with birth trauma.

Double hemiplegia results in bilateral spastic weakness of face, arm and leg. The arms are severely affected in contrast to spastic diplegia.

Congenital choreoathetosis

Double athetosis is characterised by involuntary movements, usually chorea, athetosis and dystonia of the limbs, trunk, face and bulbar muscles (see p. 161). The onset can be delayed for some months after birth and the severity can vary from mild incoordinate movements to complete helplessness. The intellect can be normal but communication may be difficult because of marked dysarthria. Pathologically, cell-loss, gliosis and abnormal myelination are seen in the basal ganglia, which appear marble-like (status marmoratus).

Kernicterus is caused by high levels of unconjugated bilirubin (above 300 μmol/l) damaging the neonatal brain, which is stained yellow. Death can occur in the acute phase and surviving infants may exhibit permanent disability consisting of mental retardation, deafness, impaired eye movements and involuntary movements including choreoathetosis, dystonia and rigidity. The pathology is neuronal loss and gliosis of the subthalamic nucleus, globus pallidus, thalamus, oculo-motor and cochlear nuclei. The cause is Rhesus or ABO incompatibility, where maternal antibodies cross the placenta and cause haemolysis of fetal red cells. All pregnant women should be routinely screened and maternal sensitisation can be prevented by giving the mother anti-D immunoglobulin immediately *post partum*. Phototherapy and exchange transfusions are used to prevent the bilirubin level rising excessively.

Congenital Ataxias

In the unusual ataxic type of cerebral palsy, cerebellar incoordination and hypotonia can vary from mild to severe and are often associated with speech disturbance and mental retardation. The usual pathology is sclerosis of the cerebellum. A combination of cerebellar ataxia and cerebral diplegia can exist together.

INTRAUTERINE INFECTIONS

The permeability of the placenta to invading organisms and the immune status of the mother are the major determinants for fetal infection. With very few exceptions, the placenta is an effective barrier against bacterial and protozoan invaders. Most fetal infections are viral but, in the vast majority of cases, a normal infant is delivered at term.

Congenital Rubella

In a non-epidemic year about 200 infants in the United Kingdom are affected. Rubella infection in the first trimester has a greater chance of causing neonatal damage (50%), and the damage is more severe. The risks in the third trimester are smaller (< 10%). The main features are cataract, deafness, mental retardation and congenital heart disease. There is no treatment for the infection itself and the aim is prevention. All girls between the ages of 10 and 13 should be immunised with live vaccine. All pregnant women should screened for rubella antibodies and seronegative cases (about

20%) should be vaccinated immediately *post partum* and warned not to become pregnant for three months. Those seronegative mothers who become exposed to rubella can be passively immunised with gamma globulin, although this practice is not universally accepted. If, during pregnancy, there is a seroconversion from negative to positive, or if specific IgM antibodies appear, rubella infection has occurred and termination of pregnancy may be justified.

Congenital Neurosyphilis

Syphilis can be transmitted to the fetus from the fourth month. The patterns of neurosyphilis are similar to those in adults but with a shortened time-course. If the fetus does not abort, the child is born with florid manifestations of secondary syphilis and *Treponema pallidum* may be found throughout the body. Asymptomatic and symptomatic meningitis occurs in the first weeks, meningovascular symptoms from one to six years, and general paralysis from nine to fifteen years. Specific features of congenital syphilis are bilateral deafness, interstitial keratitis and deformed teeth. Congenital syphilis should be prevented by serologically screening all pregnant women. If there is a possible exposure, the tests should be repeated in the 36th week of pregnancy. In positive cases, treatment of the mother with penicillin usually leads to a healthy baby. An infant suspected of harbouring the disease will require serological testing, examination of the CSF, and appropriate penicillin treatment. In all cases it is important to check for infection in the parents, siblings and other possible contacts.

Cytomegalic Inclusion Disease

Cytomegalovirus infection *in utero* occurs in about 1 in 4000 live births in the US; in the United Kindgom, about 400 babies annually have significant mental retardation associated with the condition. The neonate may show microcephaly, mental retardation and fits, as well as thrombocytopenia, purpura, jaundice, hepatosplenomegaly and gastrointestinal bleeding. In the brain there are disseminated foci of inflammatory cells containing viral inclusion bodies, which may calcify and show on x-ray in severe cases. About 50% of women of childbearing age are seronegative with specific comple-ment-fixing tests and are susceptible. The disease is usually asymptomatic and the only diagnostic test is seroconversion on serial testing, which is not a practical screening procedure. The excretion of virus from the cervix does not imply fetal infection. For the infant, the infection can be identified by virus isolation in human fibroblast cultures, finding large number of nuclear inclusion bodies in cells in the urine, and a specific IgM antibody in cord blood. At the present time there is no means of protecting the mother, or of preventing *in utero* infection or treating the infant.

Toxoplasmosis

This is a protozoal infection most commonly con-tracted from uncooked meat and excreta of domestic cats. The maternal infection is usually inapparent and can only be detected by conversion from negative to positive on specific serological tests. About 0.5% of pregnant women show such a conversion, and the *in utero* infection rate is about 40%. About half of these will show clinical signs of neonatal toxoplasmosis. The neonate can develop fits, spastic quadriparesis, hydro-cephalus and chorioretinitis. The organism is abundant and foci of granulation tissue in the brain may calcify

and be seen on x-ray. The diagnosis in the infant is verified by the persistence of high toxoplasma titres, when the maternal levels in the infant should be falling, or by the presence of a specific IgM antibody. Treat-ment, a combination of pyrimethamine and sulfadia-zine, should be given early and will not be effective in severe or late cases.

Varicella-Zoster

Congenital varicella is extremely rare and can be recognised by mental retardation, fits, microcephaly and hypoplasia of limbs. Infection near term can produce an infant with typical varicella, which may be fatal. Maternal infection is not, in itself, grounds for a termination.

Herpes simplex

A viraemia following a primary infection in the first trimester can very occasionally damage the fetus. More commonly infection is transmitted to the infant, during vaginal delivery, from genital herpes. In this case CNS involvement can occur, with mental retardation, fits, blindness and microcephaly.

13

Degenerative Disorders

INTRODUCTION

The aetiology of many of the diseases described in this chapter is not known. A number of them have eponymic labels, or are described as atrophies of various types. For unknown reasons, nerve cells of a particular type or location successively shrink and die. Neuronal death results in neurotransmitter dysfunction, which has been demonstrated to be closely correlated with the severity of the clinical syndrome in some instances. Degenerative disorders of the nervous system tend selectively and symmetrically to affect one or more systems of neurones. They usually lead to gradually progressive disability and may shorten life expectancy. Their clinical and pathological features often vary considerably from patient to patient.

Histologically the affected part of the nervous system may show only loss of neurones with reactive gliosis, although some disorders have special features, such as the Lewy bodies seen in Parkinson's disease and the neurofibrillary tangles of Alzheimer's disease. There is frequently evidence of a pathological process known as 'dying-back'; neuronal atrophy begins at the end of the axis cylinder and proceeds centripetally towards the cell body (Fig. 13.1). The cell body itself may be histologically normal, but appears incapable of maintaining normal function at the end of a long axon. In many degenerative conditions there is degeneration of two or more 'linked' groups of neurones, for example the alpha-motor neurones and corticobulbar/corticospinal tracts in motor neurone disease. This has been explained on the basis of trans-synaptic degeneration, although the mechanism is unclear.

It is possible only to speculate about the cause of many degenerative neurological conditions. Some are genetically determined but many are not. A few, such as Friedreich's ataxia and some of the spinal muscular atrophies, are monogenically inherited, although their exact genetic defect is unknown. A number of autosomal recessive disorders are characterised by deficiency of an enzyme which may produce neuronal dysfunction, and ultimately death, either by failure of production of essential metabolic products or deposition of accumulated neurotoxic substances. The latter applies to Tay–Sachs disease, in which hexosaminidase deficiency results in intraneuronal accumulation of ganglioside (see p. 218). Dominantly inherited diseases are rarely associated with a known specific metabolic defect. Polygenic inheritance is probable in some degenerative syndromes, including Alzheimer's disease, where occasionally more than one member of a family is affected but the pedigree does not conform to Mendelian patterns of transmission. Development of the disease appears to be dependent on a combination of environmental and genetic factors.

Probably the simplest explanation for the mechanism of system degenerations, and one often given to patients or their relatives, is one of premature ageing of specific groups of neurones. Most degenerative neurological disorders are encountered more frequently in the elderly, and tend to affect the same groups of neurones which degenerate in 'normal' ageing. Some of the neuropathological changes of Alzheimer's disease, for instance, are found at autopsy in intellectually normal old people. Loss of Purkinje cells is a prominent feature of most of the cerebellar degenerations; these cells also decline in number with advancing age. The mechanisms of natural cell death may offer clues as to why neurones die prematurely. Human fibroblasts in tissue culture will only divide for a limited period of time, and this time is inversely

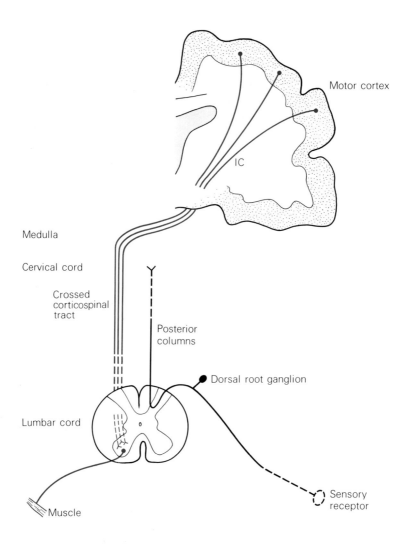

IC = internal capsule

Fig. 13.1 *Diagrammatic representation of the 'dying-back' process. The distal part of the descending corticospinal tract has degenerated while the cell bodies and proximal tract remain intact. Cells in the dorsal root ganglia are bipolar; as a result,* *'dying back' affecting the first sensory neurone gives rise to degeneration of the rostral parts of the fibres ascending in the dorsal columns, and the distal sensory fibres in the peripheral nerves.*

proportional to the donor's age. Transfer experiments have shown that this phenomenon is dependent on the nuclear constituents of the cell. Errors in duplication of DNA are likely to increase with age because of damage from external agents, such as radiation, infection and toxins. These will eventually result in abnormal RNA and protein synthesis, cellular dysfunction and death. Two genetically-determined diseases characterised by defective DNA repair, ataxia telangiectasia and xero-

derma pigmentosum, are associated with degenerative neurological syndromes. Why degeneration is confined to certain systems is unknown. We are also ignorant about the external factors which may accelerate cell death. It is of interest that a condition which was initially thought to have many of the clinical and pathological hallmarks of a degenerative disorder, Creutzfeldt–Jakob disease, is now known to be caused by a transmissible agent (see pp. 193, 238).

DEMENTIA

Dementia is defined as a global impairment of higher intellectual function in an alert patient. It has been estimated that 5–10% of the population aged over 65 years suffer from some degree of dementia, and this proportion rises to 20% over the age of 80. The dementias of adult life are often divided into senile and presenile types, based on whether the age of onset is before or after the age of 65, but this distinction is artificial as the causes of dementia (Table 13.1) are the same, albeit different in relative frequency, in the two age groups.

Table 13.1

Causes of Dementia

Alzheimer's disease
Multi-infarct dementia
Parkinson's disease
Huntington's chorea
Hydrocephalus
Tumours
Metabolic and deficiency states
Creutzfeldt–Jakob disease
Syphilis
Pick's disease

Alzheimer's Disease

Clinical features

About 60% of demented patients have Alzheimer's disease and the proportion increases with age. The onset is insidious, usually after the age of 40, with loss of recent memory and lack of interest in personal care and surroundings. The early signs of the disease may go unnoticed by the patient's family and be observed first by his employers when work performance declines. The intellectual deficit, gradually becomes severe, with disinhibition, slovenliness, disorientation, and restlessness. Focal deficits such as dysphasia and dyspraxia are often present. Myoclonic jerks and generalised seizures may occur. The patient eventually becomes mute and helpless, and death occurs at any time from 2 to 15 years after onset.

Pathophysiology of Alzheimer's disease

The condition is characterised by loss of neurones together with widespread senile plaques and neuro-fibrillary tangles in the certebral cortex (Fig. 13.2). There is also cell loss in the nucleus basalis in the diencephalon and the locus caeruleus in the pons. The significance of these latter findings has become apparent with the recent demonstration of the neurochemical basis of Alzheimer's disease.

Activity of choline acetyltransferase (ChAT) is significantly reduced in the cerebral cortex of patients with this disorder. ChAT synthesises acetylcholine and is only found in cholinergic neurones. Not all cholinergic neurone systems are depleted of ChAT in Alzheimer's disease. The most marked reduction in activity is seen in the temporal neocortex, hippocampus, and amygdala. The major contribution to ChAT activity in the cortex is not from intrinsic cholinergic cortical neurones, but from nerve terminals which project from elsewhere, particularly from the nucleus basalis in the diencephalon (Fig. 13.3). ChAT activity is low in the nucleus basalis and this is paralleled by loss of cells. Activity of the enzyme dopamine-B-hydroxylase, a marker of noradrenergic neurones, is also reduced in the cerebral cortex in Alzheimer's disease. Noradrenergic nerve terminals in the cortex project from cells in the locus caeruleus (blue structure) which is located in the rostral part of the pons (Fig. 13.3). The relative importance of the noradrenergic and cholinergic pathways in Alzheimer's disease is not clear, but ChAT activity is significantly correlated with the density of senile plaques and severity of dementia. It appears that degeneration of the ascending cholinergic system is an important factor in the development of Alzheimer's disease, but whether this is a primary event or not is unclear.

Therapy

The neurotransmitter deficits described above do offer a rational basis on which to treat patients with Alzheimer's disease. However, clinical trials of therapy with choline chloride and lecithin (phosphatidylcholine) have been disappointing. These substances are

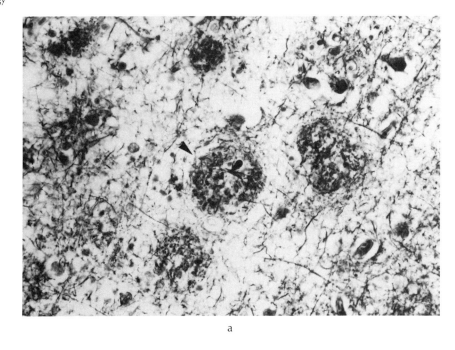

a

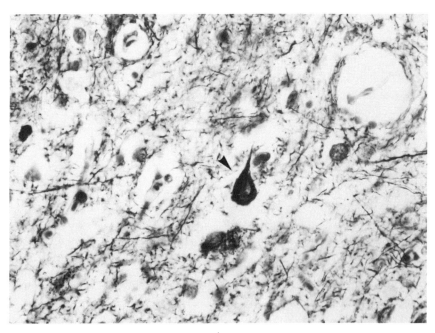

b

Fig. 13.2 (a) *Senile argyrophilic plaques (example arrowed) in the cerebral cortex in Alzheimer's disease. There is degeneration of the neurofibrils in several neurones with formation of neurofibrillary tangles, seen at higher magnification in (b) (Courtesy of Dr F Scaravilli.)*

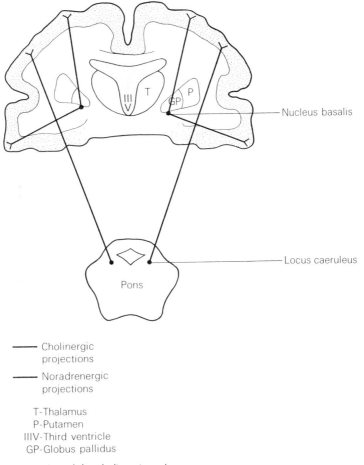

Fig. 13.3 *Diagrammatic representation of the cholinergic and noradrenergic projections to the cerebral cortex. (Not to scale.)*

precursors of acetylcholine and may require a certain amount of ChAT activity in order to increase brain acetylcholine. The use of selective direct cholinergic agonists may be of value but these have not as yet been developed.

The management of patients with dementia is currently largely confined to the provision of nursing care. Treatment of concurrent depression is important. Sedation may be required for the agitated, restless patient. Care should be taken in prescribing drugs, including sedatives, as many increase confusion, particularly in the elderly. If possible, the demented patient should be looked after at home where his or her surroundings are familiar. Admission to hospital often precipitates a severe confusional state. This should be

borne in mind at the time of first assessment; the majority of demented patients can be investigated on an out-patient basis. The care of these patients is both emotionally and physically demanding for their relatives, who may be elderly spouses or children with their own families. It is essential to provide as much support as possible for them from hospital- and community-based services. The home should be visited by an occupational therapist to assess the need for structural adaptations or other aids to accommodate nursing a physically handicapped patient. Simple aids such as handrails on the stairs, non-slip mats in the bath, and special feeding implements can be very helpful. Regular visits from the district nurse to help with bathing, skin and bladder care are essential in the late stages of the disease. In some areas laundry services are available for incontinent patients. The relatives of demented patients need intermittent respite from their onerous duties. Day centres provide this regularly, and it should be possible to arrange short-term hospital or Local Authority Home admission to cover holidays. The provision of this sort of support will generally result in longer home care for the patient. Nevertheless, most require hospital admission in the terminal phase of their illness. The management of patients with Alzheimer's disease outlined above is not specific, and patients with other degenerative disorders of the nervous system have similar needs.

Differential diagnosis of dementia

Although Alzheimer's disease is statistically the most likely cause of dementia developing in middle life or later, it is essential that each case is investigated for other causes of intellectual deterioration (Table 13.1) as some are treatable. Degenerative dementias such as Alzheimer's disease, and another more rare condition known as Pick's disease which is clinically indistinguishable and characterised by circumscribed frontal and temporal cortical atrophy, are diagnosed by exclusion. Neither can be diagnosed with certainty during life except by cortical biopsy and this is rarely justifiable. The CT scan shows cortical atrophy and ventricular enlargement in the degenerative dementias (Fig. 13.4). The increased ventricular size reflects brain shrinkage and does not imply obstruction to cerebrospinal fluid (CSF) drainage.

Hydrocephalus can give rise to dementia (see p. 81). The same is true of intracranial tumours, either by causing hydrocephalus or by a more direct effect on the cerebral cortex. This particularly applies to slow-growing tumours such as meningiomas compressing the frontal lobes. Tumours of the corpus callosum and subdural haematomas can also present with mental changes, but the history is usually short (weeks or months) and focal neurological signs may be present.

Diffuse cerebrovascular disease is probably the second most common cause of dementia after Alzheimer's disease; the two conditions may be indistinguishable and often coexist. Multi-infarct dementia is commonly associated with hypertension and multiple small deep infarctions (lacunes) rather than major vessel occlusions (Fig. 13.5). The history often reveals

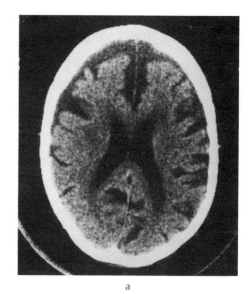

a

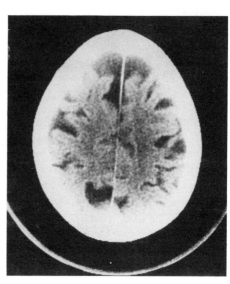

b

Fig. 13.4 CT brain scan in Alzheimer's disease showing enlarged lateral ventricles (a) and widening of the cortical sulci (a and b). (Courtesy of Dr Brian Kendall.)

stepwise deterioration rather than a gradually progressive decline. Depending on the areas of brain involved, dysarthria, dysphasia, dyspraxia, and other focal signs and symptoms may occur. Frontal lobe involvement can give rise to incontinence and a slow shuffling gait (marche a petits pas) accompanying intellectual deter-

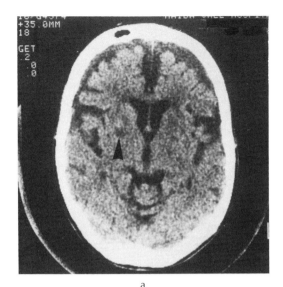

a

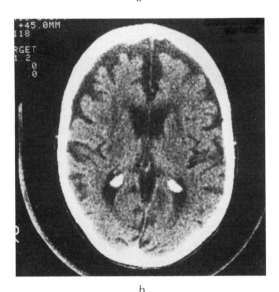

b

Fig. 13.5 *CT brain scan in multi-infarct dementia. There are several small areas of low attenuation (lacunes) deep within the cerebral hemispheres (arrowed in a) and more diffuse low attenuation around the anterior horns of the lateral ventricles (b), as well as generalised cortical atrophy.*

ioration. The existence of multi-infarct dementia demonstrates the importance of treating hypertension in the prevention of stroke (see also p. 138).

Metabolic disorders and deficiency states, such as hypothyroidism, alcoholism with or without Korsakoff's syndrome, and B$_{12}$ deficiency are causes of dementia

and these should be excluded. Neurosyphilis is now rare but treatable (see p. 235); normal blood serology makes this diagnosis unlikely but the CSF should be examined in younger demented patients. Creutzfeldt–Jakob disease is a rare dementing illness which is thought to be caused by an infective agent with a long incubation period. It can be difficult to distinguish from Alzheimer's disease but the evolution is more rapid, focal neurological deficits are common, particularly cortical visual problems, and myoclonic jerks are frequent. The EEG characteristically shows paroxysmal generalised sharp wave complexes with widespread slow background activity. Pathologically there is widespread loss of neurones in the cerebral cortex and subcortical grey matter, with astrocytic proliferation and spongiform changes.

Huntington's chorea, an autosomal dominant disorder which gives rise to dementia and chorea, has been discussed in Chapter 10, as have other degenerative diseases of the basal ganglia.

The clinical presentation of depression in the elderly often mimics dementia; this is sometimes called pseudodementia. Apathy, motor retardation, delusions, confusion, impaired concentration and complaints of memory-loss in depressed patients may readily suggest dementia. The situation is made more complex by the fact that dementia tends to be associated with depression. Psychometric testing may indicate that the intellectual deficit is far smaller than would be expected from the patient's complaints, but severe psychomotor retardation can make assessment difficult.

PROGRESSIVE SUPRANUCLEAR PALSY

Progressive supranuclear palsy (the Steele–Richardson–Olszewski syndrome) is a relatively rare disease of unknown aetiology which affects males more frequently than females, gives rise to symptoms between the ages of 45 and 70 years, and usually leads to death in five to ten years. The presenting symptoms include unexplained falls, mental disturbances, and slurring of speech. The clinical syndrome comprises mild dementia, nuchal rigidity and mask-like facies, a supranuclear vertical gaze palsy, and pseudobulbar palsy. Mild extrapyramidal rigidity may be present in the limbs, the tendon reflexes are usually increased, and the plantar responses are often extensor.

Autopsy studies show widespread symmetrical neuronal loss with gliosis, mainly affecting the globus pallidus, red nucleus, subthalamic nucleus, substantia nigra, tectum and periaqueductal grey matter, and the dentate nucleus. Neurofibrillary tangles are seen in these structures, and in other parts of the brainstem where cell loss is not evident. These neurofibrillary tangles are ultrastructurally different from those of Alzheimer's disease, and the cerebral cortex is unaffected. There is no effective therapy for progressive supranuclear palsy, and the parkinsonian features of the disease do not usually respond to L-dopa or anticholinergic drugs.

MULTIPLE SYSTEM ATROPHY AND PROGRESSIVE AUTONOMIC FAILURE

Primary degeneration of the autonomic nervous system may either occur in isolation, or be combined with other degenerative diseases of the nervous system. In the latter, there are two groups of cases, those with progressive autonomic failure (PAF) associated with Parkinson's disease, and others in which autonomic failure occurs together with 'multiple system atrophy' (MSA) comprising a disorder known as the Shy–Drager syndrome. The clinical features of PAF are common to all three groups (Table 13.2). Autonomic function can be assessed at the bedside by using a few simple tests (see p. 56).

Parkinson's disease with PAF develops later in life than PAF alone or MSA, and the degree of autonomic failure tends to be less severe. The pathological

---

Table 13.2

Clinical Features of Progressive Autonomic Failure

Abnormal pupillary responses
Sleep apnoea
Laryngeal stridor
Postural hypotension
Fixed heart rate
Defective sweating
Impotence
Complex, variable bladder dysfunction
Intermittent diarrhoea

---

abnormalities underlying this syndrome are those of idiopathic Parkinson's disease (loss of pigmented cells in the substantia nigra and Lewy inclusion bodies) with additional degeneration of central autonomic neurones. The age of onset of MSA is usually between 35 and 60 years, and postural hypotension is a common presenting symptom. The neurological features observed are variable but include parkinsonism, truncal ataxia, corticospinal tract signs in the limbs, and neurogenic muscular atrophy. The parkinsonism is unresponsive to L-dopa, which tends to exacerbate the postural hypotension. This can be controlled by tilting the patient (head up) at night and by the administration of fludrocortisone but the other features of MSA are progressive and unresponsive to therapy. Death usually occurs within five to ten years of onset. Pathologically, cases of MSA show lesions in the corpus striatum and the pontine and olivary nuclei as well as the changes found in Parkinson's disease with PAF.

CEREBELLAR AND SPINOCEREBELLAR DEGENERATIONS

The cerebellar and spinocerebellar degenerations are a complex group of disorders which comprises more than 50 distinct syndromes. Many of these are extremely rare and will not be dealt with in detail here.

Late Onset Cerebellar Ataxia

Probably about half of the degenerative ataxic syndromes with an age of onset of symptoms over 20 years are genetically determined, and nearly all of these are of autosomal dominant inheritance. Most patients with dominantly inherited late onset cerebellar ataxia do not have a pure cerebellar syndrome; many have additional associated clinical features, including dementia, supranuclear ophthalmoplegia, optic atrophy, pigmentary retinal degeneration, and extrapyramidal involvement such as impassive facies, rigidity, dystonia or chorea in variable combinations. The age of first symptoms, usually progressive unsteadiness, is in the third to fifth decades of life, and life expectancy is shortened.

Patients such as these who do not have similarly

affected relatives are not uncommon. Singleton cases tend to have a later age of onset and associated additional features are less prominent, especially those involving the visual and oculomotor systems. The aetiology of this 'idiopathic' late onset cerebellar syndrome is unclear, but it is possible that some represent fresh dominant mutation. A small number of cases have recently been found to have a deficiency of the enzyme glutamate dehydrogenase. The CT scan may show striking atrophy of the brainstem and cerebellum in late onset degenerative cerebellar disorders (Fig. 13.6). In the absence of a family history, it is important to distinguish these degenerative syndromes from other conditions which may be treatable, including hypothyroidism, alcoholism, hydrocephalus, posterior fossa mass lesions, and the nonmetastatic effects of malignancy.

The pathological findings in late onset cerebellar degenerations are somewhat variable. Most of the dominant cases have olivopontocerebellar atrophy (OPCA) at autopsy. There is loss of cells in the pontine and olivary nuclei and also of the Purkinje cells in the

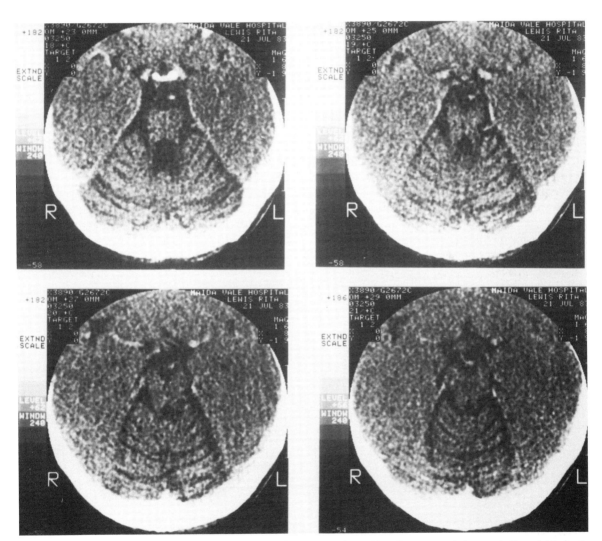

Fig. 13.6 *CT scan of the posterior fossa in a patient with 'idiopathic' late-onset cerebellar ataxia. The serial cuts show enlargement of the fourth ventricle and brainstem atrophy, together with enlargement of the cerebellar sulci indicating atrophy of the cerebellar hemispheres. (Courtesy of Dr Brian Kendall.)*

cerebellum. The pathological name for this condition is somewhat misleading as accompanying degeneration of anterior horn cells, the long tracts in the spinal cord, and the basal ganglia is frequent. OPCA is also found in some singleton cases but others have cerebello-olivary atrophy or, rarely, pure cerebellar cortical atrophy. No treatment is known to be effective in either familial or singleton cases. Genetic counselling is important if inheritance is dominant, as the children of affected individuals have a 50% chance of developing the disease.

Early Onset Cerebellar Ataxia: Friedreich's Ataxia

Degenerative ataxic disorders with onset in childhood or adolescence are nearly always genetically determined and are usually of autosomal recessive inheritance. The commonest of these is Friedreich's ataxia, which has a prevalence of 1–2 per 100 000 in Europe. Symptoms develop between the ages of 8 and 16 years in most cases. The cardinal features of the disease are progressive limb and gait ataxia, dysarthria, and absence of the tendon reflexes. Pyramidal weakness, extensor plantar responses, and loss of joint position and vibration sense appear eventually in all patients. Scoliosis and electrocardiographic evidence of heart disease (Fig. 13.7) occur in about 70%; pes cavus, optic atrophy, nystagmus, and distal wasting of the limbs are

less common. Patients becomes chairbound, on average, 15 years after the onset of symptoms, and death tends to occur in the fourth and fifth decades of life.

Cardiac failure, often precipitated by arrhythmias, is common in the few months or years prior to death. About 10% of patients also develop diabetes mellitus. The aetiology of the cardiac and metabolic complications of Friedreich's ataxia is unknown, as is that of the neurological disorder. Some, but not all, cases have been found to have a deficiency of mitochondrial malic enzyme which converts pyruvate to malate in the mitochondrial matrix.

Pathologically, the spinal cord shows degeneration of the posterior columns, most prominent rostrally, and also of the corticospinal tracts which is more marked caudally (Fig. 13.8). This is a good example of 'dying-back' (Fig. 13.1). There is also degeneration of Clarke's columns and the spinocerebellar tracts. Changes in the brain are largely confined to gliosis of the cerebellar white matter. The dorsal root ganglia show widespread loss of neurones and there is degeneration of the large myelinated fibres in the peripheral nerves. This can be documented during life by the use of nerve conduction studies. Motor nerve conduction is normal but sensory action potentials are either greatly reduced in amplitude or absent. Interstitial myocardial fibrosis is seen in the heart. There is no known effective treatment for Friedreich's ataxia, although effective therapy for cardiac failure and diabetes is important, and orthopaedic management of skeletal deformity may be helpful. As

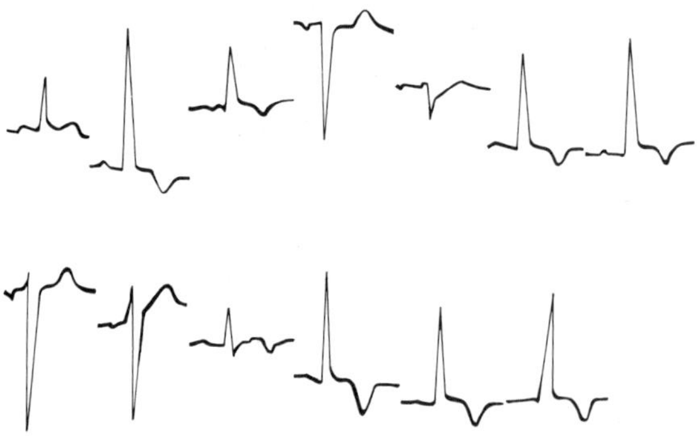

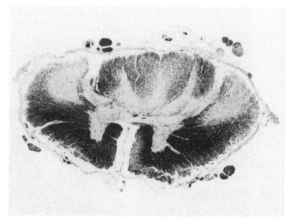

Fig. 13.7 *Electrocardiogram from a 25-year-old patient with Friedreich's ataxia. There is widespread T-wave inversion and ventricular hypertrophy. (Leads arranged, left to right, I–aVF (above), and V1–V6 (below). (From Harding AE, The Hereditary Ataxias and Related Disorders, Churchill Livingstone, 1984.)*

Fig. 13.8 *Transverse section of the thoracic spinal cord in Friedreich's ataxia, showing myelin pallor of the posterior columns and corticospinal tracts. (Courtesy of Dr F Scaravilli).*

the disorder is of autosomal recessive inheritance, the recurrence risk to subsequent children of the patient's parents is 25%.

Other Syndromes

There are a number of other autosomal recessive conditions which give rise to early onset progressive ataxia. Ataxia may be associated with hypogonadism, deafness, pigmentary retinopathy, optic atrophy or myoclonus (the Ramsay Hunt syndrome). There is also a rare X-linked form of spinocerebellar syndrome. The exact genetic defect underlying these conditions is unknown.

Metabolic ataxic disorders

The small number of ataxic disorders with known metabolic defects include deficiencies of urea cycle enzymes and some aminoacidurias such as Hartnup disease. Abetalipoproteinaemia is characterised by failure to synthesise apoprotein B, the carrier protein which transports some lipids out of the intestinal cell.

This disorder may be complicated by a neurological syndrome resembling Friedreich's ataxia but can be distinguished by the presence of hypocholesterolaemia and the presence of thorny deformed erythrocytes (acanthocytes) on peripheral blood film. The distinction is important, as there is good evidence that the neurological complications of abetalipoproteinaemia are secondary to vitamin E deficiency and they can be prevented or improved by vitamin E therapy.

Ataxia telangiectasia

The association of ataxia telangiectasia with a defect of DNA repair was mentioned in the *Introduction*. This autosomal recessive disorder gives rise to symptoms in early childhood, with delay of motor milestones and mild mental retardation. Progressive ataxia is often accompanied by athetoid movements of the limbs and a complex disorder of eye movements. The skin lesions which give the disease its name (Fig. 13.9) are not usually seen until the child is five or older. Telangiectases develop on the conjunctivae, nose, ears, and flexion creases of the limbs. Ataxia telangiectasia is associated with defects of both cell-mediated and

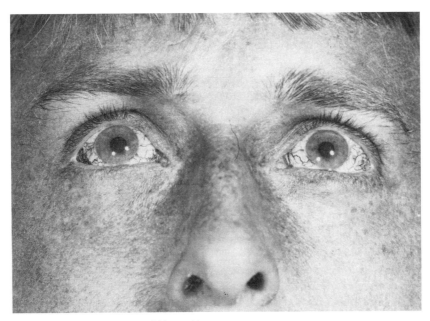

Fig. 13.9 *Conjunctival telangiectases in a 16-year-old boy with ataxia telangiectasia. (Courtesy of the Photographic Department, National Hospital for Nervous Diseases.)*

humoral immunity, leading to chronic bronchopul-monary infection in childhood. Death occurs in the teens, and is often precipitated by the development of lymphoid malignancy. Patients and their cells are abnormally sensitive to x-ray irradiation because of defective DNA repair. Autopsy shows extensive loss of the Purkinje and granule cells in the cerebellum, variable degeneration of the posterior columns, and rudimentary thymic and lymphoid tissue.

Hereditary spastic paraplegia

The hereditary spastic paraplegias are often classified together with the hereditary ataxias because there is some clinical and pathological overlap between the two groups of conditions. A disorder comprising signs and symptoms confined to those of a spastic paraplegia can be inherited as an autosomal dominant trait. It is most frequently of early onset and sometimes gives rise to delayed motor development. Spasticity of the lower limbs is more marked than weakness. Disability is only very slowly progressive and somewhat variable. Degeneration of the corticospinal tracts, most marked caudally, is seen in the spinal cord, and there is also 'dying-back' of the posterior columns.

DISORDERS OF THE MOTOR NEURONE

Motor Neurone Disease

The commonest degenerative disorder of motor neurones is known as motor neurone disease in the UK and amyotrophic lateral sclerosis in the USA. The essential histological abnormality is asymmetrical loss of large motor neurones together with gliosis in the anterior horn cells in the spinal cord (Fig. 13.10), and similar changes in some motor cranial nerve nuclei. Of the latter, the hypoglossal nuclei are commonly affected and the facial, trigeminal and vagal motor nuclei less frequently so; the nuclei of the oculomotor, trochlear, and abducents nerves are rarely involved. There is accompanying degeneration of the corticospinal tracts in the spinal cord which, if severe, can be traced upwards into the white matter of the cerebral hemi-spheres.

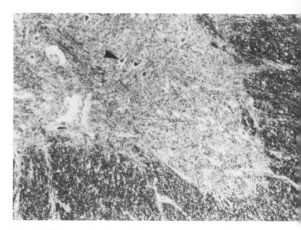

Fig. 13.10 *Anterior horn (transverse section) from a patient with motor neurone disease. There is only a small number of surviving neurones (arrow). (Courtesy of Dr F Scaravilli.)*

Clinical features

Onset of symptoms is usually in the fifth to seventh decades of life with loss of function in the limb or bulbar muscles. Four types of clinical presentation are recognised, progressive muscular atrophy, amyotrophic lateral sclerosis, bulbar palsy, and pseudobulbar palsy, although their distinction is somewhat artificial as most patients will eventually show the features of all four. Asymmetrical weakness and wasting of the hands is the commonest presentation (Fig. 13.11). Muscle cramps are common, as are symptoms of fatigue and sensitivity to cold. Examination at this stage often shows evidence of more widespread denervation, with wasting, weakness and fasciculation of other muscles. This can be confirmed by the use of electromyography (see p. 60). Motor and sensory nerve conduction is normal.

The neurogenic atrophy progresses over weeks, months, or rarely one or two years, to involve all four limbs. It is not confined to muscles innervated by one or more peripheral nerves. The tendon reflexes in involved limbs are often increased. The presence of a pathologically brisk reflex in a weak and wasted muscle is virtually pathognomonic, and it is not possible to diagnose motor neurone disease with any degree of certainty unless there is a combination of upper and lower motor neurone deficits in a single limb. Spasticity may develop in the legs, and the plantar responses are extensor in the majority of established cases.

Bulbar weakness, comprising slurred speech or

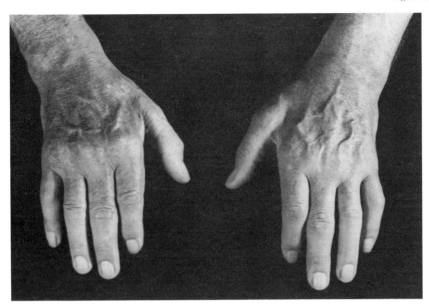

Fig. 13.11 *Bilateral wasting of the dorsal interossei, more marked on the left, in a 58-year-old male with motor neurone disease. (Courtesy of the Photographic Department, National Hospital for Nervous Diseases.)*

difficulties with chewing and swallowing, is the present-ing symptom in about one quarter of patients, particu-larly in older age groups. Weakness may be due to reduced voluntary movement of the palate, pharynx, and tongue (bulbar palsy), with wasting and fascicula-tion of the latter (Fig. 13.12). Dysphonia occurs, as well as dysarthria, as a result of laryngeal weakness. More commonly, there is a mixed deficit in the bulbar muscles due to involvement of the corticobulbar fibres at or above the level of the brainstem (pseudobulbar palsy, see p. 48). No objective evidence of sensory involvement is found in patients with motor neurone disease, although many have sensory symptoms. These can largely be explained on the basis of painful muscle cramps, and difficulties in differentiating numbness from weakness, although muscle weakness is occa-sionally evident at an early stage. Eye movement disorders are rarely seen, and sphincter function is unaffected.

The clinical course of motor neurone disease is a distressingly progressive one, with eventual involve-ment of all striated muscles other than those mediating eye movements. The commonest cause of death is

aspiration pneumonia, resulting from a combination of bulbar palsy and weakness of the intercostal muscles and diaphragm. Fifty per cent of patients die within three years of onset of symptoms, but a small propor-tion survive for ten years or even longer. Presentation with bulbar weakness implies a particularly poor prognosis. Cases with long survival often have the syndrome of progressive muscular atrophy, with little or any bulbar or pyramidal involvement. It is probable that these represent examples of a distinct disease, which is sometimes referred to as chronic asymmetrical spinal muscular atrophy.

Aetiology

The cause of motor neurone disease is unknown. More males are affected than females, in a ratio of about 1.7:1. Five to ten per cent of patients have a family history of the disorder, although pedigrees indicating autosomal dominant inheritance with full penetrance are rare. Searches for toxic and infective causes have so far been fruitless. Early suggestions that the develop-ment of motor neurone disease is related to antecedent

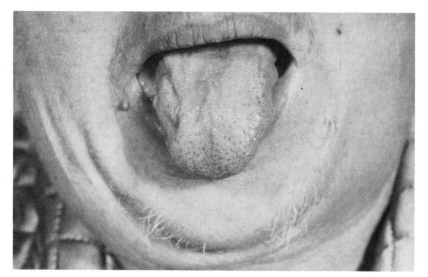

Fig. 13.12 *Asymmetrical wasting of the tongue in a 52-year-old female with motor neurone disease. (Courtesy of the Photographic Department, National Hospital for Nervous Diseases.)*

trauma or the nonmetastatic effects of malignancy were almost certainly based on observations of coincidence.

Therapy

Treatment is currently supportive only, but the responsibility for this sort of care should not necessarily be transferred to the patient's relatives and general practitioner as soon as the diagnosis has been made. Patients have special needs which change as the disease evolves. The presence of bulbar palsy may render swallowing and the production of intelligible speech virtually impossible. If swallowing difficulties give rise to malnutrition, and the patient is otherwise relatively well, a feeding gastrostomy may be required. Cricopharyngeal myotomy is helpful in a small proportion of cases, usually those with pseudobulbar palsy. A large number of electronic communication aids are now available; these are essential for the well-being of severely dysarthric or anarthric patients. The type required depends mainly on manual dexterity.

Diaphragmatic weakness may give rise to orthopnoea in the supine position, nocturnal ventilatory insufficiency, and insomnia early in the course of the disease and, at this stage, selected patients (those with adequate bulbar function) can be helped by a cuirasse ventilator at night. Patients with severe limb weakness may need walking aids, wheelchairs which can be fitted with swivelling supports for weak upper limbs, and feeding aids. The needs for these, and also for home adaptation, are best assessed by an experienced occupational therapist.

Spinal Muscular Atrophy

The genetically-determined disorders of the motor neurone which give rise to progressive symmetrical muscle weakness and wasting are conventionally called spinal muscular atrophies. These are a clinically and genetically heterogeneous group of disorders which are classified mainly on the basis of age of onset and distribution of muscle weakness. Pathologically, in the spinal muscular atrophies (SMA) there is widespread loss of anterior horn cells with preservation of the long tracts in the spinal cord, and macroscopic atrophy of the anterior nerve roots. Cell loss is seen in the cranial motor nuclei in a distribution similar to that of motor neurone disease. Electromyography and biopsy of skeletal muscle show the characteristic features of denervation. Peripheral nerve conduction is normal.

Acute infantile type

The commonest form of SMA is the acute infantile type (Werdnig–Hoffman disease). Inheritance is autosomal recessive. The diagnosis may be suspected before birth, as about one-third of cases show reduced or absent intrauterine fetal movements. Presenting features in the remainder include hypotonia and weakness, poor feeding, and delayed motor milestones, usually before the age of three months. The neonate is typically inactive and hypotonic, with profound proximal weakness. Breathing is entirely diaphragmatic as the intercostal muscles are severely affected. Bulbar weakness is prominent but the muscles of the face are spared. Fasciculations may be seen in the tongue and there is often a fine tremor of the fingers. Affected infants tend to lie in a 'frog-like' position. The tendon reflexes are absent. Death occurs in 50% of cases by the age of seven months and in 95% by 17 months.

Chronic childhood type

Chronic childhood proximal SMA (Kugelberg–Welander disease) is a more variable disorder, with onset ranging from three months to 15 years, but 95% of affected children are abnormal by the age of three. Walking is delayed or never occurs in about 50% of cases. Muscle weakness and wasting are mainly proximal but sometimes generalised. Patients with early onset often have marked skeletal deformities, such as scoliosis, lordosis, and joint contractures (Fig. 13.13). Facial weakness, wasting of the tongue, and fasciculations in limb muscles are seen in half of affected children. Only 5% are still ambulant by the age of 20, and most patients die before the fifth decade of life. Inheritance is autosomal recessive in the majority of cases.

Rare forms of SMA

There are a number of rarer forms of SMA, including two adult-onset proximal forms, one of which is dominantly inherited. The distal form of SMA superficially resembles Charcot–Marie–Tooth disease. The

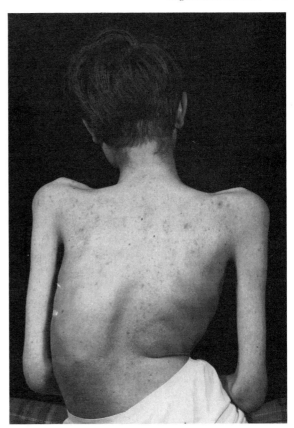

Fig. 13.13 *Generalised muscle wasting and scoliosis in a 14-year-old boy with the chronic childhood form of spinal muscular atrophy. (Courtesy of the Photographic Department, National Hospital for Nervous Diseases.)*

scapuloperoneal type affects the shoulder-girdle musculature and the muscles below the knees. There is an X-linked SMA which gives rise to bulbar involvement along with mainly proximal limb weakness, often associated with gynaecomastia, developing in adult life (bulbospinal muscular atrophy).

PERIPHERAL NEUROPATHIES

The differential diagnosis of peripheral neuropathy is discussed in Chapter 16. Even after intensive investigation, it is impossible to identify a cause for peripheral neuropathy in about 25% of patients. The majority of these have a symmetrical sensorimotor neuropathy with onset in middle life or later, and a smaller proportion have a progressive multifocal neuropathy (mononeuritis multiplex). Such patients are distinct from those with inherited neuropathies of recognised or unknown pathogenesis. The commonest of these is Charcot–Marie–Tooth disease, also known as peroneal muscular atrophy or hereditary motor and sensory neuropathy (HMSN).

Hereditary Motor and Sensory Neuropathy (HMSN)

HMSN is a group of conditions, rather than a single disease. The two major forms are known as HMSN types I and II. In type I, nerve conduction velocity is markedly slowed, and this is associated morphologically with segmental demyelination of peripheral nerves, accompanied by hypertrophic changes due to recurrent demyelination and remyelination (Fig. 13.14). Nerve conduction velocity is relatively preserved in HMSN type II, and this reflects the underlying primary axonal degeneration.

Both disorders are usually of autosomal dominant inheritance and their clinical features are similar, although the age of onset is later, on average, in type II HMSN. There is slowly progressive distal weakness and wasting, starting in the legs where the anterior tibial and peroneal muscles are most affected. The tendon reflexes are depressed or absent, particularly in type I cases. Distal sensory loss and skeletal deformities such as pes cavus (Fig. 13.15) and scoliosis are also more frequent in HMSN type I. The peripheral nerves may be palpably enlarged in this condition. Both disorders are slowly progressive but vary considerably in severity between patients. A small proportion of cases are chairbound in the sixth or seventh decades of life but 10–20% are asymptomatic.

Most of the other inherited neuropathies are rare. The hereditary sensory neuropathies are characterised by progressive distal sensory loss developing in early childhood, particularly for pain and temperature, often accompanied by painless ulcers and neuropathic joint distortion. Refsum's disease is a good illustration of how a specific metabolic defect can be identified following

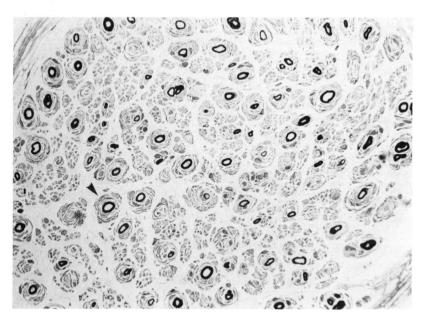

Fig. 13.14 *Transverse section of the sural nerve from a 38-year-old female with HMSN type I. There is widespread loss of myelinated fibres, and a number of 'onion bulb' formations (arrow) around axons which have undergone recurrent demyelination and remyelination. (Courtesy of Professor PK Thomas.)*

the clinical observation of a distinct syndrome. The neuropathy of Refsum's disease is similar to that of HMSN type I but it is accompanied by other features including ataxia, pigmentary retinopathy, deafness, cataract and ichthyosis. Inheritance is autosomal reces-sive. Phytanic acid is found in high concentrations in the serum; this results from a block in the alpha-oxida-tion of phytanic acid derived from dietary phytols. Improvement or arrest in progression of the disorder may be achieved by a low phytol diet.

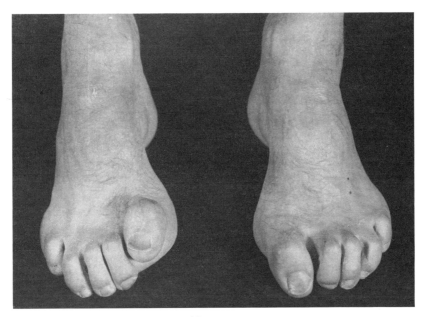

Fig. 13.15 *Pes cavus and clawing of the toes in a 24-year-old male with HMSN type I.*

14

Metabolic Disorders

GENERAL PRINCIPLES

Membrane Structure

Neurones and glia are complex membrane structures: the axons are invested in a membranous myelin sheath formed by oligodendroglia or Schwann cells. These membranes all have a lipid bi-layer structure, with protein between the layers.

Cellular and myelin membrane lipids are composed of phospholipids, the sphingolipids (derived from sphingosine), the gangliosides (in which lipid is combined with carbohydrate and sialic acid), and cholesterol. Fatty acids forming the elementary basis of the complex membrane lipids are synthesised with neuronal mitochondria from acetyl co-enzyme A so that the brain is not dependent on a supply of free fatty acids in the diet and blood supply.

Instructions for protein synthesis lie in the nuclear DNA, and the proteins themselves are manufactured in cytoplasmic ribosomes. Some proteins function as enzymes, others form structural components of cells and myelin. Structural proteins are combined with lipids (lipoproteins) in cellular membranes and myelin, and with carbohydrate (glycoproteins) in cellular membranes only. The carbohydrate portion of the glycoprotein may protrude from the cell surface and aid in cellular recognition interactions and immune responses. A number of genetically-determined disorders of lipids, proteins and carbohydrate resulting from specific enzyme deficiencies present in childhood (see p. 218).

The continual construction and repair of membranes requires adequate energy supply and utilisation, and is dependent on complex interactions between the nucleus and the cytoplasm and a cellular transport system. If these processes are disturbed by systemic disease, drugs or toxins (Fig. 14.1) then axonal degeneration, demyelination and irreversible neuronal autolysis may occur.

Some enzymes are dependent on cofactor availability, e.g. vitamins: longer term changes may be brought about by drugs and hormones. The major influences of hormones in altering brain cellular activity appear to be exerted during development, when deficiency or excess of thyroid hormones or sex hormones in particular may have permanent effects.

Membrane Excitability

Excitable membranes (such as neurones and muscle cells) exhibit differential permeability resulting in an uneven distribution of ions across the membrane, and hence a potential difference. Maintenance of membrane potential and its restoration following depolarisation depends on energy requiring ion transport. The 'sodium pump' is a Na^+/K^+-linked ATPase system, integral to membrane structure, utilising energy from ATP hydrolysis. Neuronal excitability depends therefore on the structural integrity of component membranes, energy supply to the membrane pumps, and an appropriate ionic distribution.

If neuronal excitability is reduced, nerve conduction and neural transmission may fail. Neurological deficit may occur depending on the site, extent and severity of the insult. The amplitude of the EEG record may fall and the dominant frequency slow down: in hypothermic or barbiturate coma it may become quite isoelectric. Alternatively, neurones may become hyperexcitable, leading to excessive discharges. In the cerebrum these manifest as epilepsy (see p. 107). The poison strychnine or the neurotoxin of the tetanus bacillus stimulate

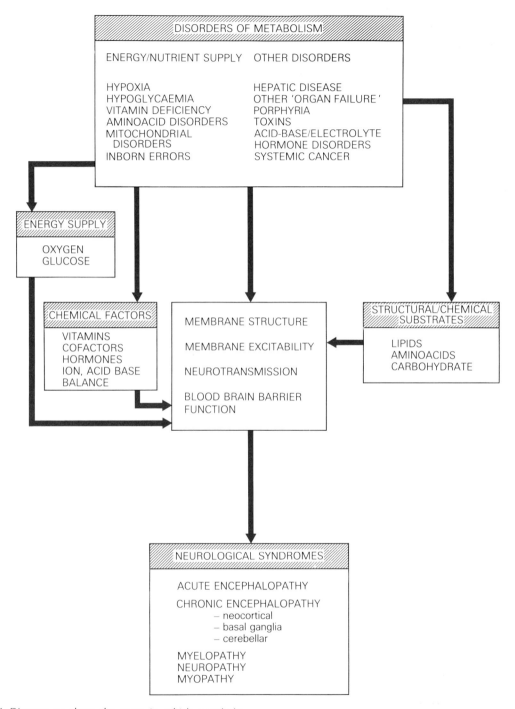

Fig. 14.1 *Diagram to show the ways in which metabolic disturbances can lead to neurological disorders.*

excessive discharge of anterior horn cells of the spinal cord and brainstem, leading to painful muscle spasms.

Neurotransmission

Neurotransmitters may be classified into three groups: (Table 14.1).

Table 14.1

Neurotransmitters

Amino acids	γ-aminobutyric acid (GABA)
	glycine
	glutamate
	aspartate
Monoamines	catecholamines noradrenaline
	adrenaline
	dopamine
	5-hydroxy-tryptamine (serotonin)
Acetylcholine	
Neuropeptides	pituitary peptides
	gut hormones e.g. substance P
	opioid peptides (endorphins)
	hypothalamic releasing hormones
	circulating hormones.

Amino acids

These transmitters are involved in fast, point-to-point chemical signalling in the nervous system.

Monoamines responsible for diffuse regulatory systems

The monoamine neurotransmitters are associated with diffuse neural pathways which have their origin in small groups of neurones within the brainstem and which project in ascending and descending pathways to large terminal fields within the brain. Most monoamine release occurs at non-synaptic sites by release of neurotransmitter capable of affecting large numbers of target cells. The monoamines appear to play a modulatory rather than direct communicatory role within the nervous system.

The neuropeptides

These consist of large groups of recently-discovered substances belonging to the endocrine and neuro-endocrine systems. The opioid peptides (endorphins) have morphine-like properties, and one of the peptides, substance P, is thought to be important in the transmission of nociceptive information in pain fibres (see p. 265).

Neurotransmitters are associated with specific types of receptors and some neurones are capable of releasing more than one form of neurotransmitter.

Systemic disease may potentially lead to disorders of neurotransmission in several ways, perhaps accounting for some aspects of the encephalopathies associated with various types of organ failure. The balance of amino acids available for cerebral uptake may be altered in renal or hepatic failure or there may competition for uptake by other organic molecules. So-called 'false transmitters' may result from abnormal hepatic function. Neuroleptic drugs and other psychiatric drugs such as the benzodiazapines and antidepressants may all have an important direct effect on transmitter function (see also p. 162). Since neurotransmission is dependent on excitable membrane function it is also susceptible to changes in ionic environment or energy availability caused through systemic disease.

Blood–Brain Barrier

The blood-brain barrier, which represents the sum of the permeabilities of the capillaries, astroglia and neurones, isolates the brain from the bloodstream and from the cerebrospinal fluid. It is highly selective, with restricted permeability, and protects the brain from fluctuations in the electrolyte and acid–base composition of plasma as well as from toxic subtances present in the bloodstream. The choroid plexus acts as a selective barrier and contributes to a stable brain environment secreting cerebrospinal fluid.

Summary

The central nervous system, although in some respects protected from the systemic environment, is acutely sensitive to changes in oxygen and glucose delivery because of a high dependence on oxidative metabolism of the latter as an energy source (see p. 209). In addition, the local chemical and ionic environment influences function. In the longer term, structure and function are influenced by aminoacid metabolism and factors affecting the synthesis and repair of membranes. Although metabolic disease may interfere with many facets of CNS function, only a limited number of clinical syndromes occur.

NEUROLOGICAL SYNDROMES

Systemic diseases may interfere with several metabolic processes, so that the changes within the nervous system are complex. The clinical manifestations depend on the rate of evolution of the disease and on the dominant site of dysfunction within the nervous system (Figs 14.1, 14.2).

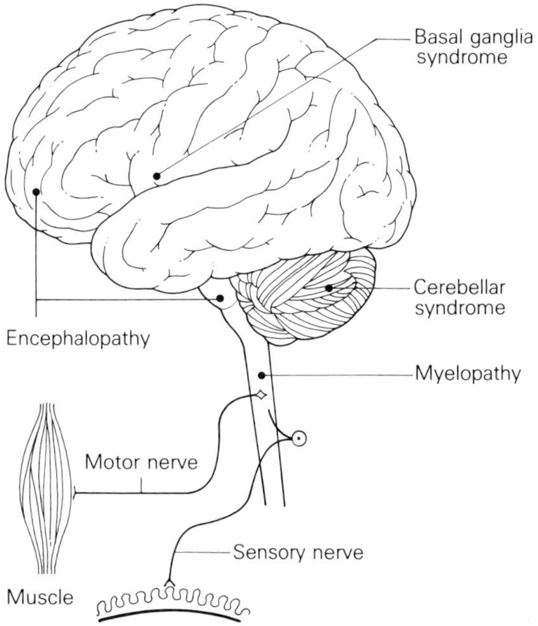

Fig. 14.2 *Sites of major impact in metabolic disorders of the nervous system.*

Acute Metabolic Encephalopathy

A rapidly-developing systemic disturbance may have widespread effects on the nervous system, and acute functional failure of the cerebrum leads to confusion, progressing to coma. The changes are more marked if the brain is immature, as in the young, or involuted, as in the elderly.

There is motor underactivity, excessive drowsiness, short attention span and distractibility, lack of a coherent train of thought, and disorientation for time (confusion). Overactivity and excitement with hallucinations (delirium) may supervene. The neurological signs of metabolic encephalopathy differ from those of progressive structural disease (e.g. expanding cerebral tumours) in that they tend to exhibit marked fluctuations.

Nonspecific findings are tremor, asterixis, and spontaneous muscle jerkings (myoclonus). Tremor combined with visual hallucinations and excitement is characteristic of alcoholic encephalopathy (delirium tremens). Asterixis which consists of episodic flexion of the wrist and fingers due to brief interruptions in muscle

tone is commonest in hepatic encephalopathy but is also seen in renal and respiratory insufficiency. Myoclonus occurs in uraemia, respiratory alkalosis, and penicillin and bismuth toxicity. In addition, epileptic seizures, choreiform and dystonic movements may occur. Muscle tone and tendon reflexes may be increased in hepatic encephalopathy and hyponatraemia; a slowed relaxation phase occurs in myxoedema and hyponatraemia. The respiratory rate may be depressed by the effects of drug intoxication or increased in states of metabolic acidosis (see also p. 52). Periodic breathing (Cheyne–Stokes respiration) is a late development.

Changes occur in the electroencephalogram which, in general, are nonspecific and consist of increased slow-wave activity. Sometimes characteristic phasic wave-forms are seen, as in hepatic encephalopathy. The amplitude of the wave-form may be severely reduced and the electroencephalographic record may become isoelectric in hypothermia, barbiturate intoxication and myxoedema.

Chronic Metabolic Disorders of the Nervous System

Some systemic diseases produced progressive structural damage to the nervous system, such as the neuronal loss and gliosis that accompany hepatic encephalopathy. Various sites may be preferentially affected (Fig. 14.2): neuropathy and myopathy are dealt with separately (see Chapters 16 and 17).

Neocortical syndrome

This is of insidious onset, not constant in its time-course, and there are fluctuations in the degree of mental and physical impairment. There is a decline in overall intellectual performance. Powers of concentration and attention fall and cause a fluctuating amnesia and temporal disorientation. There is difficulty in maintaining a coherent line of thought, leading to circumlocutory conversation. Aphasia and agnosia are rare.

If the frontal lobes are damaged, as in hepatic failure and alcohol abuse, then the patient's social behaviour may be abnormal with clowning, facetiousness and lack of insight.

Basal ganglia syndrome

The basal ganglia are damaged in hepato-lenticular degeneration (Wilson's disease, p. 162) and acquired hepatic encephalopathy in which choreic involuntary movements and dystonia occur. Parkinsonism may follow manganese and carbon monoxide intoxication. A variety of involuntary movements may occur and persist following treatment with psychotropic drugs (see p. 162).

Cerebellar syndrome

Cerebellar damage manifests in slurred speech (dysarthria), in incoordination of the arms (intention tremor), and an unsteady gait (ataxia), and is associated with myxoedema, hepatic failure, mercurial poisoning, chronic phenytoin intoxication and carcinoma (see p. 220). Chronic alcohol abuse may selectively affect the anterior lobe of the cerebellum, causing severe lower-limb ataxia.

Myelopathy

The spinal cord is preferentially affected in vitamin B_{12} (cobalamin) deficiency. Rarely, chronic hepatic failure presents with a spastic paraparesis with flexor plantar responses.

DISORDERS OF ENERGY AND NUTRIENT METABOLISM

Hypoxia

Every minute, 750 ml of blood is delivered to the brain, and oxygen is extracted from the blood at the rate of 50 ml per minute. The overall cerebral oxygen consumption remains relatively constant and is closely coupled to blood-flow. Cerebral hypoxia occurs in disease when either an adequate cerebral blood flow is associated with a decrease in arterial oxygen tension ($P\text{CO}_2$), i.e. hypoxic hypoxia, or when the cerebral blood flow is itself reduced, i.e. ischaemic hypoxia.

Anoxic hypoxia

This follows cardiac or pulmonary disease, periodic obstruction of the upper airway, neurological disorders leading to weak respiratory muscles, airways obstruction or impaired regulation of breathing. Carbon monoxide poisoning was formerly a common cause.

The brain has few energy reserves in the form of glycogen and high-energy phosphate and depends mainly on aerobic glycolysis (Fig. 14.3). Under conditions of acute hypoxia the first symptoms of metabolic encephalopathy begin to arise when the $Pa\text{O}_2$ falls to 60 mmHg. At $Pa\text{O}_2$ of 30 mmHg coma supervenes. Progressive hypoxia can, in part, be compensated for by increased anaerobic glycolysis which is, however, less efficient and results in rising lactic acid levels (Fig. 14.3). The latter, together with a further reduction in oxygen tension, inhibits glycolytic enzyme activity and causes an eventual depletion of high-energy phosphate stores. Actual neuronal damage and cell death is thought to be due to the release of free 'superoxide' radicals, which damage the cell membrane.

In *carbon monoxide poisoning* the high affinity of haemoglobin, myoglobin and cytochrome oxidase for carbon monoxide results in severe cellular and tissue

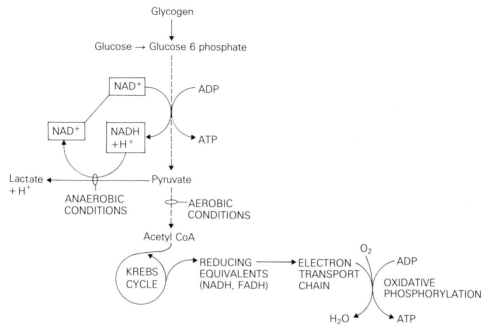

Fig. 14.3 *Aerobic and anaerobic metabolism of glycogen and glucose.*

hypoxia. Intoxication leads to acute encephalopathy, sometimes with visual field defects, papilloedema, retinal haemorrhage and death. A high proportion of survivors are left with chronic encephalopathy and basal ganglia disorders, such as Parkinsonism, which develop either immediately or after a latent period. Treatment consists of the administration of 100% oxygen in association with hyperbaric treatment if available.

Hypoventilation leads not only to *hypoxia* but also to *hypercapnia*. This in itself does not reduce the brain energy resources but leads to vasodilatation, an increase in cerebral blood-flow, and a rise in the intracranial pressure. A rise in $PaCO_2$ due to hypoventilation also causes cerebral acidosis and a depression of cerebral electrical excitability.

The treatment of hypoventilation consists essentially of maintaining adequate oxygenation, if necessary with assisted ventilation, whilst attempting to treat the underlying cause.

Ischaemic hypoxia

This most commonly follows cardiorespiratory arrest.

Consciousness is lost after 10 seconds, and irreversible brain damage occurs after a few minutes of complete circulatory arrest at normal body temperatures. During the period of circulatory arrest the brain suffers the effects of hypoxia and acidosis. Following resumption of the circulation the intravascular accumulation of aggregates of red blood cells, together with an increase in the blood viscosity, may lead to regions of ischaemia, particularly in the border zones between territories supplied by major vessels (p. 135).

Acute circulatory arrest such as that following myocardial infarction requires immediate restitution of the circulation, oxygenation, and the correction of acidosis.

Hypoglycaemia

The brain consumes 75 mg of glucose each minute which requires 50 ml of oxygen for oxidation via pyruvate and the tricarboxylic acid cycle (TCA) (Fig. 14.3). Under normal conditions only 15% of glucose is metabolised anaerobically with the formation of lactic acid. Oxidative phosphorylation takes place within neuronal mitochondria, which are able to travel through the cytoplasm to sites of high metabolic activity. Anaerobic glycolysis occurs in the cytoplasm.

In severe hypoglycaemia, all glucose reserves within the brain are exhausted after 1–2 hours and irreversible neuronal damage occurs due to autolysis of proteins and lipids. Hypoglycaemia thus presents with an acute encephalopathy which, if severe or recurrent, can lead to irreversible brain damage and dementia. Convulsions and coma may be the only symptoms but sometimes hypoglycaemia presents with the focal symptoms and signs together with preservation of consciousness. This is due to a differential glucose demand in different areas of the brain. The grey matter of the cortex and the hippocampi appears to have a selectively high glucose uptake. The cerebral features of glucose deficiency (neuroglycopenia) are not necessarily associated with obvious peripheral signs of sympathetic activity such as sweating and tachycardia.

The treatment of hypoglycaemia is by rapid infusion of high concentrations of glucose.

Deficiency of Vitamins (Table 14.2)

Nutritional deficiency in developed countries is usually seen only in socially isolated individuals such as the mentally ill and the elderly, and in those with chronic alcoholism. However, gastrointestinal disease and hepatic disorders also lead to malabsorption and abnormal utilisation of a normal dietary intake, whilst loss of protein, amino acids and salts may occur in chronic renal disease. In these conditions, deficiencies are usually multiple. Fortunately, the nervous system is able to synthesise necessary carbohydrate from glucose and can manufacture most proteins and complex lipids; it is therefore relatively protected in many deficiency states. Nevertheless, some exogenous source of certain vitamins, amino acids and fatty acids is essential.

Deficiencies of the B vitamins lead to acute and chronic disorders of the central nervous system as well as chronic polyneuropathy (Table 14.2).

Table 14.2

Vitamin Deficiencies

Vitamin	Function	Neurological syndrome
B$_1$ (thiamine)	Pyruvate metabolism	Wernicke's encephalopathy, Korsakoff psychosis Neuropathy
B$_3$ (nicotinic acid)	Component of coenzymes NAD, NADP (see Fig. 14.3)	Acute or chronic encephalopathy Brainstem or cerebellar syndrome Myelopathy
B$_6$ (pyridoxine)	Cofactor in protein metabolism	Neuropathy associated with isoniazid administration
B$_{12}$ (cobalamin)	Purine synthesis: Conversion of methyl-malonate to succinate: ?cyanide metabolism	Chronic encephalopathy (dementia) Myelopathy Neuropathy
Folic acid	Defective thymidylate (and hence DNA) synthesis	?Myelopathy ?Neuropathy ?Neural tube defect
D	Calcium/bone metabolism	Myopathy
E	Antioxidant Protects CNS membrane against 'free radicals'	Myelopathy (spinocerebellar degeneration) Neuropathy ?Myopathy

Thiamine (B₁) acts as a coenzyme for gamma ketoacid dehydrogenase and transketolase, and may form a component of membranes: deficiency may impair oxidative decarboxylation of pyruvate, causing increased blood levels of the latter. Thiamine deficiency is usually a result of a high metabolic demand for thiamine coexisting with dietary insufficiency, as in chronic alcohol abuse or starvation. Neuropathy and Wernicke's encephalopathy (see p. 213) are the main neurological features.

Nicotinic acid deficiency leads to abnormalities of intracellular energy utilisation; acute and chronic central and peripheral nervous dysfunction accompany the mucosal changes of pellagra.

'Vitamin B₁₂' (as methylcobalamin) is essential for the conversion of homocystine to methionine, permitting purine synthesis and (as adenosylcobalamin) for the conversion of methylmalonate to succinate. Cobalamin deficiency is most commonly due to lack of intrinisic factor secretion in the stomach, occasionally due to malabsorption in the terminal ileum and, more rarely, to strict vegetarianism. Haematological features of B₁₂ deficiency may or may not coexist with the neurological manifestations of deficiency, which include peripheral neuropathy, subacute combined degeneration of the spinal cord (see p. 171), optic atrophy, and dementia.

Deficiency of folic acid has been associated with neurological manifestations in dietary deficiencies, gastrointestinal disorders, and drug toxicity (e.g. anticonvulsant drugs), but its primary causal role is still the subject of debate.

Vitamin D deficiency is associated with muscle weakness (see p. 260) and through its effect on calcium metabolism may affect the nervous system (see p. 215).

Vitamin E deficiency may be associated with a neuropathy and spinocerebellar degeneration.

Amino Acid Disorders

Several inborn errors of metabolism effect amino-acid metabolism, e.g. phenylketonuria (see p. 218). Amino acids are taken up into the brain by specific uptake mechanisms common to various groups. The brain amino-acid concentration reflects the relative concentration of competing amino acids in the plasma rather than a specific plamsa amino acid itself. Since amino acids are the precursors of neurotransmitters, a major disturbance of supply may be expected to have severe effects, e.g. dopamine excess with ingestion of L-dopa (see p. 158). Alterations in brain amino acids may also be an important factor in acquired metabolic encephalopathy, e.g. due to liver disease.

Mitochondrial Disorders

Mitochondria are the major sites of energy production in the cell. Failure of mitochondrial function leads to reduced ATP synthesis, accumulation of reducing equivalents, and acidosis. Such failure is more likely to affect organs with a high energy turnover such as the retina, nervous system, skeletal muscle, heart and liver. A number of rare, probably genetic, disorders are recognised (see p. 261), but it seems likely that various acquired disorders and toxins may impair some aspect of mitochondrial function although the precise mechanism remains ill-defined.

Other Specific Disorders (Fig. 14.1)

Hepatic encephalopathy

This may present in acute and chronic forms when porto-systemic shunting of blood occurs secondary to chronic liver disease. The effects of shunting may alter the supply of glucose and nutrients to the brain, disrupt acid–base and electrolyte homeostasis, prevent structural membrane maintenance, and induce disorders of neurotransmission.

In chronic hepatic failure, branch-chain amino acids in both brain and cerebrospinal fluid are increased, although the plasma concentrations are normal, suggesting an increased brain uptake. By contrast, in acute hepatic failure the plasma aromatic amino acids are increased. The hyperammonaemia associated with hepatic failure and porto-systemic shunting is thought not to be the primary cause of encephalopathy.

The treatment of hepatic encephalopathy is directed

towards the treatment of the primary hepatic disease, reducing dietary nitrogen intake and sparing protein catabolism, preventing hypoglycaemia and, possibly, administering catecholamine neurotransmitter precursors such as L-dopa.

Hepatic porphyria

Three forms of hepatic porphyria affect the nervous system: porphyria variegata; copro-porphyria; and the commonest, acute intermittent porphyria, in which recurrent encephalopathy, peripheral neuropathy and abdominal crises occur. The encephalopathy may be of the confusional or psychotic form. A basic and inherited deficiency of the enzyme uroporphyrinogen-1-synthetase underlies porphyria and, in acute attacks, increases in circulating delta amino laevulinic acid (ALA) and porphobilinogen (PBG) occur. Drugs which induce ALA synthetase, such as barbiturates and phenytoin, can precipitate acute attacks of encephalopathy.

Precisely how the metabolic abnormality of porphyria disrupts nervous function is unknown. Acute porphyric crises do, however, have clinical features akin to known cases of mitochondrial dysfunction, including episodic occurrence of hyperthermia, weight-loss, tachycardia and encephalopathy. It is also of interest that drugs which interfere with mitochondrial metabolism (barbiturates, benzodiazepines, chloramphenicol, progesterone) may precipitate porphyric crises.

Toxins

Carbon monoxide, cyanide and carbon disulphide

These cause major disturbances of oxidative metabolism (see p. 208).

Lead poisoning

Plumbism results from the ingestion and inhalation of excessive amounts of lead occurring in industrial plants, paints, the fluids contained in lead piping and in the exhaust fumes from vehicles using petrol containing high concentrations of lead tetraethyl.

Acute encephalopathy is seen largely in children and is accompanied by seizures, papilloedema and meningitis. Pathologically, the brain is oedematous. Chronic encephalopathy is a more common manifestation, with dementia and epilepsy.

Lead intoxication also leads to chronic motor neuropathy, typically presenting with wrist drop and finger extensor weakness, abdominal colic and anaemia.

Treatment with chelating agents (Calcium EDTA, BAL, and penicillamine) leads to improvement in encephalopathy and neuropathy.

Mercury poisoning

Organic (methyl, ethyl mercury) mercury poisoning causes a chronic encephalopathy with ataxia, dysarthria and tremors as well as a neuropathy: outbreaks have occurred in the past due to the use on wheat of a mercury-containing fungicide in Iraq and due to the conversion of inorganic mercuric chloride to methyl mercury by marine organisms with subsequent entry into shellfish and hence the food cycle in Japan (Minamata Bay outbreak). Elemental mercury may be ingested or the vapour inhaled causing personality and behavioural changes, limb and head tremors (hatter's shakes). Pathologically the granular cells of the cerebral and cerebellar cortices are selectively damaged.

Manganese poisoning

Industrial inhalation of manganese dust (e.g. in miners) may lead to a chronic encephalopathy and Parkinsonism.

Whether intoxication with the heavy metals mercury and manganese may interfere with enzymatic activity, as may be the case with lead, is not known. Treatment, however, is by administration of chelating agents.

Alcohol intoxication

Chronic ethanol ingestion may be associated with complex changes in systemic and cerebral chemistry, perhaps accompanied by alcoholic cirrhosis or hepatic encephalopathy (see above). Essential nutrients such as thiamine may be reduced by malnutrition, and hypoglycaemia may occur. Acid–base and electrolyte homeostasis are disturbed and ketoacidosis, hyponatraemia, hypokalaemia, hypophosphataemia, hypocal-caemia and hypomagnesaemia have been associated with acute alcoholic encephalopathy. Cell membranes, especially those of cerebral capillaries, are defective possibly due to acetaldehyde formation.

Chronic alcoholism produces a number of acute and chronic neurological syndromes.

Acute syndromes: i. *Delirium tremens* is an acute encephalopathy often following alcohol withdrawal, in which frightening visual hallucinations, tremors and sometimes seizures occur, with a confusional state but with no depression of consciousness.

ii. *Wernicke's encephalopathy* is associated with alcohol abuse, malnutrition and thiamine deficiency. Acute capillary haemorrhages, astrocytosis and neuronal death in the upper brainstem and diencephalon lead to a reduced conscious level (sometimes coma), opthal-moplegia and ataxia. Rarely, the syndrome follows malnutrition and prolonged vomiting or diarrhoea due to gastrointestinal disease or in pregnancy.

iii. *Central pontine myelinolysis* consists of demyelination of fibre tracts within the pons, leading to the rapid development of paralysis of the face, bulbar muscles and limbs. Malnutrition and liver disease are common accompaniments. Hyponatraemia is frequently present and may be involved in the pathogenesis of the condition.

The treatment of the acute alcoholic encephalopathies consists of correcting fluid balance, acid–base and electrolyte disturbance, and administration of calories – usually as glucose initially – together with high doses of intravenous thiamine and other B vitamins. Systemic infection is common and requires exclusion. Anticonvulsant drugs and tranquillisers may be required in the epileptic and delirious patient. Head trauma with skull fracture and subdural haematoma is much commoner in the alcoholic and should be considered as a contributory factor in all such patients.

Chronic syndromes: i. *Cerebral atrophy and dementia.* Often the frontal lobes are severely affected and social misconduct, change in personality and lack of insight are prominent symptoms along with failure of memory. Dysarthria, nystagmus and tremor may coexist. Wer-

nicke's encephalopathy may lead on to a chronic amnesic syndrome with loss of short-term memory and confabulation (Korsakoff's psychosis)

ii. *Cerebellar syndrome*: The cells of the cerebellar cortex, especially the Purkinje cells of the anterior lobes, may be selectively damaged in chronic alcoholism, leading to progressive ataxia and loss of balance.

iii. *Peripheral disorders*: Peripheral neuropathy (see p. 246) and a range of muscle disorders, including acute rhabdomyolysis and a proximal myopathy with type II fibre atrophy, also occur.

The treatment of these chronic neurological disorders consists of the withdrawal of alcohol, reversal of malnutrition, and the administration of high doses of vitamins including thiamine. After 'drying out', treatment of the underlying disease of alcoholism can begin.

Tropical conditions

In the Tropics, chronic optic atrophy, myelopathy and peripheral neuropathy are seen in undernourished populations, who may also be exposed to toxins contained in vegetables and bush teas. In India a chronic myelopathy has been linked to the consumption of lathyrus peas.

Disorders of Acid–Base, Electrolyte or Hormone Balance

Impaired water and electrolyte balance occurs commonly in gastrointestinal, renal, hepatic and endocrine disease, or as a result of intravenous fluid or diuretic therapy. Vomiting may result in metabolic alkalosis, and severe diarrhoea or enteric fluid-loss may cause potassium and bicarbonate depletion. In renal failure metabolic acidosis, sodium, potassium and water retention, an accumulation of urea and other nitrogenous compounds occurs: hypertension and altered vitamin D and calcium homeostasis are further features, all of which may prejudice cerebral function. Disorders of the neurohypophysis and hypothalamus have a particular influence on water balance, whilst abnormalities of adrenal and adrenocorticotrophic hormone function affect salt balance.

Acid–base

According to the Henderson–Hasselbach equation pH is determined principally by the ratio log $[HCO_2^-]/[CO_2]$. Changes in this ratio in the brain and CSF do not precisely parallel those in blood, because CO_2 diffuses more rapidly across the blood–brain barrier than does bicarbonate. For example, in treating metabolic acidosis with a bicarbonate infusion, the blood $PaCO_2$ may rise: CO_2 diffuses into the CSF ahead of bicarbonate thus reducing the ratio and paradoxically increasing acidosis initially. Severe acidosis has a deleterious effect on brain metabolism by causing inhibition of glycolysis, reducing red cell 2'3 diphosphoglycerate resulting in lowered tissue oxygen availability and causing secondary hyperventilation which gives reduced cerebral blood-flow.

Disorders of water balance

Water intoxication/hyponatraemia (Table 14.3): When plasma water increases inappropriately, sodium concentration and plasma osmolality fall. Water enters the brain by osmosis and this may result in acute encephalopathy with fits. The commonest cause of this situation is the inappropriate use of intravenous fluids (notably 5% dextrose), particularly when renal handling of water may be (albeit temporarily) impaired, e.g. following surgery or other major stress. Many neurological disorders cause inappropriate water retention, notably head injury, meningitis, encephalitis or acute stroke, or acute Gullain–Barré syndrome: compulsive water-drinking is rare. A variety of systemic diseases, particularly carcinoma of lung, and various chronic lung, liver and gastrointestinal disorders, may cause or even present with neurological features due to inappropriate water retention and hyponatraemia.

The diagnosis is confirmed by measurement of plasma and urine osmolalities and electrolytes. Initial treatment is water restriction with careful monitoring of fluid and electrolyte balance. Occasionally, hypertonic saline solutions are given to raise sodium concentration rapidly, or pharmacological means of inhibiting renal water retention, e.g. lithium or demeclocycline, are used.

Hyperosmolality: This results either from excess solute accumulation or inappropriate loss of plasma water. Solute excess occurs as glucose in diabetes or as urea (and other compounds) in renal failure. The brain may shrink due to osmotic loss of fluid and an encephalopathy can develop, with muscle twitching and fits. Brain osmolality gradually increases and only slowly equilibrates with blood. The precise composition of the

---

Table 14.3

Hyponatraemia

Mechanism	Example
a. Dilutional	Excessive inappropriate intravenous fluids Compulsive water drinking
b. Inappropriate ADH secretion	Systemic: Carcinoma 　　　　　Chronic infective lung disease 　　　　　Liver/gastrointestinal disease
	Drugs: Vincristine 　　　　Carbamazepine 　　　　Phenothiazines 　　　　Tranylcypromine
	Neurological: Head injury 　　　　　　Infection 　　　　　　Stroke 　　　　　　Guillain–Barré syndrome 　　　　　　Acute intermittent porphyria

solute in such brain in these conditions is uncertain and it is postulated that, in addition to potassium, chloride and sodium, there is intracellular production of 'idiogenic osmoles'.

Hyperosmolality characterised by hypernatraemia (Table 14.4) also results from failure of renal water retention, due to reduced or absent secretion of antidiuretic hormone by the neurohypophysis or to reduced renal sensitivity to the latter as a consequence of, e.g., hypokalaemia or hypercalcaemia. Rarely, severe hypernatraemia is caused by failure of the thirst mechanism due to hypothalamic disease – usually vascular damage or tumour – and, if combined with impaired ADH secretion, very high plasma sodium levels result, causing encephalopathy and muscle weakness.

In disorders where hypertonicity is due to prolonged accumulation of abnormal solute, e.g. diabetes or renal failure, excessively rapid corection of plasma osmolality may lead to water uptake by the relatively hypertonic brain, causing cerebral oedema and worsening encephalopathy. This is a particular risk in renal dialysis (dialysis disequilibrium). In children, brain shrinkage associated with severe water loss may cause small haemorrhages or venous thrombosis.

Treatment of diabetes insipidus can be anticipated and prevented or minimised by careful observation of patients at risk, e.g. following pituitary surgery or head trauma. Incontinence may cause the diagnosis to be missed in its early stages of development. Appropriate investigation for the underlying cause, and fluid balance correction, possibly with supplementary vasopressin, is then carried out.

Disorders of Calcium and Phosphate Metabolism

Hypo- and hypercalcaemia

In the central nervous system, calcium is particularly involved in the control of neurotransmitter release and reuptake. In the peripheral nervous system it takes part in acetylcholine release at the neuromuscular junction and excitation–contraction coupling in muscle. Changes in serum calcium, particularly ionised calcium, may therefore produce nervous and muscular disorders. Serum calcium and parathyroid hormone are intimately related and it is thought that high levels of either may be neurotoxic. Raised levels of parathyroid hormone in renal failure have been correlated with abnormalities of the electroencephalogram and motor nerve conduction. Disturbances of vitamin D metabolism and several other causes of hypo- or hypercalcaemia have an effect on the nervous system or on muscle.

Table 14.4

Hypernatraemia

Mechanism	Examples
a. Solute excess	Diabetes mellitus, renal failure, hyperosmolar intravenous fluids
b. Water depletion	
i. Reduced intake	Impaired thirst mechanism
ii. Increased extra renal loss	Burns, skin loss Diarrhoea, vomiting
iii. Increased renal loss	Reduced antidiuretic hormone secretion (pituitary surgery, hypothalamic disease, trauma)
	Reduced renal response to ADH (nephrogenic diabetes insipidus, hypokalaemia, hypercalcaemia)

Both hypo- and hypercalacemia may lead to mild chronic encephalopathy, often with psychiatric features such as depression. Seizures, both generalised and partial, are more likely to occur in hypocalcaemia than in hypercalcaemia but the electroencephalogram is abnormal in both states. Chronic hypocalcaemia (usually due to pseudohypo- or hypoparathyroidism) may be associated with raised intracranial pressure and papilloedema, thus mimicking a cerebral tumour. Frank tetany or a positive Trousseau or Chvostek sign point to hypocalcaemia in the absence of acute respiratory alkalosis due to hyperventilation. Muscular weakness and limb pains occur in several conditions causing hypo- or hypercalcaemia. The tendon reflexes are increased in hypercalcaemia and decreased in hypocalcaemia. Hypocalcaemia requires investigation and treatment of the underlying cause. Rarely, a low serum calcium requires urgent parenteral correction if, for example, intractable fits are occurring. Hypercalcaemia, whilst needing investigation, also more frequently requires symptomatic treatment. Rehydration is the most important aspect of this in the acute stages.

Hypophosphataemia

Encephalopathy occurs when the plasma phosphate level falls to less than 1 mg per 100 ml. Often a chronic inadequate intake of phosphate is associated with an acute depression of levels following the administration of glucose, insulin or lipid.

When hypophosphataemia occurs during hyperalimentation, 2'3 diphosphoglycerate in red blood cells in lowered, causing reduced tissue oxygen availability. The alcoholic patient is particularly vulnerable during treatment for alcoholic withdrawal when, in addition to hypophosphataemia, metabolic acidosis causes hyperventilation with a consequent reduction in cerebral blood-flow.

The treatment of hypophosphataemia consists of supplementary phosphate together with treatment of the associated conditions giving rise to the acute change in phosphate levels. Severe hypophosphataemia may require acute correction with intravenous potassium phosphate.

Potassium

Perhaps surprisingly, plasma potassium levels have little overt effect on cerebral function. The predominant effect of hypokalaemia is muscle weakness (see p. 261). Hyperkalaemia causes major cardiac dysrhythmias before it affects muscle function, although weakness and myotonia do occur in rare genetically-determined disorders marked by hyperkalaemia.

Hormone Disorders

It is relatively common for disorders of the central or peripheral nervous system to be the presenting feature of an endocrine disorder. The major associations are summarised in Table 14.5.

Thyroid

Thyrotoxicosis may cause an acute encephalopathy with fits and, rarely, chorea. Much more commonly it causes anxiety, marked postural tremor and muscle weakness (see p. 260). Hypothyroidism may present with coma associated with hypothermia. Many adults with the condition notice impaired memory and may have a dementia: deafness, cerebellar ataxia and complaints of muscle weakness, cramps and aches are frequent (see p. 260). In infants, hypothyroidism is an important cause of retarded development.

Corticosteroids

Therapeutic corticosteroids may occasionally precipitate a severe encephalopathy with psychotic features. Psychiatric disturbance with depression is common in Cushing's disease, and muscle weakness is common in many cases of corticosteroid excess, either due to hypokalaemia or muscle-fibre atrophy. Addison's disease may cause an encephalopathy and muscle weakness.

Pituitary

Acromegaly is usually associated with a significantly-sized growth-hormone-secreting tumour of the anterior pituitary gland. Apart from visual field disturbances due to chiasmal compression (and other local effects), mental change in the myopathy are recognised features of this endocrinological disturbance.

Table 14.5

Endocrine Disorders – Metabolic Effects

Disease	Major biochemical abnormalities	Neurological syndrome
Hypopituitarism	Hypoglycaemia Hyponatremia Hypothermia	Acute or chronic encephalopathy Individual hormone deficiencies
Thyrotoxicosis	Hyperthyroidism	Acute encephalopathy, chorea Anxiety, tremor, muscle wasting
Myxoedema	Hypothyroidism	Acute encephelopathy (coma) Chronic encephalopathy (-dementia, cerebellar syndrome, deafness,) Hypothermia, Neuropathy, Myopathy
Cushing's syndrome	Corticosteroid excess	Acute encephalopathy (psychosis) Chronic encephalopathy (depression) Myopathy
Addison's disease	Corticosteroid deficiency	Acute encephalopathy Myopathy
Acromegaly	Growth hormone excess	Chronic encephalopathy Myopathy
Hyperparathyroidism Hypoparathyroidism	Hypercalcaemia (1° type) Hypocalcaemia (Hypo-para or 2° hyperparathyroidism)	Acute or chronic encephalopathy Myopathy
Insulinoma	Hyperinsulinism/hypoglycaemia	Acute or chronic encephalopathy (focal or generalised features)
Diabetes mellitus	Hyperglycaemia, ketoacidosis Electrolyte imbalance	Acute encephalopathy (focal or generalised features) Neuropathy

Parathyroid hormone (see p. 215)

Insulin

Episodes of hypoglycaemia are the presenting feature of insulin-secreting tumours of the pancreas but the presentation may be odd 'giddy spells' or 'blackouts' which require distinction from epilepsy, syncope and vertigo (see p. 118). In a known diabetic on insulin any odd 'turn' should be suspected of being hypoglycaemic in the first instance.

Hyperglycaemia may be associated with coma in diabetic ketoacidosis or a non-ketotic hyperosmolar state. Diabetes mellitus may present with a focal neurological deficit due to cranial nerve palsy, a cerebrovascular event or symptoms due to a peripheral neuropathy.

Other disorders

Phaeochromocytoma may present with severe paroxysmal headaches associated with raised blood pressure, and occasionally subarachnoid haemorrhage.

INBORN ERRORS OF METABOLISM

Inborn errors of metabolism are genetically-determined diseases which usually give rise to symptoms in childhood. Many of them are caused by a specific enzyme deficiency which results in blocking of a metabolic pathway and disruption of normal cell function. Inheritance is autosomal recessive in the majority of enzyme deficiencies, although a small number are X-linked. In autosomal recessive disorders, affected individuals (homozygotes) usually have virtually undetectable levels of enzyme activity. Enzyme assay can thus be used in antenatal diagnosis for fetuses known to be at risk of inheriting a specific disorder. Heterozygote (carrier) parents tend to have levels of activity midway between normal and the homozygous state. Populations in which a particular disorder has a high prevalence can therefore be screened for carriers.

The symptoms and signs of inborn errors of metabolism vary enormously and their pathogenesis is often poorly understood. Mental retardation is the commonest neurological feature. A summary of the clinical and genetic features of some of the more important inborn errors of metabolism affecting the nervous system is shown in Table 14.6. Two examples are described in more detail below.

Phenylketonuria

Phenylketonuria (PKU) is the second (after cystic fibrosis) most frequent autosomal recessive disorder in the UK; the incidence is about 1 in 10 000 live births. Affected children are normal at birth and in the neonatal period. Developmental delay becomes apparent at around the age of three months. The child then fails to sit, walk, or talk at the appropriate times. The IQ of untreated patients is usually under 50. Behavioural abnormalities and microcephaly are common, and seizures occur in one-quarter. At autopsy the brain is small and shows loss of myelin accompanied by fibrillary gliosis.

The normal conversion of phenylalanine to tyrosine does not occur in children with PKU, due to a deficiency of hepatic phenylalanine hydroxylase. Circulating levels of phenylalanine are high, and excess amounts of phenylalanine and phenylpyruvic acid are excreted in the urine. If a low-phenylalanine diet is instituted before the end of the first month of life, intellectual development is normal. The diet can be relaxed or discontinued in late childhood, as the hyperphenylalaninaemia does not seen to affect the mature nervous system. However, female patients contemplating pregnancy must return to dietary restriction because the increased circulating phenylalanine has an adverse affect on the fetus and gives rise to retarded, microcephalic offspring. Antenatal diagnosis of PKU is not currently available. Neonatal screening of blood for excess phenylalanine is performed in most countries where the disorder has a high prevalence.

Tay–Sachs Disease

Tay–Sachs disease is particularly common in the Ashkenazi Jewish population, where it has an incidence of 1 in 3–4 000 live births. It is a hundred times less frequent in other racial groups. Inheritance is autosomal recessive. The first sign of the disease is usually an abnormal startle reflex to sound, consisting of limb extension and myoclonus, in the first few weeks of life. Early development is normal but psychomotor regression becomes manifest between the ages of four to six months. The child does not sit up, loses head control, and takes no interest in its environment. By the end of the first year blindness is obvious. This is associated with the finding of a cherry-red spot at the macula. This appearance is caused by the normally red macula contrasting with a surrounding pale area of retina containing abnormal amounts of stored lipid. Lipid storage in the brain results in enlargement of the head. By the third year the child is demented, blind, cachectic, and assumes a decerebrate posture. Death occurs between the ages of three and five years.

The enzyme hexosaminidase A, which splits the terminal N-acetylgalactosamine residue from GM_2 ganglioside, is deficient in patients with Tay–Sachs disease. This results in accumulation of ganglioside (a type of glycolipid) and distension of neurones in the central nervous system and autonomic ganglia, as well as the ganglion cells in the retina.

Tay–Sachs disease can be diagnosed antenatally by measuring hexosaminidase A activity in cultured amniotic fluid cells. Carriers can be detected with a fairly high degree of accuracy using leucocytes for the

Table 14.6

Inborn Errors of Metabolism

Disorder	Clinical Features	Inheritance	Deficiency
Lipid metabolism			
Leucodystrophies: e.g. metachromatic (late infantile)	Dementia, ataxia, areflexia, spasticity, in first decade	AR	Aryl sulphatase A
Gangliosidoses: e.g. Tay–Sachs disease	see text		
Sphingolipidoses: e.g. Niemann–Pick disease	Failure to thrive, dementia, cherry-red spot, hepatosplenomegaly, death by age of 3	AR	Sphingomyelinase
Mucopolysaccharidoses			
e.g. Hurler's disease	Dementia, corneal opacities, skeletal dysplasia, coarse facies, hepatomegaly, before the age of 3	AR	α-L-iduronidase
Carbohydrate metabolism			
e.g. Pompe's disease	Myopathy, cardiomegaly, macroglossia, in infancy	AR	Acid maltase
Amino acid metabolism			
e.g. Phenylketonuria	see text		
Purine & pyrimidine metabolism			
e.g. Lesch–Nyhan syndrome	Athetosis, mental retardation, self-mutilation, gout in first decade	X-L	Hypoxanthine guanine phosphoribosyl transferase
Urea cycle defects			
e.g. ornithine trancarbamylase deficiency	Intermittent ataxia, vomiting, mental retardation in females. Neonatal death in males	X-L transcarbamylase	Ornithine
Trace metal metabolism			
e.g. Wilson's disease (see p. 162)	Tremor, ataxia, parkinsonism, cirrhosis, usually before age of 20	AR	Unknown. low serum Cu and caeruloplasmin

AR = autosomal recessive; X-L = linked

assay; this allows screening in high-risk populations such as the Ashkenazi Jewish population in the eastern United States. The risk of two carrier parents having an affected child is 25%.

There is no known treatment for this disease, nor for many other inborn errors of metabolism. Prevention, by means of antenatal diagnosis, is an important aspect of management. Children with neurodegenerative disorders require much supportive care from both medical and community services, as do their parents. This topic has been dealt with in depth by Brett (see p. 280).

THE EFFECTS OF SYSTEMIC CANCER ON THE NERVOUS SYSTEM

The nervous system may be involved by primary cancer elsewhere in the body through several mechanisms (Table 14.7).

Table 14.7

Effects of Systemic Cancer on the Nervous System

Direct invasion from adjacent structures
Metastatic disease
Non-metastatic 'remote' effects
Secondary effects due to immunosuppression, effects on bone marrow, biochemical effects
The effects of treatment

Metastatic Disease (Fig. 14.4)

Metastases in the brain are common with primary carcinoma of lung, breast, kidney, thyroid, prostate and, to a lesser extent, stomach and bowel. Only rarely is the spinal cord a site for mestastases, although it is commonly compressed by carcinoma or lymphoma arising in the spinal meninges or vertebral column. Metastases may involve the bones of the skull, particularly the base, to cause single or multiple cranial nerve palsies or orbital lesions. The meninges are sometimes infiltrated (see p. 225), with or without involvement of cranial nerves, spinal cord, or nerve roots. The brachial and lumbosacral plexuses can be directly invaded by carcinoma of the apex of the lung in the former case or by gynaecological, prostatic or large-bowel cancers in the latter (see p. 243).

Non-metastatic Effects of Cancer (Fig. 14.4)

The cause of many of the remote 'non-metastatic' effects of cancer remains unknown. A variety of mechanisms probably act to cause a wide variety of clinical syndromes.

Encephalopathy

A cerebral disturbance, with or without focal neurological signs or seizures, can result from hyponatraemia due to inappropriate ADH secretion (oat cell carcinoma of the lung probably causes a low sodium concentration most frequently), hypercalcaemia as a result of secretion of parathormone-like substances by tumour (or from metastatic bone disease), or hypoglycaemia. A diffuse inflammatory infiltration of the limbic system occasionally causes an amnesic syndrome or dementia. Patients with leukaemia or lymphomas are susceptible to a unusual viral infection caused by 'JC virus' and known as progressive multifocal leukoencephalopathy (PML). Multiple white-matter lesions result in visual field defects, hemiplegia, dysphasia, coma and death over the course of a few months. Antiviral drugs have been effective in some cases.

Hyperviscosity of the blood, as in Waldenstrom's macroglobulinaemia, may cause headaches, confusion, papilloedema, focal signs and retinopathy. Other haematological disturbances include coagulation problems resulting in intracranial haemorrhage or disseminated intravascular coagulation causing thrombotic events and stroke.

Brainstem/cranial nerves

A rare subacute cerebellar degeneration occurs in association with carcinoma and often precedes its clinical appearance. The features are a severe and progressive ataxia, dysarthria, nystagmus and, not infrequently, corticospinal tract signs. The cranial nerves may be affected as part of a non-metastatic subacute polyneuritis, particularly in lymphomas.

Myelopathy/spinal roots

Compression by extradural tumour is the commonest cause of involvement of these structures (see p. 166), but occasionally the cauda equina may be coated with a thin layer of metastatic cells and no abnormality is seen on radiculography. Less commonly a degenerative and necrotic process may affect the spinal cord, selectively affecting the anterior horn cells to cause a syndrome superficially resembling motor neurone disease (see Chapter 13). Immunosuppression associated with lymphoma or its treatment may be a precipitating cause for herpes zoster affecting the nerve roots or causing a myelopathy (see p. 233).

Peripheral nerve/muscle

A neuromyopathy causing weakness, wasting and sensory disturbance occurs in about 14% of patients with lung cancer, 4–5% of those with breast cancer and 2–8% of those with lymphoma. It may precede the manifestations of the tumour by up to three years. The sensory features are painful paraesthesiae, numbness and ataxia but, less commonly, wasting and weakness are the major feature. The presentation may be acute, akin to Guillain–Barré syndrome, or subacute over weeks or months. A clue to the diagnosis in these patients may be the presence of lymphocytes in the CSF and a raised CSF protein. Nerve conduction studies indicate a predominant axonal degeneration, or segmental demyelination, or a mixture of both (see pp. 58 and 239).

Occasionally a paraprotein band in the blood may represent a discrete immunoglobulin band with specific activity against the myelin sheaths of peripheral nerves (see also p. 246).

The Lambert–Eaton myasthenic syndrome may result in ocular, bulbar and limb muscle weakness and is most often associated with oatcell carcinoma of the lung; there may be immunological damage to a presynaptic antigen. Polymyositis is sometimes associated with carcinoma, and muscle weakness may also result from excess corticosteroid secretion or hypokalaemia promoted by the secretion of ACTH-like substances from some tumours, notably oatcell carcinoma of the lung.

Effects of Treatment of Cancer (Fig. 14.5)

An active approach to the treatment of malignant disease has resulted in increased numbers of neurologi-

cal complications caused by the effects of irradiation, drugs and opportunistic infection.

Irradiation (see also p. 172)

The effect of therapeutic irradiation depends on the site, size of field, dose, fractionation of the dose, and susceptibility (tolerance threshold) of the particular type of neural tissue. Although acute swelling of the brain may accompany radiation treatment for intracranial tumour there is usually a latent period between the end of irradiation and the onset of symptoms which may vary from a few months to many years.

Radiation myelopathy (see p. 172)

Brachial plexus injury

Symptoms usually develop a year or so after treatment for breast carcinoma, and radiogenic skin changes are commonly present. Pain in the shoulder and arm and progressive sensory and motor deficits occur. The principal differential diagnosis is carcinomatous infiltration of the plexus; symptoms less than six months after the end of treatment, very severe pain, a palpable mass, or a Horner's syndrome tend to favour this possiblility.

Lumbosacral plexus

Irradiation to the lymph nodes in the para-aortic or inguinal regions, or to structures in the pelvic cavity or lumbosacral spine may be associated, again after a latent period of more than a year, with neurogenic lesions. The motor fibres may be selectively involved and occasionally severe weakness occurs in the legs whilst sensory loss and sphincter dysfunction are less prominent.

Immunosuppression

Craniospinal irradiation for leukaemia or lymphoma may cause bone-marrow suppression. This may also follow the use of cytotoxic drugs, and opportunistic infection may involve the nervous system, causing encephalitis or meningitis (see p. 224). Immunosuppressant drugs may have a wide range of side-effects, notably the neuropathy associated with vincristine or cisplatinum treatment. Corticosteroid treatment may result in muscle weakness due to fibre atrophy or hypokalaemia (see p. 261).

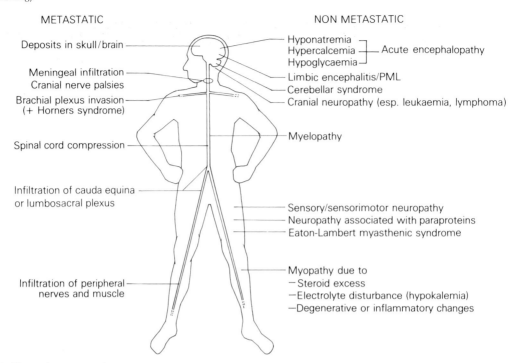

Fig. 14.4 *Effects of cancer on the nervous system.*

METASTATIC

- Deposits in skull/brain
- Meningeal infiltration Cranial nerve palsies
- Brachial plexus invasion (+ Horners syndrome)
- Spinal cord compression
- Infiltration of cauda equina or lumbosacral plexus
- Infiltration of peripheral nerves and muscle

NON METASTATIC

- Hyponatremia
- Hypercalcemia ⎤— Acute encephalopathy
- Hypoglycaemia
- Limbic encephalitis/PML
- Cerebellar syndrome
- Cranial neuropathy (esp. leukaemia, lymphoma)
- Myelopathy
- Sensory/sensorimotor neuropathy
- Neuropathy associated with paraproteins
- Eaton-Lambert myasthenic syndrome
- Myopathy due to
  —Steroid excess
  —Electrolyte disturbance (hypokalemia)
  —Degenerative or inflammatory changes

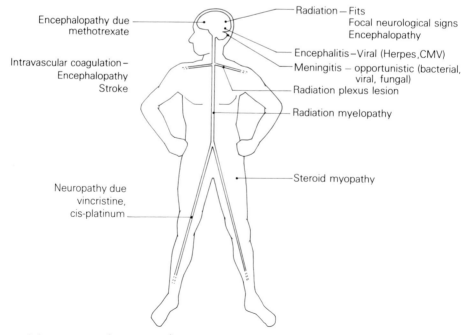

Fig. 14.5 *Effects of the treatment of cancer on the nervous system.*

- Encephalopathy due methotrexate
- Intravascular coagulation — Encephalopathy Stroke
- Neuropathy due vincristine, cis-platinum
- Radiation — Fits
  Focal neurological signs
  Encephalopathy
- Encephalitis – Viral (Herpes, CMV)
- Meningitis — opportunistic (bacterial, viral, fungal)
- Radiation plexus lesion
- Radiation myelopathy
- Steroid myopathy

15

Infective and Inflammatory Disorders

MENINGITIS

In infective meningitis there is inflammation of the pial and arachnoid membranes caused by viruses, bacteria, fungi or other organisms.

Routes of Infection and Main Organisms

Microorganisms reach the meninges either by direct extension – from the ears, from the nasopharynx, through a dural tear after injury or surgery, or through a congenital sinus communicating with the subarach-

noid space – or by spread in the bloodstream. Extension of a parameningeal infective process within the brain may also cause meningitis. A very wide spectrum of organisms can infect the meninges. The commoner organisms are listed in Table 15.1.

These organisms produce a variety of clinical events, from the self-limiting benign condition of *acute aseptic meningitis*, caused by viruses, to the lethal *acute pyogenic meningitis* caused by many bacteria; chronic meningitic illnesses may be produced by tuberculosis, fungi and other processes – neoplastic cells, contrast media, blood from subarachnoid haemorrhage, and drugs.

Table 15.1

Infective Causes of Meningitis in Britain

Bacteria and Mycoplasma	Viruses	Fungi and Other
Neisseria meningitidis	ECHO	Cryptococcus neoformans
Haemophilus influenzae	Coxsackie	
Streptococcus pneumoniae	Infectious mononucleosis	(Coccidioides immitis,
	Mumps	Histoplasma capsulatum,
		Blastomyces dermatididis, in USA)
Escherichia coli		
Streptococci (Groups B and C)	Poliomyelitis	
Staphylococcus aureus		
Treponema pallidum		
Listeria monocytogenes		
Staphylococcus epidermis		
Acinetobacter spp.		
Mycobacterium tuberculosis		
Leptospira spp.		
Mycoplasma pneumoniae		
Salmonella spp.		

For practical purposes, outside the neonatal period, 70% of acute pyogenic meningitis in Britain is caused by *Neisseria meningitidis*, *Haemophilus influenzae* and *Streptococcus pneumoniae*, all of which colonise the nasopharynx. *H. influenzae* tends to be rare after the age of six and *S. pneumoniae* becomes the commonest organism after the age of 50.

The Meningitic Syndrome

The meningitic syndrome is frequently heralded by sudden intense malaise, severe headache, and high fever. Usually during the first hours of infection signs of meningeal irritation appear – neck rigidity or retraction and Kernig's sign. Vomiting and photophobia are common. When all these features are prominent, the diagnosis is straightforward but in milder or atypical cases it may be easy to overlook meningitis if the characteristic signs are not sought. Whilst there may be delirium in meningitis, consciousness is not impaired in the early stages, nor are there focal neurological signs such as aphasia or hemiparesis. These signify either a complication of meningitis (hydrocephalus, venous sinus thrombosis) or an alternative diagnosis such as meningo-encephalitis or cerebral abscess.

In the clinical examination, particular attention should be paid to the presence of rashes or septic foci, especially in the ears, paranasal sinuses or heart. In suspected meningitis a number of clinical features may be helpful in the diagnosis of the cause. These are discussed below.

Investigations

If the diagnosis of meningitis is suspected it is of the utmost importance that the cause is established quickly. The reason for this is that pyogenic meningitis has a high mortality without treatment. There is widespread agreement among experienced physicians that delay in the recognition of a pyogenic meningitis for even a few hours is a prominent reason why the mortality for these infections remains between 5 and 15%.

Assuming that there are no focal neurological signs, and that consciousness is unimpaired (when CT scanning is indicated first), it is reasonable to proceed directly to lumbar puncture. The changes in the cerebrospinal fluid require clear understanding if rapid and logical treatment is to be instituted (Table 15.2). Two simple and practical points at lumbar puncture in this serious situation are to make sure that the CSF containers are firmly closed *before* the LP needle is withdrawn, and to ensure *personally* that the samples reach the laboratory promptly.

After macroscopic examination, cell-count and an estimation of protein and glucose, a careful Gram stain should be carried out by a skilled observer (Fig. 15.1). Ziehl–Nielsen stain for TB and Indian Ink for fungi may be necessary, depending on the clinical indications and CSF findings. Other rapid methods of diagnosis have been developed in recent years – counterimmunoelectrophoresis, latex co-agglutination, enzyme-linked immunoabsorbent assay and CSF lactate determination. These methods may be valuable (especially for cryptococcal disease) but they are rarely available as routine procedures in a District General Hospital, particularly outside normal daytime hours.

Other baseline investigations – blood film, blood cultures, urinalysis, simultaneous blood sugar, electrolytes, syphilitic and viral serology, chest and skull x-rays – should also be carried out without delay.

Differential Diagnosis

Meningitis requires distinction from other conditions in which headache, vomiting and neck stiffness occur. Subarachnoid haemorrhage, migraine and meningism during a childhood fever, or lobar pneumonia in adults, may cause diagnostic difficulty. A meningitic syndrome frequently follows myelography and certain drugs given intrathecally (for example methotrexate).

Aseptic meningitis may be clinically distinguishable from acute pyogenic meningitis, but to place undue reliability on the clinical impression of severity is at best unwise and may be dangerous.

In the differential diagnosis of meningitis, a useful check list (modified from Lambert, 1983) is as follows:

Clinical Feature	Probable Organism
Petechial rash	meningococcus
Fractured skull	pneumococcus
Ear disease	pneumococcus
Congenital CNS lesion	pneumococcus or coliform
Previous antimicrobial drugs	partially treated pyogenic infection

Rash or pleurodynia — enterovirus

Foreign travel or immunisation — possible poliomyelitis

Occupational history (infected water), prostration, myalgia, conjunctivitis and jaundice — leptospirosis

With the clinical picture and cerebrospinal fluid examination it should be possible to make a presumptive diagnosis of the cause of the meningitis within a few hours of admission to hospital. Antibiotic therapy should be started without delay if pyogenic infection is suspected.

Particular difficulties occur when an organism cannot be identified by staining or when the CSF contains a mixed picture of mononuclear cells and polymorphs, or mononuclear cells alone. The following conditions require consideration:

Partially-treated bacterial meningitis
Viral meningitis

Tuberculosis
Neoplastic meningitis
Parameningeal foci, e.g. occult paranasal sinus disease
Syphilitic meningitis
Fungal meningitis
Chemical meningitis (myelography or drugs)
Intracranial abscess
Cerebral infarction (uninfected)
Endocarditis (with cerebral embolism)
Cerebral venous thrombosis
Meningitic presentation of an encephalitic illness e.g. *Listeria monocytogenes,*
Herpes simplex.
Leptospirosis
Cerebral malaria

A long history (over five days) may cause diagnostic difficulties too. Ensure first whether or not the patient has had antibiotics recently (which may modify but not eradicate an acute pyogenic infection). Chronicity or

Table 15.2

Cerebrospinal Fluid in Meningitis

	Normal	Acute pyogenic meningitis	Virus meningitis	TB meningitis
Pressure	80–160 mm fluid	Raised	Raised	Raised
Appearance	Clear and colourless	Cloudy, maybe purulent	Clear or cloudy	Cloudy yellow, may clot on standing
Cells ($\times 10^6$/l)	less than 5 (mononuclears only)	Many (usually over 200, often several thousand, mainly polymorphs; organisms on Gram stain). Occasionally less than 10 polymorphs: this has v. poor prognosis	Many, usually several hundred to 1000, mononuclears though polymorphs do occur in early stages	Many, usually several hundred *mixed* polymorphs and mononuclears. Organisms on Ziehl–Nielsen stain
Glucose	$\frac{1}{2}$ to $\frac{2}{3}$ of blood glucose	Less than $\frac{1}{2}$ blood glucose, usually much less or absent	Almost always normal	Less than $\frac{1}{2}$ blood glucose, usually much less
Protein	0.2–0.4 g/l	Raised above 0.8 g/l	Raised or normal	Raised

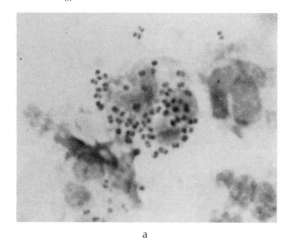

a

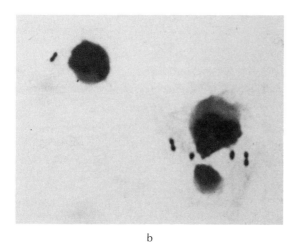

b

Fig. 15.1 (a) *Intracellular* N. meningitidis *in CSF*.
(b) *Intracellular* S. pneumoniae *in CSF*.

encephalitic signs suggest tuberculous infection, fungi, or infection with an unusual organism such as *Listeria monocytogenes*. An alternative explanation is an intracerebral disease simulating a meningitis: cerebral abscess, neoplasm or infarction should be considered.

Management and Specific Treatment

Immediate and specific therapy is vital. A scheme of antimicrobial agents is given in Table 15.3. In addition, hydration must be maintained, high fever controlled, and a careful watch maintained for the appearance of complications (see p. 228). Powerful analgesics and sedative drugs should be avoided if possible, as either may cloud the clinical course of the disease.

Prophylaxis

In epidemic meningococcal disease chemoprophylaxis with either sulphadiazine or rifampicin is recommended, although the emergence of drug-resistant strains of bacteria is an increasing problem.

In recurrent bacterial meningitis, which is sometimes associated with congenital dural defects or follows head injury, the usual infecting organism is *Pneumococcus* (Fig. 15.2). Pneumococcal vaccines may be indicated in this situation if it is not possible to localise and/or repair the defect.

Viral meningitis is usually self-limiting without sequelae, though headache may persist for some weeks or longer.

Tuberculous Meningitis, Fungi and other Forms of Chronic Meningitis

Meningitic illnesses which are truly chronic are rare but they may be caused by tubercle or by fungi such as *Cryptococcus neoformans* – or by other inflammatory disease which may or may not have an infective basis, such Behçet's disease or sarcoidosis. Neoplastic cells in the CSF may also cause a meningitic illness. In these conditions persistent headache, seizures and other encephalitic symptoms, cranial nerve palsies and hydrocephalus may be present. Diagnosis is often difficult on clinical grounds alone. Illustrative cases are given below:

Case 1

A 49-year-old Gujurati male who had lived in Britain for 15 years developed headaches and general malaise over the course of four weeks. His speech became slow and the right limbs weak. On examination he was drowsy with neck stiffness, aphasia, mild right hemiparesis and a fever of 39°C. A CT head scan was normal and other baseline investigations unhelpful. The CSF was at a pressure of 300 mm water, cloudy, and contained 146 cells, 40% of which were polymorphs.

Table 15.3

Treatment of meningitis and Encephalitis

Organism	Drugs	Comment
N. meningitidis meningitis	benzyl penicillin	penicillin 2 megaunits initially 2 hourly.
H. influenzae meningitis	chloramphenicol (caution in neonates!)l	Penicillin-allergic subjects should receive chloramphenicol.
S. pneumoniae meningitis	benzyl penicillin	All drugs must be given in high dosage and (initially) I-V.
Undiagnosed pyogenic meningitis	chloramphenicol or double therapy, = penicillin + chloramphenicol	Intrathecal penicillin sometimes used in pneumococcal NOT more than 10 000 u
M. tuberculosis meningitis and meningo-encephalitis	isoniazid rifampicin pyrazinamide streptomycin ethionamide ethambutol	Treatment is still controversial and complex. Isoniazid (with pyridoxine supplement) and rifampicin for at least 12 months plus pyrazinamide for the initial 2 months. The role of intrathecal streptomycin is still in dispute
Listeria monocytogenes meningo-encephalitis	ampicillin or ampicillin + chloramphenicol	
Neonatal bacterial meningitis	ampicillin plus gentamicin or chloramphenicol plus both	Monitor levels of gentamicin and chloramphenicol. Recent work suggesting monotherapy with either cefuroxine, moxalactam or cefotaxime appears promising but needs confirmation
Cryptococcus neoformans meningitis	oral 5-fluorocytosine and I-V amphotericin B	continue for 6 weeks, monitor antigen levels in blood and CSF. Intrathecal drugs (reservoir) may be used. Miconazole sometimes used
Herpes encephalitis	acyclovir vidarabine	

Treatment given here is only outlined for guidance. Antibiotic and antiviral therapy is still frequently complex in these diseases and reference should be made to specialised texts on infective diseases and individual problems discussed with the microbiologist supervising the laboratory investigations of the case.

CSF protein was 1.4 g/l, glucose 1.1 mmol/l, with blood glucose 3.4 mmol/l. No organisms were seen. Treatment for suspected tuberculous meningitis was started immediately. Acid-fast organisms were seen on a third CSF specimen taken two weeks later and TB bacilli confirmed by culture. The course was protracted over many months and complicated by fits and intracranial tuberculoma formation.

Case 2

A 28-year-old man with disseminated non-Hodgkin lymphoma developed the signs of a meningitic illness gradually over 10 days. A CT scan was normal. The CSF, initially normal, was repeated on the 10th day after admission and found to contain 300 cells, 80% lymphocytes, with protein: 1.8 g/l and glucose: 1.2

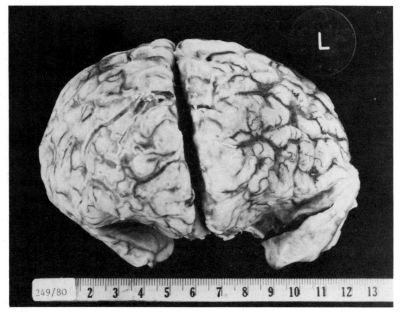

Fig. 15.2 *Meningeal exudate in pneumococcal meningitis – may be associated with cranial nerve palsies and hydrocephalus.*

mmol/l when the blood glucose was 5.4 mmol/l. Papilloedema developed. Fungi were seen on Indian Ink staining of CSF and a CSF cryptococcal antigen test was positive at 1:128. He was treated with amphotericin B and 5-fluocytosine. He became drowsy and unresponsive. Papilloedema developed. He died on the 20th day. Autopsy revealed widespread cryptococcal infection.

Case 3

A 24-year-old white male developed headaches and confused behaviour over several months. He had two grand mal fits. On examination he was sleepy and confused. Drug abuse was suspected. Investigation showed mild hydrocephalus on CT scan, and cloudy CSF at a pressure of 320 mm containing 98 cells, of which 24% were polymorphs. Protein was 3.4 g/l, glucose 1.0 mmol/l, with blood glucose 5.4 mmol/l. No organisms were found on repeated examinations and serological tests for fungi were negative. A Kveim test was positive. Hilar lymphadenopathy developed. Sarcoidosis was diagnosed. The illness has run a fluctuating course over 4 years with fits, dementia and further hydrocephalus. Steroid therapy has not been helpful.

Sequelae

Although viral meningitis is very largely a benign and self-limiting condition, bacterial and fungal infections carry a considerable mortality despite advances in antibiotic therapy. In 1981 in England and Wales the death rates for the three commonest bacterial infections were:

N. meningitidis	5.1%	(390 cases)
H. influenzae	4.3%	(374 cases)
S. pneumoniae	16.3%	(320 cases)

Survivors may be completely cured by appropriate therapy but there is still an overall prevalence of late sequelae in bacterial meningitis of 15%. These include cranial nerve palsies, hydrocephalus (Fig. 15.3), intracranial abscess formation, venous sinus thrombosis or cortical venous thrombosis. Cranial nerve involvement may cause papilloedema, sometimes with consecutive optic atrophy and visual loss. Chiasmal compression may occur, particularly in chronic meningitic processes. Deafness may follow either from VIIIth nerve involvement or extension to the middle ear. Subdural effusion or empyema may occur during treatment. Late epilepsy sometimes follows.

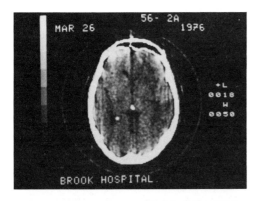
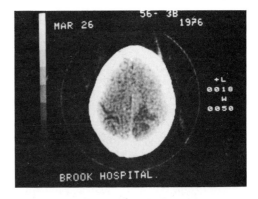
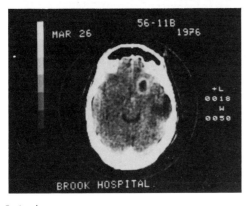
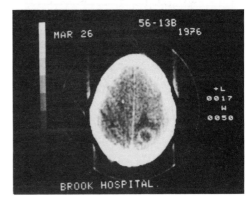

Fig. 15.3 *Brain abscess.*

BRAIN ABSCESS

A focal collection of pus within the cerebrum or cerebellum presents as an expanding mass lesion with evidence of raised intracranial pressure, headache and later vomiting and papilloedema. Focal signs of brain dysfunction – aphasia, hemiparesis, incoordination – may be present and seizures, either focal or grand mal, may occur. Fever is a usual, but by no means constant, feature. The presentation of brain abscess is frequently remarkably similar to a cerebral neoplasm, with symptoms developing over several weeks. As in meningitis, organisms may enter by direct spread from a parameningeal source, or they may be metastatic from suppurative lung disease, pelvic infection, or infected valves or congenital lesions within the heart. Abscesses also arise even when there is no known source of infection, local or distant.

The common organisms of meningitis are relatively rare causes of brain abscess. *Streptococcus* spp. (aerobic, anaerobic and microaerophilic), the anaerobic *Bacteroides* spp., staphylococci and enterobacteria are among the more common. Infections may be mixed and sometimes the causative organism is not found. Fungi also cause brain abscesses. Tubercle bacilli cause chronic caseating granulomata – tuberculomas; these may develop during the course of TB meningitis but they also arise as a primary manifestation of tuberculosis, particularly in regions with a very high prevalence of the disease. In the Indian subcontinent tuberculomas are the single commonest intracranial mass lesion.

When brain abscess is suspected, CT scanning is the most important investigation following blood picture (leucocytosis), ESR (raised), urinalysis, blood cultures and skull films. *Lumbar puncture is contra-indicated in suspected brain abscess* and contributes little to the management. The CSF is abnormal with pleocytosis, raised protein, usually with a normal glucose, but it is not diagnostic.

The treatment of brain abscess should be carried out in close liaison with a neurosurgeon. Decompression and drainage may be necessary, either to establish the diagnosis or to relieve the symptoms and signs of the expanding cerebral lesion. The choice of an appropriate antibiotic may be difficult but in general, if an abscess is of sinusitic origin (commonly metronidazole-resistant Streptococci), penicillin (16–24 megaunits per day) should be used; abscesses of otitic origin (commonly mixed organisms) usually require multiple antibiotics, e.g. chloramphenicol and metronidazole, with or without penicillin, ampicillin or co-trimoxazole. Spinal and post-traumatic abscesses are usually caused by *Staphylococcus aureus*; fusidic acid is the usual drug of choice. Abscesses of metastatic or cryptogenic origin may be streptococcal or mixed, and multiple therapy is indicated until the bacteriological results are known. Steroids are often indicated in cerebral abscess since there is usually a zone of cerebral oedema surrounding the lesion.

Despite treatment, the mortality of cerebral abscess remains high – around 30% in most series. Sequelae (seizures and focal deficits) are frequent.

PARAMENINGEAL INFECTIONS

Spinal epidural abscess is usually caused by bloodstream spread of *Staph. aureus* from a distant boil or other site of infection. The commonest presentation is lower dorsal pain, fever, and the speedy development of a paraparesis. Urgent myelography is indicated if the diagnosis is suspected. These abscesses are treated by early surgical decompression and antibiotics. Very rarely epidural abscesses occur intracranially. The signs are of local infection and cranial nerve palsies, e.g. a facial, trigeminal or oculomotor nerve lesion with pain and a high fever.

Subdural empyema is likewise secondary to local infection. The presentation is of an expanding mass lesion with fever. Differentiation from intracranial abscess may be difficult on clinical grounds. Drainage and antibiotics are indicated.

Intracranial venous-sinus thrombosis and *cortical-venous thrombosis* occur as non-infective complications of cachexia or dehydration, or of a disorder of blood coagulation, or secondary to local parameningeal infection or meningitis.

Cavernous sinus thrombosis causes severe pain, proptosis, chemosis, ophthalmoplegia and sometimes involvement of the optic nerve and trigeminal nerves. When associated with diabetic ketoacidosis, infection with the fungus *Mucor* should be suspected.

Lateral sinus thrombosis is usually secondary to suppurative ear disease. There is raised intracranial pressure, fever, and earache. The thrombosis may extend caudally to involve the nerves of the jugular foramen, IX, X and XI. *Superior sagittal sinus thrombosis* is a complication of paranasal sinus infection or cavernous sinus thrombosis, or it may occur as a metastatic infection. Cortical venous infarction causes convulsions and damage to the parasagittal areas which control the lower limbs and bladder. Fever, convulsions and a spastic paraparesis form the usual clinical picture. Signs of raised intracranial pressure develop when the sinus obstructs.

Cortical venous thrombosis should be suspected in patients with meningeal or parameningeal infection who deteriorate with high fever, progressive focal signs and convulsions. Diagnosis may be difficult and whilst the CSF is often abnormal with pleocytosis and a raised protein these changes are by no means diagnostic. CT scanning may show areas of oedema and infarction; angiography with late views of the venous phase may be necessary to establish the diagnosis and to exclude other pathology.

The treatment of venous thrombosis in infective disease is primarily to treat the underlying infection. Rehydration, supportive therapy and anticonvulsants are also indicated. The place of anticoagulants is controversial.

ENCEPHALITIS, ENCEPHALOMYELITIS AND MYELITIS

Direct invasion of the central nervous system by pathogenic viruses causes the clinical picture of *acute virus encephalitis*. Of these viruses, herpesvirus hominis Type I is the single most common cause of serious disease, although mumps (which usually causes a milder condition) is the single most common cause identified in Britain. Varicella zoster, influenza, infectious mononucleosis, measles, rubella and arbo viruses also cause the condition. There are many named varieties of encephalitis; for example, western equine encephalitis, eastern equine encephalitis, St Louis encephalitis, California virus encephalitis and Venezualan equine encephalitis are the five commonest arbo virus encephalitides in the USA.

Encephalomyelitis, an encephalitic illness with spinal cord involvement, characterised by perivascular infiltration and demyelination, is a rare sequel of all the infective viral exanthemata of childhood. It may be clinically very similar to the acute virus encephalitis described above. *Myelitis*, inflammation of the spinal cord alone causing paraparesis or paraplegia may occur after these fevers, particularly varicella and rubella. Other conditions of post-infective type include a transient cerebellar syndrome in childhood, Sydenham's chorea following streptococcal infection, and post-infective polyneuropathy (Landry–Guillain–Barré syndrome see p. 244).

Herpes simplex encephalitis, one of the commoner identified causes of viral encephalitis in Britain, has become of clinical importance since the development of specific antiviral therapy. The illness is usually a primary infection with *Herpesvirus hominis* Type I and presents with headache, fever, and general malaise. There is a disturbance of higher cerebral function with irritability, change in affect and confusion. Focal signs – aphasia, hemianopia or hemiparesis – may occur and the clinical picture may resemble an intracranial mass lesion. The pattern of the disease varies from a relatively mild meningo-encephalitic illness which is self-limiting to a severe form with coma. Seizures, particularly of temporal lobe origin, occur in either. Rarely, the infection involves the brainstem, causing oculomotor disorders, bulbar dysfunction and ataxia. The overall mortality without treatment is about 70%. In the investigation of herpes simplex infection, CT head scanning in established encephalitis may show patchy cerebral oedema particularly in the temporal lobes. EEG studies are usually helpful, showing high-voltage slow-wave changes which are characteristic but not diagnostic of the condition. The CSF, which should only be examined after CT scanning, shows an inflammatory response, usually mononuclear but sometimes with a mixed cell pattern. Antibody studies

may be difficult to interpret, but a reliable indicator of current infection is an HSV Index > 2.

$$\text{HSV Index} = \frac{\text{CSF HSV titre}}{\text{Serum HSV titre}} \Big/ \frac{\text{CSF albumin}}{\text{Serum albumin}}$$

Brain biopsy is now widely advocated in North America, but has found little favour as a measure frequently employed in Britain although the procedure is probably the most certain way of making the diagnosis – by electron microscopy, immunofluorescent staining and virus isolation from tissue.

Treatment

The recommended treatment of proven herpes simplex encephalitis has in the last decade seemed to follow the most recent trends in antiviral chemotherapy. The current treatment of choice is acyclovir, the active form of which (acyclovir triphosphate) inhibits DNA synthesis. Phosphorylation of acyclovir is dependent upon the presence of viral thymidine kinase and the drug is thus specific for certain viral infections, e.g. herpes simplex and varicella zoster. In most neurological units in Britain at the present time, intravenous acyclovir is the treatment recommended both for proven simplex infection and in cases where there is a high index of suspicion. Vidarabine (adenine arabinoside) is also of proven value in treating the disease. Management of cerebral oedema with steroids, mannitol and sometimes intracranial pressure monitoring is essential.

The results of therapy are difficult to assess. Whilst there is the suggestion that early treatment of the mild case limits the disease, severe cases in coma at the onset of therapy have a poor prognosis, with a mortality of some 40%. In the survivors, full recovery occurs in under 15% of cases and the late sequelae of epilepsy, memory disturbance and intellectual impairment are common.

OTHER SPECIFIC INFECTIONS

Poliomyelitis

Invasion of the central nervous system by the pathogenic strains of an enterovirus excreted in the faeces causes in epidemics a spectrum of clinical events, one of which is paralytic poliomyelitis. In this condition there is replication of the virus within the anterior horn cells of the spinal cord and motor nuclei of the brainstem, with subsequent cell death.

After gaining access to the body through the gut or nasopharynx there is an incubation period of seven to fourteen days. A prodromal illness occurs with headache, fever, and vomiting. Viraemia occurs at this stage. A preparalytic stage follows as the virus gains access to the nervous system. There are signs of meningitis, particularly with spinal pains and severe pains in the limbs. After several days many patients recover, but some enter the paralytic stage. Weakness of muscles progresses for three to five days. The extent and degree of paralysis is very variable, usually asymmetrical and patchy. Fasciculation occurs commonly in the muscles which are about to become paralysed, and is an important sign. Reflex loss and wasting appear. There is no sensory loss and upper motor neurone signs do not occur. In about 15% of patients the muscles of the face, pharynx, tongue and respiration are affected, causing bulbar and respiratory failure. Recovery begins after the end of the paralytic stage and is very variable, but it may be expected to continue for over one year. The overall mortality is about 7–10%. Symptomless and unrecognised infection is common.

Only in poliomyelitis has prophylactic immunisation largely eradicated a formerly widespread crippling neurological disease. The trivalent live oral vaccine contains three strains of poliovirus. In Britain it is given routinely in childhood. It is strongly recommended for adults who are visiting countries where the disease remains endemic. It is one of the safest vaccines known. The killed vaccine is probably equally effective; it is given parenterally and is used in several countries.

Rabies

Any warm-blooded animal can be infected with the rabies rhabdovirus which causes in man an almost uniformly fatal illness. Rabies is endemic in many countries but was eradicated in Britain in 1902 and does not at present occur in Scandinavia (excluding Denmark), Taiwan, Japan, Australia and New Zealand, Hawaii and Antarctica. Infection from domestic dogs is the single most important cause of the disease in man but foxes, skunks, cats, bats and other carnivorous mammals transmit the disease.

In dogs there is an incubation period of between five days and fourteen months, but it is usually less than four months. The clinical features include a change in temperament, snapping (often at imaginary objects), and a tendency to wander. Dysphagia and other paralytic symptoms appear, and the animal usually dies within a week. There are occasional reports of virus excretion by apparently healthy animals.

Transmission occurs when virus from the saliva of the dog penetrates broken skin or intact mucosa. Very rarely, infection by aerosol (e.g. bat droppings) may have occurred. The virus multiplies locally in muscle fibres close to the bite and after an uncertain interval (days or weeks) migrates along peripheral nerves to the dorsal root ganglia and to the central nervous system. Here there is an inflammatory reaction, most marked in the midbrain and medulla in 'furious' rabies and in the spinal cord in 'paralytic' rabies. Diagnostic cytoplasmic inclusion bodies (Negri bodies) are seen within neurones at autopsy.

In man the incubation period is from four days to several *years* but in over 80% of cases it is between 20 and 90 days. It tends to be shorter with bites on the face than on the limbs. A prodromal stage of malaise, fever and irritability, sometimes with intense anxiety, depression, or even psychosis, lasts several days and is followed by either 'furious' or 'paralytic' rabies. In the former, hydrophobia – laryngeal spasm, terror and uncontrollable arousal produced by attempting to drink fluids – is common. In paralytic rabies (dumb rabies) a flaccid paralysis develops. All forms of established rabies were until the last decade uniformly fatal, usually within three weeks.

The prevention and control of rabies depends upon the prevalence of endemic disease in a community. In high-risk regions (for example there are believed to be some 15 000 human deaths annually in India), domestic animals should be immunised and the keeping of wild carnivores as pets discouraged. Attempts should be made to eliminate stray dogs although this is not feasible in many countries.

Prophylactic immunisation in man with a human diploid cell strain vaccine (HDCSV) is now possible and the incidence of allergic complications is negligible. Those handling potentially infected animals should be immunised annually but there is no indication for 'routine' immunisation before foreign travel.

Following a bite or contact with a potentially rabid animal, active immunisation should commence without delay. The post-exposure course of HDCSV is 1.0 ml intramuscularly on days 0, 3, 7, 14, 30 and 90. (It was traditional to suggest that the animal be captured, chained and caged, and the brain examined for Negri bodies if it died: If not dead within 10–15 days, the animal was not rabid.) For the patient, wound toilet should also be carried out urgently – scrubbing with soap or detergent followed by liberal douching in water. 70% alcohol, tincture of iodine or 0.01% aqueous iodine should then be used. Suturing should be avoided.

Passive immunisation with anti-rabies serum is recommended following a bite by a rabid animal, and human anti-rabies immunoglobulin is now available in limited quantities.

In practice in Britain, the management of a patient in whom rabies is suspected should be discussed with the Central (or a Regional) Public Health Laboratory. Immediate advice on the diagnosis of rabies is always available from the Duty Officer, the Central Public Health Laboratory, Colindale, London, NW9 5HT. (Telephone number 01–205 7041.)

The management of established rabies is beyond the scope of this chapter. With scrupulous prolonged intensive care there have to date been three occasions when patients with rabies have survived and recovered but it remains a disease with an almost universal mortality once symptoms have commenced.

Herpes Zoster: Shingles

This common condition occurs when there is recrudescence of varicella zoster virus in the dorsal root ganglia, the virus having been acquired in an attack of chickenpox many years previously. Precipitating factors are injury and generalised diseases, particularly where there is immunosuppression. Shingles becomes more common with increasing age, perhaps because of decline in the immunity acquired following chickenpox.

Severe pain in several adjacent dermatomes precedes a vesicular eruption in the distribution of one or two dermatomes (Fig. 15.4). A few scattered lesions

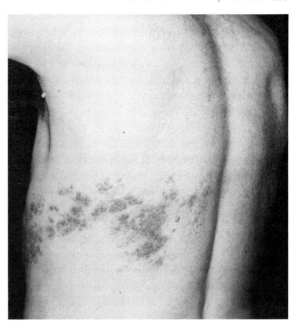

Fig. 15.4 *Herpes Zoster: vesicular rash T₆.*

appear in other parts of the body but the main eruption is unilateral and localised. There is local lymphadenopathy. The vesicles, which are often intensely irritating (identical to chicken pox) and painful, last for 7–10 days and dry into crusts. These heal gradually, leaving depigmented scars which are initially anaesthetic.

Zoster may also affect any cranial nerve, especially V and VII. In 'Gasserian herpes' the ophthalmic division of the Vth is infected and, this may lead to corneal scarring and secondary pan-ophthalmitis. In 'geniculate herpes' (the Ramsay–Hunt syndrome) a lower motor-neurone VIIth nerve palsy follows pain and a vesicular eruption (often transient and sparse) on the pinna, external auditory meatus, or fauces.

A myelitis, a meningo-encephalitis or radiculitis may be caused by zoster. The complications are secondary bacterial infection, very rarely 'purpura fulminans' (severe purpura and necrosis in the affected segment), generalised zoster in the debilitated or immunosuppressed, and the late sequel of post-herpetic neuralgia.

The neuralgic pain which follows zoster in some 10% of cases persists in over half of the patients for longer than two years. It is a burning dysaesthetic constant pain responding poorly to all analgesics. Depression is almost universal, and may be so severe as to involve the risk of suicide. Treatment is unsatisfactory and, before the introduction of antiviral therapy, there were suggestions that the early use of steroids in acute localised zoster reduced the pain. The overall prognosis is, however, towards gradual recovery within three years; a sign of recovery welcomed by the patient is the appearance of pain-free intervals.

These complications, and the emergence of effective antiviral therapy, have initiated a change in attitude towards treatment which is being reflected in current practice. Topical idoxuridine is now used routinely (care must be taken around the eye) and many physicians recommend systemic antiviral therapy. This is certainly indicated for zoster in the immunosuppressed, in severe cases of herpes zoster ophthalmicus, and in purpura fulminans. Intravenous vidarabine or, more recently, acyclovir are the current drugs of choice.

Neurosyphilis

A very wide variety of neurological syndromes follow infection with the flagellate spirochaete *Treponema pallidum*. A self-limiting aseptic meningitis may occur during secondary syphilis; the more common progressive syndromes occurring in tertiary disease are described here, and are the result of either a meningovascular arteritic process or a parenchymatous meningoencephalitis with spirochaetes within the substance of the brain.

Meningovascular syphilis

This presents either as a diffuse subacute meningitis, often with cranial nerve palsies (and sometimes with papilloedema), or as a focal form in which an intracranial gumma causes the features common to many expanding intracranial mass lesions, i.e. epilepsy, focal deficits, and raised intracranial pressure. Meningo-vascular syphilis is a cause of hemiplegia, particularly in young persons. A spinal meningovasculitis also occurs, causing acute paraparesis with lesions most common in the thoracic cord. Rarely a chronic cervical meningomyelitis (cervical pachymeningitis) causes paraparesis and wasting of the small hand muscles.

Tabes dorsalis (see p. 170)

Dementia: general paralysis of the insane (Fig. 15.5)

This chronic meningo-encephalitis causes profound cerebral atrophy, with a low-grade inflammatory meningeal reaction. Dementia is the prominent feature, with progressive loss of memory and intellect, and development of socially unacceptable behaviour. The 'delusions of grandeur' of the early descriptions of the disease reflect this process, but frequently the patient is apathetic, morbid and depressed. Epilepsy may occur. As the disease progresses, characteristic features of dysarthria, tremulousness and spastic paraparesis appear. Argyll Robertson pupils and optic atrophy may be present. Untreated GPI is usually fatal within two years.

The syndromes described above are frequently incomplete, mixed or atypical, leading to a confusing clinical picture in a disease less common in Britain now than in the first half of the twentieth century. There is, however, a resurgence of syphilis at the present time, particularly among the homosexual population, and unusual presentations of the disease continue to occur.

Congenital neurosyphilis (see p. 185)

Diagnosis

Although the clinical picture may be highly suggestive, the serological tests for syphilis are of great importance. In both blood and CSF, nonspecific reaginic antibodies are demonstrated by the VDRL test. This is a quantitative test and a rising titre indicates activity of the infection. Specific antitreponemal tests are the *T. pallidum* haemagglutination (TPHA) test and the fluorescent treponema antigen–absorbent (FTA–ABS) test. The latter can detect both IgG and IgM antibodies. Raised IgM titres suggest current infection.

In the CSF, a mononuclear pleocytosis occurs of 20–100 cells, and a raised protein of 0.5–1.5 G/l, with an increased gammaglobulin, oligoclonal bands, and positive specific antibody tests. Very occasionally in late tabes, even these tests may be negative in the CSF.

Two further problems confound the interpretation of tests. First, biological false positive reactions occur in pregnancy, systemic lupus erythematosus, infectious mononucleosis, varicella zoster, and other acute infec-

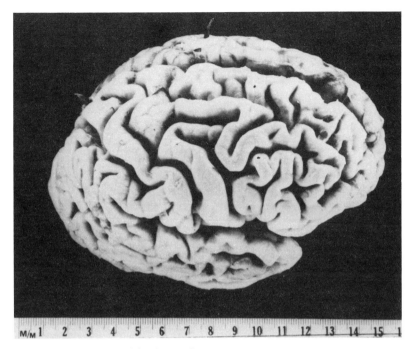

Fig. 15.5 *Cerebral atrophy due to neurosyphilis (General Paralysis of Insane).*

tions. The more specific tests are usually negative in this situation but even the FTA–ABS may be weakly positive. Secondly, *all* the serological tests for syphilis may be positive in yaws, a particular problem in patients of West Indian origin.

Treatment

Intramuscular procaine penicillin, one million units daily for 14–21 days, is the treatment of choice in all forms of active disease and usually arrests further progression. Steroid cover is usually advised in all forms CNS syphilis to reduce the allergic reactions which occur in the course of therapy (Herxheimer reactions). These may on occasion be severe and cause further and permanent neurological damage. Follow-up is important; repeat lumbar puncture is usually carried out regularly.

Tetanus and Botulism

Clostridium tetani, a ubiquitous anaerobic bacterium, is a normal inhabitant of cattle faeces and soil and its spores are therefore common. Even trivial wounds may become infected and, following incubation from a few days to several weeks, the organism multiplies and liberates a powerful toxin which travels within motor nerves to reach the CNS, where it binds irreversibly with certain sialic acid-containing gangliosides. The principal effect of the toxin is to block inhibition of spinal reflexes, resulting in the spasms of tetanus which occur either spontaneously or as a result of external stimuli.

Clinically, a previous wound may have been forgotten and the patient presents with weakness, often near the site of infection. This proceeds to tonic spasm of the jaw (trismus) which then spreads to the trunk causing opisthotonos and a rigid abdomen. Fever is usual. The paroxysmal stage follows, in which the body is thrown into painful spasms with arching of the back, clenching of the teeth and extension of the limbs. Noise and other stimuli precipitate these spasms. Death occurs in severe cases, following spasms of increasing severity and frequency.

The treatment of tetanus involves intensive care, muscle relaxant drugs and often assisted ventilation. Human antitetanus immunoglobulin is given intramuscularly, and parenteral penicillin. Wound toilet should also be carried out.

Active immunisation, if generally adopted, would eradicate this disease. Adsorbed tetanus toxoid is given as a course in Britain in childhood but the immunity gained is not lifelong and booster doses are required every five years, or following wounds. Passive immunisation with human tetanus immunoglobulin is necessary following injury if patients have not previously received toxoid. A course of active immunisation should be commenced at the same time.

Botulism

Exotoxin from various subtypes of another spore-bearing anaerobe, *Clostridium botulinum* causes a presynaptic block in neuromuscular transmission which leads to the paralytic symptoms of botulism. The organisms are most commonly found and multiply in canned foods which have been incompletely sterilised. Gastrointestinal symptoms – diarrhoea, cramps, vomiting and occasionally constipation – occur early, but the paralytic symptoms usually develop 12–48 hours after ingestion of toxin. Visual symptoms – loss of accommodation, drooping of the lids and diplopia – occur first, and are followed by a general extreme fatiguability with severe weakness of the limbs and bulbar muscles. Tendon reflexes are usually preserved and there is usually no sensory disturbance. Fever is absent.

A milder condition occurs in infants and is associated with colonisation of the bowel by the organism. Rarely botulism follows contamination of wounds.

The diagnosis may be suspected on clinical grounds, but can be confirmed by the laboratory finding of exotoxin in the remains of food or vomit and the patient's serum. The disease may occur concurrently in family members or in domestic animals who have shared the same food. Repetitive nerve stimulation shows a decrement in the evoked muscle action potential at slow rates of stimulation, but an increase in amplititude during stimulation at faster frequencies (typical of presynaptic defect).

Treatment of the established disease is largely supportive and often requires the facilities of an Intensive Therapy Unit. Ventilation may be required and a careful watch for respiratory failure is necessary at all stages of the condition. A polyvalent antiserum is also used. Complete recovery occurs if the patient survives the severe stages of the condition.

Prophylaxis by the careful scrutiny of the packing of all tinned foods has virtually eliminated this disease in Britain. Cooking for ten minutes abolishes the risk of botulism by inactivating the toxin.

Leprosy

Mycobacterium leprae is an acid-fast organism which is believed to infect 15 to 20 million of the world's population. It causes a chronic inflammatory disease which involves skin, mucous membranes, and the peripheral nerves causing disorders of sensation. The inflammatory reaction to *M. leprae* varies widely between individuals and has led to a complex classification of the forms of this disease, which is now extremely rare in Europe and North America.

In 'tuberculoid leprosy' – a benign variety of the disease in which small numbers of organisms stimulate a brisk inflammatory response in the peripheral nerves – the patient complains of numbness, tingling and loss of pain and temperature sense in a patchy distribution over the head and distal parts of the limbs. The affected nerves become enlarged and may be palpated as hard cords. In the skin, depigmented anaesthetic areas appear. The disease usually runs a self-limiting course over months or years, and the patient is thought to be non-infectious.

In 'lepromatous leprosy' – the infectious and more malignant variety of the disease in which many organisms are present in the lesions – the peripheral nerves are also affected but the organisms spread to cause granulomatous lesions in the skin and mucous membranes. A progressive disease follows, with patchy sensory loss, often in a bizarre distribution. Ulceration and necrosis occurs in the face and limbs. After many years death follows usually from intercurrent infection.

The diagnosis is established by identifying the bacteria in skin lesions or by biopsy of an affected nerve. Dapsone, rifampicin, clofamizine and thiambutazone are used in the treatment. Allergic reactions, erythema nodosum, peripheral neuropathy, and encephalopathy complicate therapy; the detailed management is beyond the scope of this chapter but steroids are of value during short reactions and thalidomide has a place in the treatment of prolonged reactions in selected patients.

Other Infective Conditions

Organisms causing the Rickettsial diseases of typhus, scrub typhus, Rocky Mountain spotted fever and Q fever may all cause meningo-encephalitis. This may also follow cat scratch fever.

Protozoa

Malaria

Plasmodium falciparum malaria causes a haemorrhagic encephalitis with intravascular clotting. The presentation is similar to other severe forms of encephalitis, with headache, disturbance of consciousness, fits and focal signs. Treatment is with appropriate supportive measures and antimalarials, but not with corticosteroids, which may be harmful. Malaria must always be considered in a febrile person who has recently returned to the UK from a malarious area, and be formally excluded.

Toxoplasmosis

This is a rare cause of meningo-encephalitis in adults, although it is seen in the acquired immunodeficiency syndrome (AIDS). It is the antenatal infection which is more common, causing hydrocephalus, intracranial calcification, and chorioretinitis (see also p. 186).

Amoebae

The fresh-water flagellate *Naegleria fowleri* causes a severe haemorrhagic meningo-encephalitis which is frequently fatal. Very rarely *Entamoeba histolytica* causes brain abscess, which carries a particularly poor prognosis.

Trypanosomiasis

The trypanosomes of tropical Africa, *T. rhodesiense* and *T. gambiense*, cause a low-grade encephalitis with lassitude, fits, somnolence and dysarthria.

Metazoa

Cestodes (tapeworms)

The larval forms of *Echinococcus granulosus* (hydatid disease) and *Taenia solium* (cysticercosis) may form cerebral lesions. Both are rare. In hydatid disease, cysts behave initially as expanding lesions but may rupture to cause a chemical meningitis. In cysticercosis a low-grade meningitis occurs around multiple cysts, which may themselves cause epilepsy or obstruct CSF pathways and cause hydrocephalus. Treatment of cysticercosis with praziquantel, often with concomitant steroids, is helpful.

Trematodes (flukeworms)

In schistosomiasis an acute encephalopathy is caused by massive invasion of ova. A chronic granulomatous reaction follows, causing low-grade inflammatory disease in brain and spinal cord.

Other Infective and Inflammatory Conditions

A number of other conditions that cause inflammatory disease of the central nervous system are difficult to classify.

Progressive rubella encephalitis

Some 10 years after the primary infection, and exceedingly rarely, there is a progressive syndrome of mental impairment, fits, optic atrophy and cerebellar and pyramidal signs. There is evidence of local antibody production against rubella viral antigen within the CNS.

Subacute sclerosing panencephalitis

The persistence of measles antigen in the CNS is believed to be the cause of this rare sequel to measles infection. Mental deterioration, fits, myoclonus and pyramidal signs occur. Death is common, but long periods of survival have been reported. Diagnosis is confirmed by demonstrating a high titre of measles antibody in blood and CSF.

Creutzfeldt–Jakob disease

This condition causes a rapidly-progressive dementia commonly resulting in death within two years of onset. Ataxia, dysphasia, visual disturbance and cerebellar features are common, and the EEG may show typical periodic complexes. Less common forms of the condition appear to be only slowly progressive and may be associated with muscle wasting and fasciculation.

The condition is caused by an agent ('slow virus') which is transmissible to primates in the laboratory and, in rare accidental cases, to man. The incubation period is long, sometimes several years, and the agent appears resistant to many physical agents commonly used to destroy microorganisms. In the common variety, neuronal loss and spongiform degeneration are seen in the brain.

Progressive multifocal leucoencephalopathy

This is an opportunistic infection with the papova viruses JC and SV–40 (and others), in patients who are immunosuppressed. Multifocal demyelinating hemisphere lesions develop, which contain virus particles. Death is usual over several years but treatment with antiviral agents has been attempted.

Reye's syndrome

This is a severe encephalitic illness of children, accompanied by fatty infiltration of the liver. Hypoglycaemia is common. A viral cause has been postulated and some outbreaks have appeared to follow influenza or varicella infection.

Mollaret's meningitis

Occasionally patients present with recurrent episodes of aseptic meningitis over many years. A viral cause is postulated. Some of these patients are helped by treatment with colchicine.

Vogt–Koyanagi–Harada syndrome

This recurrent inflammatory disease of cells of neural crest origin causes uveitis, meningo-encephalitis, vitiligo, deafness and alopecia. Steroids and immunosuppressant drugs are sometimes of value.

Epidemic neuromyasthenia

The very existence of this disorder is doubted by sceptics, who believe the headache, fever, lassitude, torpor, myalgia and depression to be an example of an outbreak of an hysterical illness, often in young women. Some patients do however seem to develop physical signs such as transient ocular palsies and muscle weakness, and vacuolar changes in peripheral lymphocytes have sometimes been noted.

Sarcoidosis

This condition may cause a chronic meningo-encephalitis with sarcoid lesions within the brain and spinal cord, a peripheral neuropathy, cranial nerve palsies (particularly bilateral seventh nerve palsies), or rarely a myopathy. The cause of the condition remains unknown.

Behçet's syndrome

The three principal features are recurrent oral and genital ulceration, inflammatory ocular disease and neurological syndromes due to a very variable and patchy meningo-encephalitis. Brainstem encephalitis, aseptic meningitis, encephalitis and cord lesions occur.

16

Peripheral Nerve Disease

INTRODUCTION

Peripheral nerve trunks contain motor, sensory and autonomic fibres. Motor axons branch in their course down the nerve trunk and within the muscles so that a single motor neurone may innervate as many as several hundred muscle fibres (the motor unit). Sensory neurones are pseudo-unipolar and their cell bodies lie in the dorsal root ganglion. Nerve fibres may be myelinated, with diameters ranging from 2 to 15 μm., or non-myelinated, with diameters ranging from 0.2 to 3 μm. Impulses travel faster in myelinated than in non-mye-

linated fibres, with the velocity depending on the fibre diameter and whether conduction is saltatory or continuous in nature (Table 16.1). The largest, fastest-conducting myelinated fibres are from alpha motor neurones and the primary sensory endings in the muscle spindles. Non-myelinated fibres consist mainly of nociceptive afferents and postganglionic autonomic fibres (see also Chapter 2).

Two types of pathological process affect myelinated nerve fibres – axonal degeneration and demyelination (Fig. 16.1) and, although some neuropathies are characteristically associated with one or other of these processes, most show a mixture of the two. Axonal or

Table 16.1
Conduction Velocity and Function of Different Nerve Fibre Types

Fibre Diameter μm	Type	Myelinated	Conduction Velocity (m/sec)	Function
10–18	A	YES	90	Primary spindle afferents, α-motor neurones
6–12	A	YES	50	Touch and pressure afferents
4–8	A	YES	30	γ-efferents, secondary spindle afferents
2–6	B	YES	10	Autonomic preganglionic
0.2–3	C	NO	2	Nociceptive afferents, postganglionic autonomic

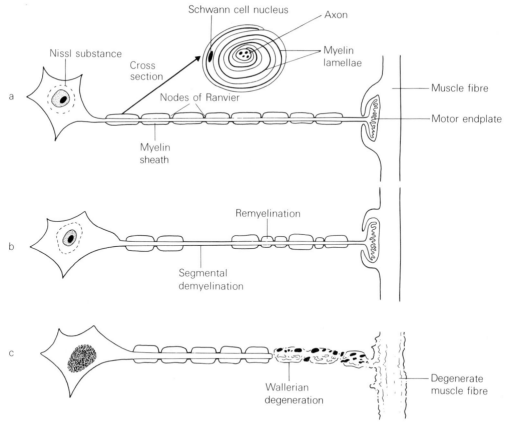

Fig. 16.1 (a) *Diagram of structure of normal anterior horn cell and myelinated fibre. (b) Nerve fibre showing segmental demyelination, and the remyelination which appears. Note the* short thinly-myelinated internodes. (c) Wallerian degeneration. Note accompanying migration of nucleus of cell-body and loss of Nissl substance (central chromatolysis).

Wallerian degeneration typically occurs after a nerve has been divided. Within about a week of injury, the axons distal to the site of injury break down and their myelin sheaths fragment. These changes coincide with loss of the electrical excitability of the degenerating nerve fibres. In axonal neuropathies only the distal portion of the axon degenerates and the more proximal, unaffected parts of the nerves conduct electrical impulses normally. Regeneration of axons occurs by growth of one of several 'sprouts' from the axon stump. In ideal conditions the rate of growth is approximately 1 mm per day. Degeneration of a motor axon or cell body results in denervation and atrophy of the muscle fibres in the motor unit and, when this process is extensive, will produce clinical muscle wasting with or without fasciculation. Denervation may be detected electromyographically by inserting a needle electrode into an affected muscle and recording the spontaneous electrical discharges of individual denervated muscle fibres (fibrillation). In chronic neuropathies, denervated muscle fibres are often reinnervated by sprouting of the terminal branches of normal motor axons from adjacent motor units. The resultant increase in the size of individual motor units may be recognised electromyographically as giant polyphasic potentials and results in fibre type grouping on muscle biopsy (Fig. 16.2).

In traumatic neuropathies with Wallerian degeneration, recovery occurs by regrowth of axon sprouts down the portion of nerve distal to the point of injury. Proximal nerve lesions will therefore recover more slowly than distal ones. Successful reinnervation is prejudiced by loss of anatomical continuity of the nerve, by the presence of infection, and by increasing age. Where disorganisation of the nerve is present,

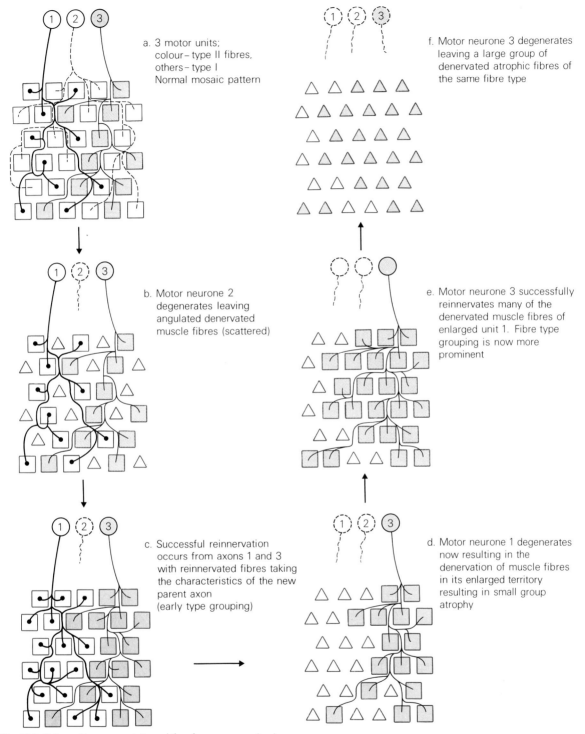

a. 3 motor units;
   colour – type II fibres,
   others – type I
   Normal mosaic pattern

b. Motor neurone 2
   degenerates leaving
   angulated denervated
   muscle fibres (scattered)

c. Successful reinnervation
   occurs from axons 1 and 3
   with reinnervated fibres taking
   the characteristics of the new
   parent axon
   (early type grouping)

d. Motor neurone 1 degenerates
   now resulting in the
   denervation of muscle fibres
   in its enlarged territory
   resulting in small group
   atrophy

e. Motor neurone 3 successfully
   reinnervates many of the
   denervated muscle fibres of
   enlarged unit 1. Fibre type
   grouping is now more
   prominent

f. Motor neurone 3 degenerates
   leaving a large group of
   denervated atrophic fibres of
   the same fibre type

Fig. 16.2 *Schematic representation of the changes occurring in
muscle during chronic denervation with reinnervation.*

axons may regrow along the wrong branch of a nerve, resulting in anomalous reinnervation. A muscle usually undergoes irreversible degeneration if denervated for two years.

In demyelination, conduction of electrical impulses is affected by loss of the myelin sheath, but the axon may not degenerate; muscle wasting is usually slight. Demyelinated nerve fibres may show conduction block or may conduct impulses at a greatly reduced velocity; measurement of nerve conduction velocity may therefore distinguish between fibre degeneration and demyelination. Local demyelination may be caused by compression, and nerve conduction studies can demonstrate the site of damage by showing a segment of the nerve where the onduction velocity is greatly reduced (See also p. 58).

Recovery from demyelination takes approximately 3–6 weeks and occurs more rapidly than in axonal degeneration, where the nerve fibre has to regrow from the point of damage to its end organ.

CLINICAL FEATURES OF NEUROPATHY

Neuropathies may present as involvement of single or multiple major nerve trunks (mono or multiple mononeuropathies) or as a diffuse symmetrical polyneuropathy. The process may be acute (few days), subacute (weeks), or chronic (months to years) and there may be recovery, progression, or a relapsing course.

Weakness is the commonest motor feature of neuropathies although muscle cramps, wasting and fasciculation are often evident. Respiratory muscle involvement produces dyspnoea and, where the cranial nerves are affected, there may be diplopia,

dysphagia and weakness of facial movements. Tendon reflexes are usually reduced or absent, with the ankle jerks being affected first. Sensory changes include loss of one or more sensory modalities and positive phenomena such as paraesthesiae, hyperaesthesiae, shooting pains or distortions of sensation. Sensory loss may follow the distribution of one or more peripheral nerves or, in a polyneuropathy, produce a distal 'glove and stocking' pattern. Autonomic disturbances include loss of sweating and trophic skin changes in the limbs, postural hypotension, impotence, sphincter disturbances and pupillary changes.

Diseases of Nerve Roots and Plexus

Nerve roots and plexus may be damaged by several pathological processes (Table 16.2), the commonest of which are cervical and lumbar spondylosis (See Chapter 11). Trauma, especially from motorcycle accidents, may avulse cervical nerve roots from the spinal cord, causing often widespread paralysis and anaesthesia of the upper limb.

Neuralgic amyotrophy (brachial plexus neuropathy)

This is an acute condition presenting with severe shoulder pain. This is followed within a week by weakness and atrophy of muscles in the territory of a single cervical root, part of the brachial plexus or of one peripheral nerve, most commonly the nerve to serratus anterior. Recovery is slow and often incomplete and the condition may spread to the other side, but recurrence is unusual. Although the cause of neuralgic amyotrophy is unknown, it may follow viral illnesses, local trauma, or immunisation and is sometimes

Table 16.2

Diseases of Nerve Roots and Plexus

Common causes of nerve root disease	Common causes of plexus disease
Cervical and lumbar spondylosis (see p. 167)	Trauma (road accidents; laceration)
Trauma (road accidents, birth)	Neuralgic amyotrophy
Herpes Zoster (see p. 233)	Malignant infiltration
Intraspinal tumours (neurofibroma; 2°) see p. 166	Cervical rib or band
Chronic meningeal inflammation	

familial. There is no effective treatment although corticosteroids may relieve the pain. A similar clinical syndrome may rarely affect the lumbosacral plexus or its branches.

Thoracic outlet syndrome

Cervical ribs or fibrous bands between the tip of C7 transverse process and the first rib may cause stretching and angulation of the C8 and T1 roots of the brachial plexus. Typically, this causes pain along the ulnar border of the arm and forearm, weakness and wasting of the small hand muscles (initially abductor pollicis brevis), and a sensory disturbance on the medial aspect of the forearm. Major vascular symptoms related to subclavian artery stenosis or dilatation or vascular occlusion are rare in this group of patients. Oblique x-rays of the lower cervical spine show the cervical ribs or, if a fibrous band is present, an elongated, pointed transverse process of the C7 vertebra. Surgical exploration and division of the fibrous band frequently results in improvement in pain and prevents further weakness or sensory loss.

Malignancy

Malignant infiltration of the cervical or lumboscral plexus presents with painful progressive weakness and sensory loss in a limb. In the arm, carcinoma of the breast is the commonest cause; a carcinoma of the lung apex may invade the T1 root and sympathetic outflow, to produce arm pain, wasting of the hand and a Horner's syndrome. Pelvic and retroperitoneal malignancies may invade the lumbosacral plexus.

Peripheral Nerve Compression or Entrapment; Mononeuropathy

Nerve damage from compression may be acute (e.g. tourniquet paralysis) or chronic (entrapment neuropathy). Both types of compression produce mainly local demyelination with a variable amount of Wallerian degeneration. Some nerves (Table 16.3) are especially susceptible to compression because of their anatomical relationships (entrapment neuropathies) and this tendency is increased in the presence of hypothyroid-

Table 16.3

Commonest Sites of Entrapment Neuropathy

Nerve	Site of Entrapment
Median	Carpal tunnel
Ulnar	Elbow
Lateral Femoral Cutaneous	} Inguinal ligament
Posterior Tibial	} Tarsal tunnel

ism, acromegaly or diabetes mellitus. The suspected diagnosis in these cases can usually be confirmed by appropriate EMG and nerve conduction studies (see Chapter 3).

Compression of the median nerve within the carpal tunnel produces nocturnal pain in the hand or forearm and paraesthesiae in the hand followed by weakness of the thenar muscles and sensory impairment over the thumb, second and third digits. The condition may be bilateral and is common in pregnancy, when it is usually self-limiting. Treatment with night splints to the wrist or local steroid injections may temporarily relieve symptoms but surgical decompression of the carpal tunnel is usually required.

Ulnar nerve entrapment may be due to compression of the nerve at the elbow within the cubital tunnel or to deformity of the elbow joint from arthritis (tardy ulnar palsy). Occasionally the ulnar nerve may be compressed at the wrist within Guyon's canal, producing a progressive wasting of the small hand muscles which spares the thenar eminence: an ulnar paresis may follow occupational trauma to the nerve in the wrist or palm with pressure from tools, crutches, etc. The radial nerve is susceptible to acute compression against the humeral shaft, as may occur when the arm is hung over the back of a hard chair ('Saturday-night palsy'). The ensuing wrist and finger drop usually recovers within 6 to 12 weeks.

Entrapment syndromes in the legs are rarer than in the arms. The commonest lower limb entrapment neuropathy is meralgia paraesthetica where compression of the lateral cutaneous nerve of thigh at the inguinal ligament causes a burning, numb sensation over the anterolateral aspect of the thigh. The common peroneal nerve is susceptible to compression against the neck of the fibula, resulting in an acute foot drop. This may follow coma or prolonged bed rest, ill-fitting plaster casts, prolonged squatting or pressure from ganglia or cysts. The posterior tibial nerve may be entrapped where it passes medial to the Achilles tendon behind the medial malleolus and under the flexor retinaculum (tarsal tunnel) causing pain and numbness of the sole of the foot; rarely, the sciatic nerve is compressed in the upper thigh.

Multiple mononeuropathies are seen in diabetes mellitus or inflammatory vascular diseases (e.g. polyarteritis nodosa), where the disturbance of function is due to areas of nerve infarction. Rarer causes of multiple mononeuropathy include malignancy, sarcoidosis, leprosy, amyloidosis and neurofibromatosis.

Hereditary Neuropathies (see Chapter 13)

Infective and Post-infective Neuropathies

Leprosy (see p. 236) is one of the few organisms which directly invades peripheral nerves.

Diphtheria

The exotoxin of *Corynebacterium diphtheriae* may cause demyelinating neuropathy. Diphtheria is a febrile illness, most commonly associated with faucial or skin inflammation, which may be followed within two to three weeks by local complications (usually palatal paralysis) and a week or so later by paralysis of accommodation, a generalised painless sensorimotor neuropathy, and cardiac dysrhythmia.

Guillain–Barré syndrome (acute inflammatory neuropathy)

The Guillain–Barré syndrome is a mainly motor demyelinating polyneuropathy occurring at any age, which commonly follows one to two weeks after a nonspecific febrile illness. Pain in the back and limbs and minor sensory symptoms precede a progressive weakness increasing over a period varying from several hours to a month. Early involvement of the proximal muscles is common and the bulbar (see p. 48), facial, and external ocular muscles may be affected. About 20% of patients develop weakness of the respiratory muscles that is sufficiently severe to require mechanical ventilation. Autonomic dysfunction commonly causes labile blood pressure and cardiac dysrhythmias, but bladder dysfunction is rare. The demyelination is caused by cell- and antibody-mediated immune responses which are often associated with an elevated concentration of protein in the cerebrospinal fluid without a pleocytosis. Nerve conduction studies usually show slowing of conduction or conduction block in the peripheral nerves; predominantly proximal involvement of nerve roots may be detected by a delayed muscle response to antidromic electrical stimulation of a peripheral motor nerve (F wave). In a proportion of severely affected patients, electromyography eventually reveals denervation.

In the acute stages, bed rest and analgesics may be required; careful observations of bulbar and respiratory function (serial vital capacity measurements) are essential in determining the need for airway protection (intubation or tracheostomy) and mechanical ventilation. Corticosteroids are of no proven value in the Guillain–Barré syndrome. The role of plasmapheresis is unproven but may possibly be beneficial if given at an early stage before the muscle weakness has begun to plateau. Physiotherapy, calipers and limb splintage are useful during the recovery phase, which commonly lasts three to six months; if extensive denervation has occurred, recovery may be incomplete after two years. Recurrent attacks are uncommon. The so-called 'Miller–Fisher' variant presents with ophthalmoplegia, ataxia and areflexia without limb weakness. Rarely, what appears at first to be the Guillain–Barré syndrome follows a chronic, relapsing course and may effectively be treated by corticosteroids and other immunosuppressants.

Metabolic and Toxic Neuropathies (Table 16.4)

Diabetes mellitus

Diabetic neuropathy may present in several different ways (Table 16.5), the commonest of which is a

Table 16.4

Metabolic/Toxic Neuropathies

Diabetes mellitus
Porphyria
Hepatic disease
Renal disease
Thyroid disease
Vitamin deficiency
Intestinal malabsorption
Alcohol (ethanol)
Drugs
Industrial toxins

Table 16.5

Types of Diabetic Neuropathy

Compression (mononeuropathy)
Multiple mononeuropathy (diabetic amyotrophy)
Symmetrical sensorimotor
Autonomic

progressive symmetrical and mainly sensory disturbance effecting the legs only with areflexia and reduced vibration sense. In the more severe cases, neuropathic foot ulcers and painless, disorganised joints (Charcot joints, see p. 171) are seen. Diabetics are more susceptible to entrapment neuropathy (e.g. ulnar and median nerves), but a subacute, painful, proximal and mainly motor multiple mononeuropathy may occur (diabetic amyotrophy); this condition usually affects maturity-onset diabetics and involves the lumbosacral plexus or, commonly, the femoral nerve, producing wasting and weakness of the quadriceps muscles with loss of the knee jerks. It is caused by areas of nerve infarction due to a microangiopathy. Recovery takes several months and may be improved by careful control of the diabetes. Diabetes mellitus is also associated with an autonomic neuropathy (see autonomic neuropathy, p 246).

Porphyria (see also p. 212)

Acute intermittent porphyria is an hereditary disorder of porphyrin metabolism in which episodes of acute,

predominantly proximal, limb weakness are associated with mental changes, abdominal pain or autonomic features. Attacks may occur spontaneously or follow the ingestion of alcohol or certain drugs (especially barbiturates).

Uraemia

Chronic uraemia may be complicated by a progressive sensory or sensorimotor symmetrical polyneuropathy. The neuropathy usually improves after renal transplantation but shows a variable response to dialysis. Pathologically, there is both demyelination and axonal degeneration but the mechanism of nerve fibre damage is unknown.

A mild sensory neuropathy is sometimes seen in chronic hepatic disorders and rarely in thyroid disease.

Vitamin deficiency

The vitamin deficiencies associated with neuropathy are mainly those of the B group (Table 16.6), the most important causes being beri-beri and pernicious anaemia.

Beri-beri is clinically similar to alcoholic neuropathy (see p. 246).

Pernicious anaemia is due to vitamn B_{12} malabsorption and causes a sensory neuropathy with spinal cord dysfunction (subacute combined degeneration of the cord, see p. 171). Pyridoxine deficiency (which may be

Table 16.6

B Group Vitamin Deficiencies Associated with Neuropathy

B_1 (thiamine)	Beri-beri	Malnutrition, alcoholism
B_6 (pyridoxine)	—	Malnutrition, isoniazid
Nicotinic Acid	Pellagra	Malnutrition
B_{12} (cobalamin)	Pernicious anaemia	Ileal disease, gastrectomy, autoimmune, nutritional
Folic Acid	—	Malabsorption, malnutrition

precipitated by isoniazid therapy for tuberculosis) and folate deficiency both cause a sensory neuropathy. Neuropathies may also occur in various types of intestinal malabsorption (e.g. coeliac disease, sprue, Crohn's disease).

Alcoholic neuropathy

Alcoholic polyneuropathy presents with painful par-aesthesiae in the legs followed by muscle weakness. The calf muscles and soles of the feet may be exquisitely tender; motor involvement can cause a severe wrist and foot drop and contractures may develop. Nerve damage is due mainly to thiamine deficiency resulting in axonal degeneration but, if thiamine treatment is started early, recovery is good.

Other toxic neuropathies

Some neuropathies are associated with a clear history of industrial exposure to a neurotoxin (e.g. acrylamide, hexane, trichlorethylene), or present a characteristic clinical picture, e.g. the motor neuropathy of lead or the associated gastrointestinal disturbance and skin pigmentation seen in arsenic poisoning.

Drugs may cause neuropathy in several ways; some are known to affect neurotubules, to interfere with vitamin or lipid metabolism, or to cause nerve ischae-mia by arteritis or vasospasm (Table 16.7). The presence of renal or hepatic disease may produce abnormally high concentrations of potentially neurotoxic drugs (e.g. nitrofurantoin).

Neoplastic Neuropathies

Nerve damage may be produced by direct infiltration of tumour, but neuropathy may also develop as a non-metastatic effect of neoplasia (see p. 221).

Myelomatosis is associated with a polyneuropathy which is sometimes caused by secondary amyloidosis. In other dysproteinaemic syndromes, nerve damage may follow impaired capillary perfusion due to the associated blood hyperviscosity or to immunological reactions within the nerve; in these cases immunosup-pression or plasmapheresis may improve nerve function.

Vascular Neuropathies

Multiple isolated peripheral nerve lesions due to areas of nerve infarction occur in the collagen vascular disorders, especially polyarteritis nodosa and rheumatoid arthritis. The subacute proximal neuropathy of diabetes mellitus is caused by a diabetic microangiopathy.

Autonomic Neuropathy

The main features of the autonomic system are summarised in Chapter 2, p. 54. Autonomic dysfunc-tion may present as postural hypotension, disturbance of bladder or bowel function, as impotence, or with altered sweating, vasomotor function, or pupillary responses, Clinical tests of autonomic function are summarised in Table 16.8.

Causalgia, a severe spontaneous pain which may occur after partial nerve lesions, has been attributed to abnormal sympathetic function and can often be relieved by sympathectomy, or pharmacologically with an adrenergic neurone blocker such as guanethidine. Many types of neuropathy affect autonomic function mildly, but some produce severe involvement due to damage to small myelinated and non-myelinated fibres (diabetes; primary amyloidosis).

Diabetes mellitus

Diabetic autonomic neuropathy presents with impo-tence, postural hypotension, diarrhoea and sphincter disturbances; cardiac denervation is also common.

Guillain–Barré syndrome

Autonomic involvement in the Guillain–Barré syn-drome usually presents with cardiac dysthythmias and labile hypertension.

Amyloidosis

In the neuropathy of primary amyloidosis there is predominant degeneration of small myelinated and non-myelinated fibres. This results in distal pain and temperature loss in the limbs, and trophic ulceration and autonomic symptoms. Other causes of autonomic failure are shown in Table 16.9.

Treatment: Symptoms of autonomic failure are difficult to treat. Autonomic diarrhoea may respond to

Table 16.7

Clinical Presentation of Some Drug-induced Neuropathies

Clinical Presentation	Drug	Site or Mode of Action
Sensory	Phenytoin	Axon
	Isoniazid	Pyridoxine metabolism
	Chloramphenicol	Axon (? B_{12} metabolism)
	Procarbazine	Axon
Motor	Dapsone	Axon
	Gold	Axon
	Amphotericin	Axon
Sensorimotor	Nitrofurantoin	Axon
	Perhexilene	Myelin
	Vincristine	Axon (neurotubules)
	Chlorambucil	Axon
	Disulfiram	Axon
Mononeuropathy	Ergotamine	Ischaemia

Table 16.8

Clinical Tests of Autonomic Function

Function	Test	Pathway
Sweating	Raise body temperature	Sympathetic
Blood pressure	B.P. response to tilt, Valsalva	Arterial baroreceptors, Efferent sympathetic
Heart rate	Beat-to-beat variation,	Parasympathetic (vagus)
Pupils	Methocholine, Hydroxyamphetamine	Parasympathetic, Sympathetic
Bladder	Pressure studies	Parasympathetic

tetracycline and daytime postural hypotension may be helped by tilting the patient's bed, head up, at night, or increasing the circulating volume with fludrocortisone.

Idiopathic Neuropathy

Despite full investigation, including nerve conduction studies and sometimes nerve biopsy, the cause of at least 50% of neuropathies remains undetermined. Most present as a chronic progressive sensorimotor distal neuropathy.

Cranial Mononeuropathies

I and II nerves (see Chapter 2)

V nerve (see p. 38)

Trigeminal neuralgia is the commonest disorder of the trigeminal nerve. It presents with stabs of severe pain in the distribution of one or more divisions (usually maxillary), often precipitated by speaking, eating, cold air on the face or by touching 'trigger areas'. The cause

Table 16.9

Causes of Autonomic Failure

1. Peripheral neuropathy	diabetes mellitus
	Guillain–Barré
	1° amyloidosis
	porphyria
	renal failure
	vincristine
2. Familial dysautonomia	Riley–Day syndrome
3. Idiopathic orthostatic hypotension	with Parkinsonism
	with multiple system atrophy
	(Shy–Drager) (see p. 157)

is uncertain but may be vascular compression of the trigeminal nerve roots: rarely, it is due to multiple sclerosis or a cerebellopontine angle lesion, when there are usually accompanying physical signs unlike the idiopathic variety.

Trigeminal neuralgia usually responds to treatment with carbamazepine but if it is intractable it may be treated with thermocoagulation of the trigeminal ganglion – which may, of course, also produce numbness of the face. Trigeminal neuropathy presents which progressive facial sensory loss together with weakness of the masseter muscle. It may be idiopathic, but compression or infiltration of the nerve must be excluded.

III, IV and VI nerves (see p. 33)

Dysfunction of the IIIrd, IVth and VIth cranial nerves causes double vision. While it is important to consider a compressive aetiology within or behind the orbit, an isolated lesion of these nerves may occur in diabetes mellitus, arteritis, syphilis, or after viral illnesses or trauma. An isolated VIth nerve palsy may be a false localising sign of raised intracranial pressure.

VII nerve (see also p. 39)

Damage to the facial nerve causes unilateral weakness of all the muscles of facial expression. If the nerve is injured proximal to its course through the middle ear,

taste to the anterior two-thirds of the tongue is affected; involvement of the branch to the stapedius muscle causes hyperacusis. The commonest facial neuropathy is known as Bell's palsy. This is an idiopathic condition presenting with pain behind the ear followed by unilateral facial weakness. Complete recovery usually occurs in a majority of patients and incomplete nerve lesion at ten days and young age are favourable prognostic factors. A proportion of cases develop Wallerian degeneration and recovery is slow, incomplete, and accompanied by aberrant reinnervation: this proportion may be reduced by early use of steroid therapy. Other causes of facial palsy are shown in Table 16.10. Herpes zoster of the geniculate ganglion causes facial paralysis, a painful vesicular eruption in the external auditory meatus or fauces, and loss of taste over the anterior two-thirds of the tongue (Ramsay

Table 16.10

Causes of Facial Palsy (Peripheral)

Bell's palsy
Ramsay Hunt syndrome (herpes zoster)
Sarcoidosis
Leprosy
Inner ear disease (cholesteatoma)
Cerebellopontine angle tumours
Basal skull fractures
Parotid gland tumours

Hunt syndrome). Bilateral facial nerve involvement is common in the Guillain–Barré syndrome and in sarcoidosis.

In hemifacial spasm, repeated shock-like contractions occur in the facial muscles of one side especially in the orbicularis oculi. The cause is presumed to be abnormal irritability of the facial nerve but in only a minority of patients can a structural lesion be found (e.g. basilar aneurysm, cholesteatoma, acoustic neuroma). Compression of the nerve by tortuous and atheromatous blood vessels may account for some cases.

The condition usually affects middle-aged females and is slowly progressive, the spasm being worse during anxiety and when talking and eating. Medical treatment is ineffective but minor mechanical or chemical injury to the facial nerve, e.g. in the middle ear, effectively reduces the spasms for months at a time.

Hemifacial spasm should be distinguished from blepharospasm, facial tics and abnormal re-innervation after Bell's palsy.

VIII nerve (see also p. 42)

VIII nerve (see also p. 42)

Common causes of damage to the VIIIth nerve incude acoustic neuroma and basal skull fractures. Nerve deafness is also seen in Refsum's disease (see p. 202), in hypothyroidism, after toxic damage from certain drugs (streptomycin, ethacrynic acid), and after viral infection (e.g. mumps).

Vestibular neuronitis presents with acute vertigo, nystagmus and vomiting. There is no disturbance of hearing and symptoms generally resolve within a few weeks. The initial attack is sometimes followed by several briefer attacks which gradually diminish in severity.

Glossopharyngeal neuralgia (see also p. 45)

Glossopharyngeal neuralgia (see also p. 45)

It is very rare for the IXth nerve to be involved in isolation, but it may be damaged by tumours in the cerebellopontine angle or at the jugular foramen. Glossopharyngeal neuralgia is the counterpart of trigeminal neuralgia and presents with brief, lancinating pains in the side of the throat, at the base of the tongue, in the neck, or deep inside the ear. Attacks may be precipitated by swallowing or touching the ear. If treatment with carbamazepine is ineffective, surgical avulsion of the nerve is indicated.

Isolated vagal or hypoglossal neuropathy is rare, but the recurrent laryngeal branch of the vagus is susceptible to damage or infiltration by tumour in the neck or mediastinum.

Polyneuritis cranialis

Patchy involvement of the cranial nerves occurs in sarcoidosis, malignant infiltration of the skull base or meninges, basal meningitis, diabetes, and lymphoma. Generalised cranial nerve motor impairment is common in Guillain–Barré syndrome.

TREATMENT OF NEUROPATHY

When a neuropathy is discovered to be due to a specific disorder then treatment is primarily directed to the cause. Neuropathies associated with collagen vascular disorders are treated with corticosteroids and/or other immunosuppressants such as cyclophosphamide. Chronic relapsing inflammatory neuropathies may respond to prednisolone in a daily or alternate-day regime, but steroids are of no proven value in the management of Guillain–Barré syndrome, dysproteinaemic neuropathy, and the neuropathies of malignancy. The place of plasmapheresis in the management of the Guillain–Barré syndrome and dysproteinaemic neuropathies is uncertain. General treatment of neuropathies include analgesics for dysaesthesiae and muscle cramps, physiotherapy and splints to improve posture and, in certain neuropathies, skin care to prevent trophic ulceration. Vitamins are of little value except when vitamin deficiency is the cause of the neuropathy.

17

Muscle Disease

INTRODUCTION

Striated muscle makes up about 40% of man's body weight. Essentially it is a biological machine which transduces stored chemical energy into useful energy forms such as work (force × distance) and heat. The force generated by muscle fibres must act through a stable system of tendons and bones in order to produce movement at joints and hence work. Work production is controlled by the selection of appropriate muscle groups and modulation of their force production by recruitment of motor neurones and adjustment of their firing rate. Coordination of work production depends on both efferent information in the motor pathways and afferent information supplied from muscle spindles, tendon organs, proprioceptive and special sense organs and cerebellar pathways.

PHYSIOLOGY

A muscle fibre is a multinucleated cell enclosed within a plasma and basement membrane (the sarcolemma). Each fibre contains myofibrils (Fig. 17.1a,b) which are in turn composed of the myofilaments or contractile, regulatory and structural proteins whose unit of structure is the sarcomere (Fig. 17.1b). An α motor neurone innervates a group of muscle fibres (the motor unit) which may be as small as six fibres (external ocular muscle) or as large as 2000 fibres (gastrocnemius). The muscle fibres of a motor unit interdigitate extensively with those of other motor units, being distributed through up to 20% of the total muscle cross-section.

Following neuromuscular transmission, a regenerative action potential spreads over the sarcolemma and reaches the myofibrils within the fibre along the transverse tubular or T system (Fig. 17.1b). Each T tubule is closely related to the terminal cisternae of the sarcoplasmic reticulum (sr). The coupling of electrical excitation to mechanical contraction occurs when the former causes the release of calcium ions (Ca^{++}) from the terminal cisternae. Ca^{++} binds to a regulatory protein – troponin – sited on the actin filament and, following a conformational change, cross-bridges form between the myosin and actin filaments. Work is performed when a further conformational change in the cross-bridges causes the filaments to slide past each other and the sarcomere to shorten. When excitation ceases, Ca^{++} is actively taken up by the sr and the reduced sarcoplasmic concentration allows dissociation from troponin and disengagement of the cross-bridges.

Energy for these processes is immediately supplied from the hydrolysis of ATP by various ATPase enzymes, one of these being part of the myosin structure (Fig. 17.2). ATP can be rapidly resynthesised in the short term from phosphocreatine (PC) or by glycogenolysis even in the absence of oxygen. These pathways are of particular importance at the start of exercise before muscle blood-flow has increased, or if high force contractions are made, since these will prevent an adequate rise in muscle blood-flow and hence oxygen delivery. In the longer term and at low contraction forces, ATP is regenerated from oxidative phosphorylation in mitochondria using a variety of substrates including blood-borne glucose, fatty acids, amino acids and lactate.

Human muscle fibres are subdivided into two essential types, the fibres of any single motor unit being homogeneous (Table 17.1). When a transverse section of muscle is stained for myosin ATPase, a chequerboard pattern of fibres is apparent. Lightly-staining fibres (low

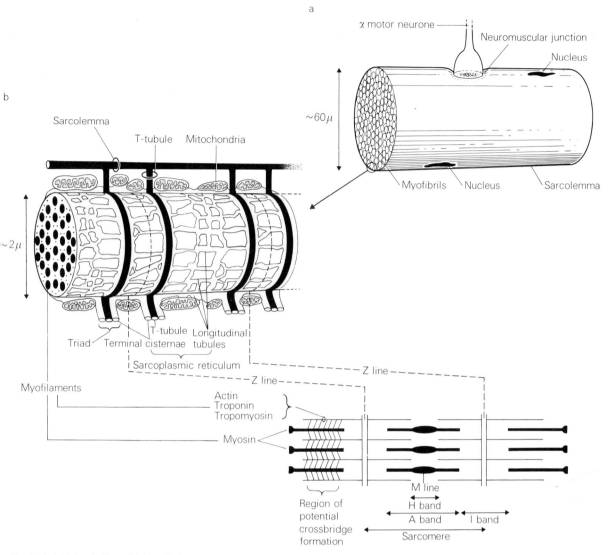

Fig. 17.1 (a) *Muscle fibre.* (b) *Myofibril.*

activity) are type I, and darkly-staining are type II. These two fibre types have characteristic properties (see Table 17.1) and may be differentially affected in a variety of muscle disorders.

PATHOPHYPHYSIOLOGY

Weakness (failure of force generation) is the principal feature of muscle disease and the cause of weakness can be analysed into a number of different components which vary from disease to disease (Table 17.2). Acute muscle-fibre necrosis may occur following exposure to certain drugs or alcohol, or when energy supply is critically reduced as in ischaemia or certain genetic disorders of metabolism, or in acute inflammation. There is massive release of intracellular electrolyte, including potassium, creatine kinase (CK), and myoglobin, which may deposit in the renal tubules and cause renal failure. Chronic degeneration of fibres is the main feature of the muscular dystrophies; a genetic mem-

a. *Immediate source.*

ATPase

Adenosine triphosphate (ATP) $\longrightarrow$ adenosine diphosphate (ADP) + inorganic phosphate (P$_i$) + **Energy**

b. *Short term (anaerobic) sources*

1. Phosphocreatine (PC) + ADP $\rightleftharpoons$ creatine + **ATP**

creatine kinase (CK)

2. Glycogen/glucose + P$_i$ + ADP $\longrightarrow$ H$^+$ + lactate$^-$ + **ATP**

glycolytic pathway (cytosol)

c. *Long term (aerobic) sources*

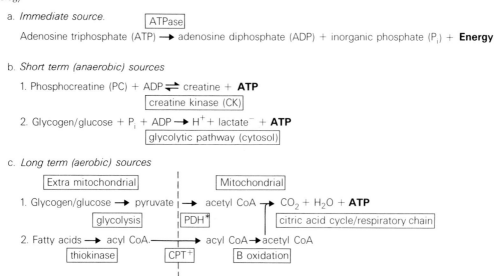

* pyruvate dehydrogenase complex
+ carnitine palmityl transferase shuttle for long chain fatty acids

Fig. 17.2 *Sources of energy in striated muscle.*

Table 17.1

Muscle Fibre Types

	Type I	Type II
Myosin ATPase	Low	High
Mitochondria and oxidative enzymes	High	Low (Type IIb) Medium–high (Type IIa)
Capillaries around muscle fibres	+ + +	+
Predominant source of energy	Oxidative metabolism	Glycogenolysis + some oxidative metabolism
Contractile properties	Slow twitch	Fast twitch
Fatigability	Resistant	Fatigable (IIb) Intermediate (IIa)
Recruitment	Low forces Tonic contractions Posture	High forces Fast contractions

---

brane defect may be the initial abnormality. In inflammatory muscle disease, damage is either directly due to an infective agent or to an abnormality of immunity or both. In both dystrophic and inflammatory disease, some fibres may regenerate, and healthy fibres hyper-trophy pari passu with necrosis in adjacent fibres. The degree of weakness will depend on the net functional cross-sectional area of remaining muscle fibres.

Muscle fibres atrophy with disuse and in response to many toxic or metabolic influences, and type II fibres

Table 17.2

Analysis of Muscle Weakness

Muscle fibre cross-section and coarse structure initially preserved	Failure of electrical excitation or excitation–contraction coupling	Reduced motoneurone recruitment (e.g. corticospinal lesion) Depletion of motoneurones (e.g. anterior horn cell loss or neuropathy) Impaired neuromuscular transmission (e.g. myasthenia gravis/myasthenic syndrome) Impaired sarcolemmal excitability (e.g. electrolyte (K^+) imbalance, periodic paralysis, myotonia) Abnormal T-tubular system (e.g. as for sarcolemma) Reduced excitation contraction coupling (e.g. acidosis, dantrolene therapy, following heavy exercise) Abnormal Ca^{++} control by sr (e.g. malignant hyperpyrexia)
	Altered or reduced energy supply for muscle fibre metabolism	Reduced glycogenolysis (e.g. myophosphorylase or phosphofructokinase deficiency) Reduced supply of substrate for oxidative metabolism (e.g. defective mitochondrial fatty acid transport – carnitine or carnityl transferase deficiency: reduced O_2 supply – vascular claudication) Impaired mitochondrial function (e.g. defective or missing respiratory chain elements including cytochromes) Impaired control of energy release (e.g. hypermetabolic myopathy, and myopathy with 'loosely coupled' mitochondria)
Muscle fibre cross-sectional area and/or number reduced early	Loss of muscle fibres due to necrosis	Toxic necrosis of muscle fibres (e.g. due to drugs, alcohol) Inflammatory myopathies Muscular dystrophies
	Atrophy of muscle fibres	Disuse Metabolic disorders (e.g. excess corticosteroids) As part of a dystrophic or inflammatory process Secondary to denervation

appear to be particularly susceptible. The consequent reduction in fibre cross-section results in weakness. Some congenital myopathies show major abnormalities of the usual proportions of type I and II fibres.

It is increasingly recognised that there are disorders of muscle where the coarse structure and fibre cross-section are initially well preserved and where weakness or other symptoms result from defective excitation, excitation–contraction coupling or energy supply (Table 17.2). Thus myasthenia gravis is associated with a reduction in available acetylcholine receptors at the neuromuscular junction, in part due to the binding of specific antibodies. The increased excitability and repetitive discharges of the sarcolemma in certain forms of myotonia (causing delay in relaxation after contraction) is found to be attributable to a specific reduction in membrane chloride conductance. The acute muscle rigidity and fibre necrosis which occurs in malignant hyperpyrexia is attributable to a genetic sensitivity of the sr to certain anaesthetics and/or muscle relaxants, resulting in massive Ca^{++} release. Enzyme defects in the glycolytic pathway have been identified (e.g. myophosphorylase and phosphofructokinase deficiency) which result in impaired force generation and contracture during high force contractions or ischaemia, in which glycolysis is essential. Parallel defects in fatty-acid transfer into mitochondria and defects in oxidative phosphorylation within the mitochondria are recognised which may result in muscle pain, weakness and necrosis under conditions where oxidative metabolism is required, such as during prolonged exercise. In many cases, however, the relationship between the biochemical defect and clinical symptoms is still ill-understood.

CLINICAL FEATURES

History

Characteristically, myopathic weakness affects the limb girdles and proximal muscles initially. The patient complains of difficulty in lifting, carrying or reaching down heavy objects, raising the arms to comb the hair or difficulty running or walking up steps, rising from a low chair or getting out of bed. Some diseases, notably myasthenia gravis, may present with complaints of drooping eyelids, double vision, inability to chew, or impaired speech or swallowing due to weakness of the cranial musculature. Breathlessness due to respiratory muscle weakness is occasionally a presenting symptom in adult-onset myopathy or neurogenic disorder (e.g. motor neurone disease). Nocturnal hypoventilation is suggested by a history of interrupted sleep, nightmares, morning headache and daytime somnolence, which is usually secondary to a lack of normal sleep. Congenital neuromuscular diseases often present as floppy hypotonic infants with breathing or sucking difficulties. Normal motor development is delayed or incomplete.

Myopathies usually cause progressive symptoms but may on occasion show short-term fluctuations, which is a point of diagnostic importance. Increasing weakness with activity followed by recovery after a brief rest suggests myasthenia gravis; severe weakness lasting hours after a night's sleep, heavy meal or exercise raises the possibility of a periodic paralysis. Symptoms specifically related to exercise, such as pain, cramps or myoglobinuria, may indicate a disorder of energy supply to the working muscles. Muscle pain and cramps at rest or on minor activity occurs in chronic denervation, in the inflammatory myopathies, in hypothyroidism, and in some toxic myopathies. Muscle stiffness and impaired relaxation of contracted muscles, particularly when worse in the cold and improving with repetition is suggestive of myotonia (impaired muscle relaxation due to repetitive sarcolemmal depolarisation).

A full family history is essential. Where a hereditary disorder such as muscular dystrophy is a possibility, it may be necessary to examine relatives fully to exclude minor or trivial features which they may not have noticed and which give a clue to the type of inheritance. Details of pregnancy such as the presence and timing of intrauterine movements, any feeding, swallowing or respiratory difficulty in early life, and developmental milestones should be obtained from the patient's mother. In adults, a description of sporting abilities at school is a useful guide with which to compare later disability. Details of any medication taken may be relevant to the cause of a myopathy (Table 17.3).

Examination

The patient should be observed performing the tasks which he or she finds difficult to do. Girdle and truncal

Table 17.3

Drug-induced Muscle Disorders

Pattern of disease	Drug	
Acute rhabdomyolysis	Diamorphine	
	Phencyclidine	
	Amphetamines	
	Alcohol	
Subacute proximal myopathy	Diamorphine	Lithium
	Alcohol	Emetine
	Clofibrate	Corticosteroids
	Chloroquine	All drugs causing
	Quinine	hypokalemia
Myasthenic syndromes	D penicillamine	
	Aminoglycosides	
	Tetracyclines	
	Phenothiazines	
	Propranolol	
	Phenytoin	
	Lithium	
Malignant hyperpyrexia	Various anaesthetic agents	
	Psychotropic drugs (acute dystonic syndrome)	

weakness is often more obvious when watching a patient walk, or get up from the floor or a low chair, than on the examination couch. Spinal posture is checked for excessive lumbar lordosis or scoliosis resulting from pelvifemoral or paraspinal muscle weakness. The cranial musculature should be particularly examined for ptosis, external ocular paresis, weakness of the jaw or face, and impairment of swallowing, tongue or palatal movements. The neck muscles are frequently affected, especially the flexors.

Selective wasting of muscle groups, together with relative preservation or even enlargement of other groups anatomically nearby, is the hallmark of the muscular dystrophies. Diffuse weakness and wasting suggests an acquired myopathy or, more rarely, a congenital myopathy. Tendon reflexes tend to be preserved until a late stage in weak muscles, and sensory changes are absent.

It is easy to miss significant respiratory muscle weakness, and therefore observation of the respiratory rate, the accessory muscles of respiration and the movements of the diaphragm are important. Major diaphragmatic weakness is suggested by inward abdominal wall movements on inspiration rather than the normal outward movement as the diaphragm actively descends: the supine vital capacity is typically much less than that in the erect posture due to the effect of gravity on the abdominal contents. Measurement of vital capacity, peak inspiratory/expiratory mouth pressures, or arterial blood gas monitoring are routine ancillary measurements in the clinical assessment of respiratory muscle weakness.

In genetically-determined myopathies, mental and cardiac function should be especially noted, whilst in acquired myopathies extra attention is given to looking for evidence of systemic disease affecting the skin, joints, endocrine system and heart.

Investigation

The purpose of investigations is, firstly, to confirm that

the clinical features are due to a primary muscle disorder and, secondly, to define the nature of the disorder. The plasma CK is usually elevated in primary muscle disease due to leakage from damaged fibres, but it may be normal in metabolic and congenital disorders and the enzyme may be mildly elevated in neurogenic muscle wasting, following exercise, intramuscular injections or needling of the muscle as in electromyography (EMG). In acquired proximal myopathy and metabolic and myasthenic disorders, appropriate specific screening tests (see p. 26 and Table 17.4) are essential, since the muscle biopsy may show only non-specific changes.

In an EMG study, a needle electrode is used to search for spontaneous electrical discharges in resting muscle and to sample the size, shape and interference pattern of motor unit potentials during contraction. Quantitative methods are also available and the examination often allows the distinction between myopathic and neurogenic weakness to be made but rarely yields a specific diagnosis. Evidence of impaired neural function or neuromuscular transmission failure is confirmed by nerve conduction studies, repetitive nerve stimulation and, when indicated, single-fibre electromyography (see Chapter 3).

In many muscle disorders a specific diagnosis can only be made by examining a muscle biopsy. A wide range of specific histochemical and biochemical techniques, in addition to routine histology and electron microscopy, are now available and are essential in the diagnosis of many metabolic disorders, enzyme defects and congenital myopathies. The extent of muscle fibre loss can be, to some extent, judged from strength measurements, from 24-hour urinary creatinine excretion, or from CT scanning of muscles (Fig. 17.3): the latter allows fat infiltration of muscle and selective muscle involvement to be clearly seen.

SPECIFIC MUSCLE DISORDERS

The classification of muscle disease is a mixed descriptive, genetic and aetiological one which reflects our incomplete knowledge. The main groupings with examples are shown in Table 17.4 and the more important disorders are outlined below.

Muscular Dystrophy

X-linked recessive

The severe form (Duchenne) has a prevalence of 1/3500 males and is usually detectable clinically at 2–5 years of age. Motor development is delayed and the gait clumsy and later waddling. Later the child can only rise from the floor by using his hands to climb up his legs (Gower's manoeuvre). The cranial musculature is initially spared, but the costal origin of the pectoralis major, triceps, brachioradialis, latissimus dorsi and pelvic girdle muscles are selectively involved early and the calf

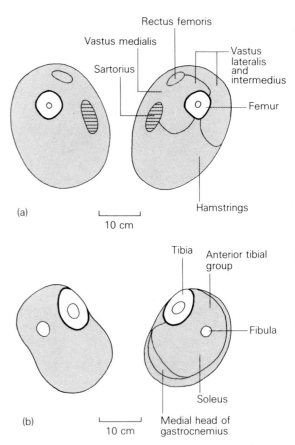

Fig. 17.3 *Mid-thigh (a) and mid-calf (b) CT scans of a man with Becker muscular dystrophy. In the thigh scan, sartorius is hypertrophied and is the only muscle of normal density. The low density of other groups is due to muscle replacement with fat and connective tissue. In the calf scan, the muscles are bulky and of normal density except for selective fat infiltration of the medial head of gastrocnemius.*

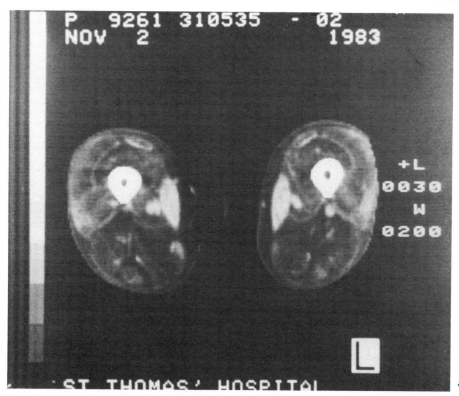

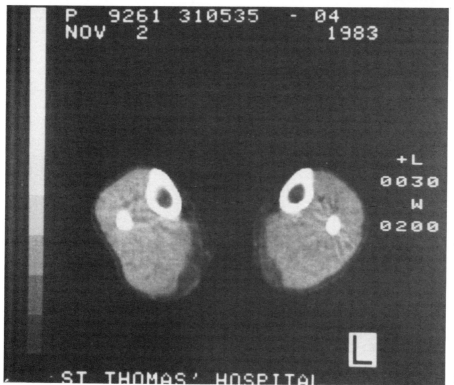

Table 17.4

Classification of Muscle Diseases

Genetically-determined myopathies	*Examples*
1. Muscular dystrophies	Duchenne, Becker, facioscapulohumeral, limb girdle, myotonic, scapulo-peroneal, oculo-pharyngeal
2. Myotonic disorders	Myotonic dystrophy, myotonia congenita, paramyotonia congenita
3. Periodic paralyses	Hypo-, hyper-, normokalemic periodic paralysis
4. Specific disorders of metabolism	Myophosphorylase deficiency and other enzyme defects of glycogen, fatty acid or mitochondrial metabolism
5. Congenital myopathies with specific anatomical features	Central core, minicore, nemaline rod diseases, congenital fibre type disproportion
6. Others	Malignant hyperpyrexia
Acquired myopathies	

1. Inflammatory myopathy	Specific viral, bacterial or parasitic infection
	Polymyositis alone
	      with skin lesions (dermatomyositis)
	      associated with collagen disease
	      associated with malignant disease

2. Metabolic myopathy	Associated with corticosteroid excess
	      thyroid disease
	      acromegaly
	      calcium/vitamin D disorders
	      electrolyte disorder – hypokalemia
	      alcohol excess
	      drugs (see Table 17.3)

3. Myasthenic disorders	Myasthenia gravis, myasthenic syndrome (Eaton–Lambert syndrome), congenital myasthenia

muscles are enlarged and of a rubbery consistency. Later most muscle groups are weak (Fig. 17.4a). Contractures of the hip flexors and ankle plantar flexors are common. By the age of 8–11 years the boy, frequently by this stage obese, becomes confined to a wheechair; respiratory muscle weakness, together with progressive scoliosis, leads to respiratory insufficiency. Death occurs in the late teens or twenties. A cardiomyopathy and a mild non-progressive intellectual deficit are common associated features.

A milder though similar pattern of muscle disease (Becker dystropy) is also seen, with the same inheritance as Duchenne. These patients become wheel-chair-bound late in the third decade, on average, and death occurs in the fifth decade, although the range is wide. In both Duchenne and Becker dystrophy the CK is high (e.g. 30–300 times normal) in the early stages but falls with age and disease progression. Female carriers may have trivial clinical features occasionally and a raised CK more usually.

Autosomal dominant

Facio-scapulohumeral dystrophy is very variable in extent and severity, even within a given family. It presents in the second or third decade with facial,

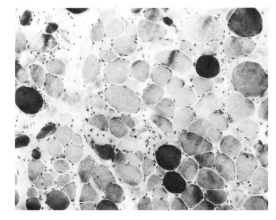

a

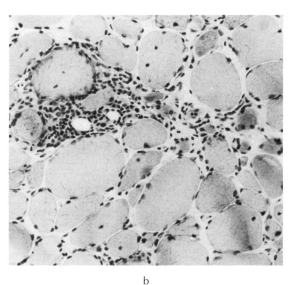

b

Fig. 17.4 (a) *Muscle biopsy (haematoxylin and eosin, transverse section) from a boy with Duchenne dystrophy. There is increased fat and connective tissue between the fibres, excessive variation in fibre size, and some fibres with internal (central) nuclei. The dark rounded fibres are eosinophilic hypercontracted fibres and some of the smaller darker fibres are basophilic and probably regenerating. There is no inflammation.*
(Courtesy of Dr B Lake in Brett, EM, Paediatric Neurology, Churchill Livingston, 1983, with permission.)
(b) *Muscle biopsy (haematoxylin and eosin, transverse section) from a woman with polymyositis. There is marked variation in fibre size, excess numbers of internal nuclei, and muscle fibre necrosis: a marked interstitial inflammatory infiltrate of cells is seen and there are some darker basophilic regenerating fibres.*

periscapular, humeral (frequently sparing the deltoid initially), and anterior tibial weakness. An early onset tends to carry a poorer prognosis but more often severe disability does not occur until the fourth or fifth decades, and sometimes weakness may be trivial and unnoticed by the patient at all. A dystrophy with a scapulo-peroneal distribution occurs, which may have either an X-linked recessive or an autosomal dominant inheritance, or alternatively it may be neurogenic in origin.

Myotonic dystrophy is associated with characteristic lens abnormalities and eventual cataract, frontal balding, intellectual deterioration, testicular atrophy and other endocrine disturbances (e.g. glucose intolerance), immunological (low serum IgG) and cardiac conduction defects: sudden death may occur from the latter. The principal muscular features are ptosis, weakness and wasting of the muscles of mastication and sternomastoids, and early distal involvement affecting the hands and causing foot drop. Generalised weakness occurs later and the extraocular, bulbar and respiratory muscles may be involved. Grip and percussion myotonia are variable features but myotonia can always be detected on EMG. The onset may be at any age and congenital cases present as floppy retarded infants with breathing and sucking difficulties. In the latter group the mother is invariably the affected parent although she may be asymptomatic apart from a bad obstetric history.

Myotonic dystrophy must be distinguished from myotonia congenita. In the dominant form of this disease the muscles are often large, not weak, myotonia is prominent, and skeletal muscle is the only organ affected: in the recessive form a moderate degree of proximal weakness occurs in later life, but overall the implications are less serious than with myotonic dystrophy. A number of rare dominantly-inherited dystrophies occur, affecting the distal muscles, external ocular and pharyngeal muscles.

Autosomal recessive

Limb girdle dystrophy usually causes progressive weakness of the pelvic and shoulder girdle muscles, sparing the cranial musculature. The condition requires careful differentiation from spinal muscular atrophy (due to anterior horn cell degeneration), chronic polymyositis, and adult-onset acid maltase deficiency (a glycogen storage disease) which is characterised by severe diaphragmatic weakness and early respiratory failure, with mild proximal limb weakness and severe pelvic girdle and trunk weakness.

Inflammatory Myopathy

Specific inflammatory disorders rarely occur in the UK and, in the common form of the disease, there is no known infective agent. Polymyositis may occur at any age (commonly 30–50 years). Proximal and later distal painful or painless weakness progresses over a period of weeks or months and may extend to facial, pharyngeal, respiratory and cardiac muscle. In the uncommon acute form there can be very rapid progression over days, severe muscle pain and myoglobinuria. The muscles alone may be affected but frequently there are associated skin lesions (dermatomyositis), notably peri-orbital violaceous rashes, erythematous zones over the extensor surfaces of the limbs and extremities, and areas of vasculitis. Polymyositis may occur in the context of a collagen vascular disease and, over the age of 50, dermatomyositis may be associated with occult malignant disease (usually carcinoma). In adults there is experimental evidence of a cell-mediated immune response directed against striated muscle, but in children there may be a vasculitis within muscles associated with immunoglobulin and complement deposition (Fig. 17.4b).

Immunosuppressive treatment with corticosteroids or cytotoxic drugs is usually effective. The pattern of medication is controversial, but high doses of cortico-steroids (e.g. prednisolone 60–100 mg/day in adults) are required initially and azathioprine is frequently started at the same time. Cyclophosphamide, methotrexate, plasma exchange, and whole-body irradiation have also been used in refractory cases but a number of patients, particularly those with a very chronic course, respond poorly or not at all.

Metabolic Myopathy

Patients presenting with acquired proximal muscle weakness should be carefully screened for endocrine disorder (see Table 17.4) and disorders of electrolyte (notably potassium), calcium, or vitamin D metabolism.

A full drug history is essential (Table 17.3), and details of alcohol intake are relevant since excess may be associated with either acute rhabdomyolysis or a subacute myopathy. Disorders of energy metabolism and enzymatic or biochemical deficiencies, though frequently genetically determined, may not present until the teens or even adult life with exercise-related symptoms or simple progressive muscle weakness. A muscle biopsy is especially helpful under these circum-stances.

Thyroid disease

i. *Hypothyroidism*: Muscular pains, stiffness and cramps are common symptoms not necessarily associated with weakness. Muscle relaxation is slowed and this is most clearly seen following a tendon jerk. The delay in relaxation is *not* due to repetitive muscle excitation (as in myotonia) but is probably the result of a reduced rate of cross-bridge uncoupling. Frank muscle weakness occurs in some patients, and the muscles may be firm and enlarged on palpation. The creatine kinase is raised and fibre atrophy is seen on muscle biopsy.

ii. *Thyrotoxicosis*: Muscle weakness and wasting often affect the limb girdles, and evidence of fibre atrophy (of both types I and II) is seen on biopsy. The creatine kinase is usually normal but experimentally there is an increased rate of muscle breakdown. In males (usually of mongoloid race) a rare form of hypokalemic periodic paralysis occurs, causing episodic truncal and limb weakness. Myasthenia gravis is associated with autoim-mune thyroiditis and occasionally complicates hyperthyroidism; conversely, myasthenia is exacer-bated by hyperthyroidism.

The ophthalmoplegia which may complicate Graves disease is caused by enlargement of the extraocular muscles due to infiltration with mucopolysaccharide, fat, inflammatory cells and eventually fibrosis. The globes may be proptosed and elevation and/or external rotation are limited due to tethering causing diplopia. Enhanced sympathetic activity causes overactivity of levator palpebrae superioris, resulting in lid lag and lid retraction. Intraocular pressure may be raised (particu-larly on upgaze) due to tethering, and the optic nerve can be compressed in the orbit, causing visual failure. CT scanning demonstrates the enlarged muscles but the results of thyroid function tests are variable and do not correlate with the severity of the opthalmopathy. Treatment is of the underlying thyroid disorder initially. Tarsorrhaphy may be required to protect the cornea if proptosis is severe, and steroids and immunosuppression are of value. Rarely, orbital decompression is required to preserve failing vision.

Corticosteroids

The administration of corticosteroids is one of the commonest causes of proximal muscle weakness but endogenous excess, as in Cushing's disease, may have similar effects. The synthetic fluorinated compounds such as dexamethasone are particularly potent in this respect, but individual susceptibility is marked. Muscle biopsy reveals selective atrophy of type IIb fibres initially, and it is thought that the steroids exert their effect through altered rates of protein turnover. Corticosteroids may also cause weakness through hypokalaemia. Treatment is aimed at minimising the necessary steroid dosage, finding alternative medication where possible, and maintaining physical activity. Primary hyperaldosteronism (Conn's syndrome) commonly presents as muscle weakness secondary to hypokalaemia.

Potassium disorder

Hypokalaemia is commonly caused by medication, notably diuretics. This is an important cause of morbidity and chronic hypokalaemia may cause structural muscle changes. Rarely, patients with an inherited membrane disorder present with episodes of weakness, usually following a period of rest after exercise or a meal. The weakness may be profound, though usually sparing bulbar and respiratory function, and is associated with the movement of potassium into cells, causing hypokalaemia. Hypokalaemic periodic paralysis may be treated by avoiding heavy carbohydrate meals, and treatment with carbonic anhydrase inhibitors and potassium supplements. A fixed myopathy occurs in some patients. Hyperkalaemic and 'normokalaemic' forms are described, and they may be associated with myotonic features.

Energy metabolism (see Fig. 17.2 and Table 17.2).

There are numerous enzymatic defects of muscle energy metabolism.

i. *Glycogenolytic*: Myophosphorylase and phosphofructokinase deficiency are the best known. During high intensity or ischaemic contractions, muscle pain occurs, with contracture (electrically silent) and rhabdomyolysis if ischaemia continues. Patients complain of pain at the start of exertion or during high intensity exercise but may exercise normally at low work loads when oxidative metabolism of fatty acids predominates. Lactate production is absent during ischaemia, indicating a block in anaerobic glycolysis (see Fig. 17.2). The diagnosis is confirmed by biopsy and enzyme assay.

ii. *Mitochondrial disorders*: Many specific defects affecting oxidative metabolism have now been characterised. In some cases there is a history of muscle pains, weakness, and fatigability at low exercise levels, punctuated by episodes of severe lactic acidosis indicating excess anaerobic glycolysis and impaired lactate metabolism. Some patients have different symptoms, including chronic progressive external ophthalmoplegia, a myopathy and, variably, other features including pigmentary retinopathy, cerebellar syndrome, dementia, neuropathy, and cardiac abnormalities. The muscle biopsies of such patients show accumulations of abnormal mitochondria ('ragged red fibres') and the precise biochemical lesion may be determined on isolates of mitochondria. Severe mitochondrial lesions may also cause an encephalopathy in childhood.

Related disorders of fatty acid metabolism cause episodic muscle weakness or pain and acidosis on prolonged exercise. Deficiency of carnitine (systemic or muscle) or the enzyme necessary for fatty acid transfer into mitochondria (CPT I or II) is responsible (see Fig. 17.2). The diagnosis may be suggested by accumulations of lipid on muscle biopsy, and some cases of carnitine deficiency may be effectively treated by oral replacement.

Myasthenia Gravis

This condition is characterised by the presence of fatigable weakness affecting (in descending order of frequency) the external ocular, jaw, facial, bulbar, respiratory and limb muscles. It is associated with a circulating IgG antibody which binds to the acetylcholine receptors of the neuromuscular junction, and there are abnormalities of the post-synaptic membrane with a reduction in the number of receptors. The antibody may be passively transferred to a fetus *in utero* and cause transient neonatal myasthenia. The immunological abnormality is associated with thymic hyperplasia in 75% of cases and thymoma in about 15%. Antibodies to striated muscle are usually present in the latter group. The condition is often associated with other autoimmune diseases and may be exacerbated or precipitated by certain drugs (Table 17.3).

Once suspected clinically, the diagnosis can be confirmed by observing an improvement in strength after administering a short-acting anticholinesterase drug e.g. edrophonium chloride. Repetitive supramaximal nerve stimulation at low frequencies (3 Hz) causes an abnormal decrement of the compound muscle action potential due to blocking of transmission to individual muscle fibres (see p. 62): excess 'jitter' and fibre-blocking can be detected using single fibre techniques. Acetylcholine receptor antibodies are present in 75% of patients with purely ocular symptoms, and in about 90% of those with generalised disease.

Oral anticholinesterase medication (usually pyridostigmine or neostigmine) results in symptomatic improvement in most cases. Diarrhoea is a common side-effect, which can be treated by dosage modification or atropine. Not all muscles are influenced to the same degree by this medication and optimal dosage for one group may be excessive or suboptimal for another; assessment should always therefore be directed to clinically relevant muscle groups such as respiration and bulbar function. Thymectomy is frequently recommended for patients with generalised myasthenia (i.e. not pure ocular disease), whose symptoms are not fully controlled by anticholinesterases, and who are fit for chest surgery (sternotomy). The presence of thymoma is an added indication for surgery since these tumours are locally invasive. Immunosuppression with corticosteroids and cytotoxic agents is also highly effective in inducing remission of disease and may be a necessary preliminary to surgery in patients with severe disease: it is also a valuable treatment in those not fit for surgery for other reasons, for persistent symptoms after surgery, or for severe isolated ophthalmoplegia. Remission may sometimes be hastened by removal of antibody by plasma exchange.

Great care must be taken to closely monitor bulbar and respiratory function in this condition. The manipulation of anticholinesterase drugs or the use of corticosteroids is always attended by the risk of deterioration in muscle strength and should only be performed where adequate facilities for control of the airway and ventilation are available.

Patients with myasthenia gravis are, in addition, sensitive to the effects of fever, and intercurrent infection and a number of drugs also exacerbate the condition (Table 17.3).

Other myasthenic disorders: myasthenic syndrome (Eaton–Lambert syndrome)

This condition is characterised by progressive proximal weakness, sometimes involving ocular and bulbar muscles. Supramaximal nerve stimulation at slow rates show a small compound muscle action potential which rapidly increments at fast rates of stimulation – a feature typical of a presynaptic transmission defect. (see p. 59). The clinical concomitant is that strength may temporarily improve after a voluntary contraction, or a depressed tendon reflex may be greatly enhanced after a voluntary contraction. The condition is associated with oat cell carcinoma of the lung, or with autoimmune disease, and probably has an immunological basis but acetylcholine receptor antibodies are not present. Treatment with agents which potentiate transmitter release may be helpful and guanidine is effective but may cause marrow suppression and renal impairment. Trials are in progress with other agents such as 3' 4' aminopyridine, immunosuppression, and plasma exchange.

GENERAL PRINCIPLES OF MANAGEMENT

Objective criteria of change in muscle strength or performance can greatly assist the long-term documentation and management of muscle disorders. The MRC scale (see p. 8) is useful in quantitating broad categories of weakness and assessing its distribution but, for the longitudinal monitoring of individual patients, more precise methods can be used. Timed tests of performance (e.g. straight-leg raising, holding the arms outstretched, raising the head from the bed) are appropriate for monitoring fatigable conditions but are less sensitive to change in strength *per se*. Maximum voluntary strength can be precisely measured using dynamometers or spring balances; this accurately reflects the functional output of a muscle group and allows change in strength to be identified independently of other factors. Tests of performance such as the ability or time taken to walk upstairs, to rise from a standard low chair, or to sit up from supine are also useful, but it should be appreciated that the ability to perform complex actions is not related in a simple manner to the strength of individual muscle groups, as such actions are influenced by skeletal stability, pain, strength of synergists and other factors.

The prevention of contractures and obesity and maintenance of joint mobility, together with instruction on posture and gait, are important facets of management, especially in advancing muscular dystropy and inflammatory myopathy. When the ability to walk is borderline, a contracture, a marked gain in weight, or an unnecessary fall resulting in injury or bedrest may result in irreversible progression of weakness and premature permanent recourse to a wheelchair.

Weakness of paraspinal muscles and scoliosis, often of great severity, occurs particularly in Duchenne dystrophy and the judicious use of spinal and limb braces and corrective surgery may permit an extra period of independent mobility.

Prompt management of chest infection, respiratory insufficiency and bulbar dysfunction is essential. Even in untreatable disease the use of tracheostomy and/or assisted ventilation, particularly at night, may greatly enhance the quality of life if symptoms of respiratory insufficiency and bulbar dysfunction are troublesome.

Genetic counselling should always be offered to patients, and relatives of patients, with muscular dystrophy where appropriate. On occasion, adequate counselling may entail the examination and investigation of relatives in order to detect carriers or mildly affected individuals. A variety of techniques are now available for both early pre- and postnatal detection of certain dystrophies, but the practical application of these in the individual patient is a highly specialised and difficult area of management.

18

Pain

For a definition of pain it is hard to beat 'Pain is what the patient says hurts'. Pain is an experience rather than just another sensation. Many factors interact to create this experience (Fig. 18.1).

NEUROLOGICAL MECHANISMS

Nociceptive receptors

A nociceptor is a receptor preferentially sensitive to tissue-damaging stimuli. There are, however, no receptor nerve endings which inevitably evoke pain when stimulated or whose frequency of discharge primarily determines the intensity of the perceived discomfort. On the other hand, there are morphologically distinct nerve endings in all tissues which when activated *may* give rise to pain, depending on a variety of modulating influences. These nerve endings constitute the nociceptive receptor system.

In most tissues (skin, adipose tissue, fascia, periosteum, joint capsule, pleura, pericardium, peritoneum, dura mater, mucous membrane), the nociceptive receptor system is represented by a continuous three-dimensional plexus of unmyelinated nerve fibres that permeates the tissue. In the cornea, teeth, joint ligaments, tendons and muscles the nociceptive receptor system is histologically more straightforward and consists simply of free nerve endings. Except in the CNS and all capillaries, the walls of blood vessels contain a plexus of encircling unmyelinated nerve fibres, embedded in the adventitial sheath.

These receptor systems are normally inactive but are excited by excessive distortion of the tissue in which they are embedded, or by marked alterations in the chemical composition of the surrounding tissue fluid. The magnitude rather than the direction of physical distortion determines the degree of excitation. Perivascular nociceptors may be stimulated by either marked vasodilation or marked vasoconstriction.

Chemical excitation may occur when a sufficient concentration of various substances accumulates in the surrounding tissue fluid, for example, lactic acid, potassium ions, bradykinin, prostaglandin E, 5-hydroxytryptamine, and histamine.

Adjectives used by patients sometimes help to determine the pathogenesis of the pain. 'Throbbing' suggests a pain of vascular origin, whereas 'pressing' or 'bursting' suggest a more diffuse interstitial cause. 'Burning' in acute pain may suggest chemical provocation, though in chronic pain it relates to the unpleasant sensations associated with nerve destruction (dysaesthesia).

Primary Afferent Neurones

Nociceptive activity is transmitted to the central nervous system through small-diameter afferent neurones. The majority of the axons travel in the peripheral nerves to the dorsal horn of the spinal cord. A minority, however, travel in autonomic nerves and enter the spinal cord by the anterior rather than the dorsal root.

The nociceptive axons, whether somatic or visceral in origin, are all less than 5 μm in diameter. Those between 2 μm and 5 μm are thinly myelinated (A-delta), and those less than 2 μm – the majority – are unmyelinated (C fibres). Their small size is responsible for their relative inexcitability, slow conduction velocity, and resistance to ischaemia. Their relative inexcitability to electrical stimulation, compared with mechanorecep-

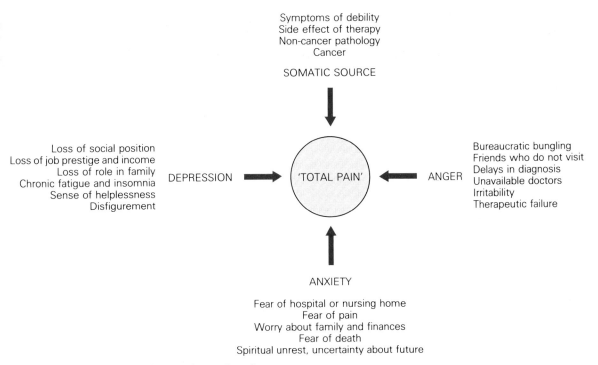

Fig. 18.1 *A diagram to illustrate the many factors that influence the patient's perception of pain, with particular reference to cancer.*

tor afferents, may account in part for the effectiveness of transcutaneous electrical nerve stimulators in the relief of certain types of chronic pain.

Central Connections

As the nociceptive afferents enter the spinal cord they give off ascending, segmental and descending collateral branches that then enter the spinal grey matter. Some form polysynaptic connections subserving reflex motor and autonomic activity whilst others synapse on secondary neurones which have axons ascending in the contralateral anterolateral (spinothalamic) tracts (see p. 21). The dorsal horn grey matter, and the substantia gelatinosa especially, contain several neurotransmitters including substance P, γ-aminobutyric acid (GABA), glycine and enkephalins.

Nociceptive impulses are subject to modulation (either inhibition or facilitation) by descending supraspinal pathways and by large myelinated sensory fibres

from the same and neighbouring spinal segments. Onward transmission into spinothalamic and other pathways is therefore potentially modified by many influences. At a higher level the posterior group of thalamic nuclei, reticular formations and periaqueductal gray matter are thought to be important in processing nociceptive information. Cortical analysis of pain is ill-understood but it seems clear that modulation of nociception occurs at all levels of the nervous system.

Opioid Peptides

An increasing number of naturally-occurring peptides with morphine-like properties have been isolated in the last decade. Three distinct families have been identified. Each stems from a different prohormone and is preferentially associated with a different class of opioid receptor. The enkephalin group has a high specificity for the delta-receptor, dynorphins for the kappa-receptor, and endorphins the the mu-receptor (morphine binding site). All three families of opioid peptides, together with their complementary receptors, are present in the brain and are concentrated in certain areas, e.g. dorsal horn and periaqueductal gray matter, midline raphenuclei in the brainstem. The opioid peptides form the chemical messengers (neurotransmitters and neurohormones) of a widespread and complex inhibitory signalling system. With respect to pain modulation, the mu-receptor is perhaps the most important. Experiments have shown that β-endorphin is by far the most potent as an analgesic agent.

PRINCIPAL PATTERNS OF PAIN

Pain Sensitivity

Pain threshold is defined as the least stimulus intensity at which a person perceives pain and *pain tolerance threshold* as the greatest stimulus intensity causing pain that a person is prepared to tolerate. Pain threshold varies between ethnic groups even under controlled conditions in the laboratory. Within a given ethnic group, however, some people are more sensitive to noxious stimuli than others. What some describe merely as warmth is reported as painful by others. Normal subjects may be divided into hypersensitive, normosensitive and hyposensitive. Hyposensitive subjects experience much less pain even, for example, after myocardial infarction.

Sensory input can be modified at successive synapses throughout its course from the spinal cord to the cortical areas of the brain responsible for the perception of pain. The central nervous system also has the ability to develop patterns of abnormal spontaneous activity. This abnormal activity can arise in the pain pathways anywhere between the dorsal horn and cerebral cortex following a peripheral nerve or root lesion. This may result in the continuing perception of pain in the absence of peripheral stimuli.

Modulation within the brain is in part of psychological origin. A person's sensitivity to pain varies according to mood or morale, and to the perceived meaning of the pain. For example, bone pain in cancer is perceived as a threat and tends to be more intense than osteoarthritic pain which, unless very bad, is normally regarded merely as a nuisance. Thus for any given noxious stimulus, the pain experienced can vary from ache to agony. In therapy, therefore, attention must be paid to a variety of factors that modulate pain intensity including anxiety, depression, and fatigue (Table 18.1) as well as to attempts to treat the source of the pain itself.

Table 18.1

Factors Affecting Pain Threshold

Lowered threshold	Raised threshold
Discomfort	Relief of symptoms
Insomnia	Sleep
Fatigue	Rest
Anxiety	Sympathy
Fear	Understanding
Anger	Companionship
Sadness	Diversional activity
Depression	Reduction in anxiety
Boredom	Elevation of mood
Introversion	
Mental isolation	
Social abandonment	Analgesics
	Anxiolytics
	Antidepressants

Referred Pain

The phrase *referred pain* is used to describe the perception of pain in the skin or other superficial structure but which is caused by a noxious stimulus in a deeper structure at some distance from the site of the pain. Patients with angina pectoris commonly experience referred pain in the upper chest, shoulder, neck and arm. This pain is the result of myocardial ischaemia but is manifested at other sites.

Referred pain from compression of peripheral nerves or spinal cord is relatively easy to understand. So is referred pain from a lesion in the region of the thalamus. Referred pain from bone and from myofascial structures is partly understandable on the basis of a 'flare' phenomenon – local nociceptive recruitment via plexus linkage. Pain referred from viscera can be explained on an embryological basis. An example is the presence of pain in the ipsilateral shoulder associated with inflammation of the diaphragm in cholecystitis.

Both the diaphragm and the shoulder are innervated by fibres derived from the primitive C4 segment. It is postulated that the brain 'misinterprets' the afferent impulses that converge on it from both visceral and somatic structures. The pain from the viscus is represented as having come from the embryologically-corresponding somatic area.

Nociceptive and Dysaesthetic Pain

Nociceptive pain, caused by physical or chemical stimulation of the nociceptors, possesses the qualities associated with, for example, cramp, bruising and toothache. In contrast, pain caused by neuronal destruction, whether peripheral or central, is dysaesthetic in quality. 'Dysaesthesia' describes an unpleasant cutaneous tingling, stinging or burning sensation. If intense, the patient calls it pain. Allodynia is such pain provoked by a non-noxious stimulus like a light touch. The patient cannot bear to have water or clothing touch the affected area. Dysaesthetic pain, with or without allodynia, is most commonly seen in post-herpetic neuralgia, after amputation or traumatic avulsion of nerve roots, and in paraplegia.

Causalgia is a term used to describe the syndrome of sustained burning pain commonly seen after a traumatic nerve lesion. It is combined with vasomotor and sudomotor dysfunction, together with trophic skin changes. *Neuralgic* pain occurs in the distribution of a nerve or nerve root. Paroxysmal neuralgia has a sharp lancinating quality: each episode of pain tends to be brief (lasting perhaps seconds) but may be frequently repeated.

Acute and Chronic Pain

Pain may be classified as either acute or chronic (Table 18.2). Chronic pain can be subdivided into:

   i. chronic pain of malignant origin
   ii. chronic pain of non-malignant origin
   iii. 'chronic pain syndrome'

The physical manifestations and the psychological concomitants vary according to type (Table 18.3). Severe acute pain is accompanied by an autonomic 'fight or flight' response, seen also in acute anxiety. The patient looks distressed and tends to protect the painful area. In contrast, vegetative features tend to predomi-

Table 18.2
Acute and Chronic Pain: Classification with Examples

Category	Examples
Acute	Acute nerve root irritation/compression Herpes zoster Trigeminal neuralgia, migrainous neuralgia Raised intracranial pressure
Chronic malignant pain	Soft-tissue distension Visceral involvement Bone metastasis Nerve compression or infiltration
Chronic pain of non-malignant origin	Degenerative spinal disease, arachnoiditis Post-herpetic neuralgia Causalgia Thalamic pain Phantom limb pain Tension headache Raised intracranial pressure
'Chronic pain syndrome'	

nate in chronic pain of non-malignant origin. These features are also commonly seen in organic depression. This implies that a patient may be in severe pain yet not look distressed. It is all too easy for a doctor with no experience of chronic pain to forget this distinction. A doctor's understanding of pain is usually taken from his own experience of acute pain – toothache, headache, etc. – all of which pass relatively quickly. In contrast, chronic pain is a situation rather than an event.

'Chronic pain syndrome'

Although most people with chronic pain of non-malignant origin have a clearly identifiable disorder, a small number do not but tend to have complex social and psychological problems. These patients have become dependent on their painful situation as a complex strategy to avoid the challenges of life. They obtain considerable 'secondary gain' from their suffering and have a vested interest in maintaining ill health. They exhibit 'pain behaviour' which has the perpetuation of the sick role as its goal. Treatment is complex and is based on 'operant conditioning'. This focuses on overt pain behaviour and seeks to reduce it by modifying the environmental consequences of the patient's actions.

ASSESSMENT OF PAIN

In the great majority of patients with pain it is possible to determine an underlying cause. The diagnosis is reached by the usual methods, in particular enquiring about the characteristics of the pain (Table 18.4) followed by examination and special investigations where indicated. The manner in which a patient reacts to pain may be influenced by several factors other than the original cause. Some patients may exaggerate their symptoms, either because they form the opinion that the doctor does not believe them or for some secondary gain such as sympathy from relatives or for compensation. At other times symptoms appear exaggerated because of associated depressive illness. By contrast, some patients may minimise their pain to an extraordinary degree or their tolerance may fluctuate.

In assessing pain, therefore, it is important to recognise the patient's total situation, since this in- fluences the perception of pain, whilst at the same time attempting to reach a diagnosis of its cause.

PAIN RELIEF

There are several facets to pain relief and frequently more than one needs to be exploited.

Explanation

The importance of *explaining* in simple terms the mechanism(s) underlying the patient's pain should not be forgotten. Pain that does not make sense or, worse, is seen as a threat is always more intense than pain which is understandable.

Modification of the Pathological Process

Whenever curative therapy is possible, this is the treatment of choice. Often therapy can to some extent modify the results of the pathological process; for example carbamazepine in trigeminal neuralgia, ergotamine in migrainous neuralgia, immobilisation of the neck in radicular pain from cervical spondylosis. In other settings, palliative treatment is of great value: non-curative radiotherapy may be very effective for pain caused by bone metastasis.

Elevation of Pain Threshold

Psychological methods

There are an increasing number of psychological and physical techniques for pain control that act largely by psychological mechanisms. These include relaxation, biofeedback, hypnosis and exercise/physiotherapy. Progressive use of a painful and sensitive limb may help to increase the pain threshold. Reduction of stress and the removal or modification of precipitating psychological factors are of great importance in many patients and should not be underestimated, even where there is a clear physical cause for the pain.

Table 18.3

Acute and Chronic Pain: Physical and Psychological Concomitants

	Acute		Chronic	
Time course	transient		persistent	
Meaning to patient	positive i.e. draws attention to injury or illness	negative i.e. serves no useful purpose		positive i.e. as patient obtains secondary gain
Accompanying features	fight or flight: 1. pupillary dilatation 2. increased sweating 3. increased respiratory rate 4. increased heart rate 5. shunting of blood from viscera to muscles		vegetative 1. sleep disturbance 2. anorexia 3. decreased libido 4. constipation 5. somatic preoccupation 6. personality change 7. work inhibition	

Table 18.4

The PQRST Characteristics of Pain

	'Tell me about your pain.' 'Where is it?'
PQRST	
P Palliative factors	'What makes it less intense?'
Provocative factors	'What makes it worse?'
Q Quality	'What is it like?'
R Radiation	'Does it spread anywhere else?'
S Severity	'How severe is it?'
T Temporal factors	'Is it there all the time, or does it come and go?'

Counter-irritant cutaneous stimulation

The relief of chronic pain by counter-irritants is a common practice in primitive cultures and is still a basic principle in the home remedies used by many people. Treatment with massage, vibration, ice packs, hot water bottles and menthol ointments are all effective in relieving the aches and pains of bedfast patients. Relief of pain may outlast the duration of the activity of the counter-irritant but, even if it does not, a short period of relief from a niggling ache may serve to improve morale.

Cold can be applied directly to the painful area with an ice pack, cold damp towels or with a reusable gel pack. Cold packs can provide relief from headache, spasticity and/or muscle spasms, and joint and back pains associated with immobility. Some people prefer hot packs, heating pads or a hot water bottle, especially for back pain and muscle spasm. A hot water bottle may also be helpful for abdominal cramp.

Many analgesic ointments contain menthol, easily detected by its strong odour. An application of menthol ointment to the skin produces a sensation of warmth or cooling that may last several hours. The mechanism by which menthol relieves pain is obscure but it is frequently effective for joint pain, muscle spasm and tension headache.

Various theories have been invoked to explain counter-irritation, most based on the gate control theory of pain and/or on the production of endogenous opioids.

Transcutaneous electrical nerve stimulation

This method of pain modulation was known to the Romans, who used electric eels as current generators. There was a revival of interest in the 19th century when more sophisticated sources of electricity became available. The use of electro-analgesia subsequently waned because the majority of patients did not benefit from it. In recent years, stimulated by the gate control theory of pain, there has been renewed interest in transcutaneous electrical nerve stimulation (TENS). TENS may work by stimulating the large fibres involved in pain conduction and thereby inhibiting the small fibre input to the dorsal horn of the spinal cord. The successful use of TENS depends on the correct positioning of the electrodes and the optimal adjustment pulse width, frequency and intensity.

Published data shows that TENS may give short-term benefit in many patients treated for various types of chronic pain but its efficacy usually declines with time. It is possible that TENS acts by suggestion, distraction, counter-irritant or placebo mechanisms.

Acupuncture

Acupuncture may be performed in several ways, including the manual rotation of needles and low-frequency or high-frequency electrical stimulation through them. Naloxone, a specific opioid-receptor antagonist, reduces or abolishes low-frequency electro-acupuncture analgesia though it has no effect on analgesia induced by high-frequency electro-acupuncture. Naturally-occurring opioid peptides are released into the cerebrospinal fluid during acupuncture. The evidence that different forms of acupuncture elicit specific neurohormonal effects gives acupuncture a certain scientific respectability. It has, however, only a limited place in clinical practice as an adjunct in the management of chronic pain of non-malignant origin.

Interruption of Pain Pathways

Nerve block

Nociception may be blocked by use of a local anaesthetic or one of several destructive (neurolytic) techniques. Theoretically, local anaesthetic blocks are temporary but, in practice, they may provide partial or complete pain relief for a prolonged period.

A number of local anaesthetic agents are available, notably lignocaine and bupivacaine. The former is short-acting (1–2 hours); the latter relatively long-lasting (8–12 hours). Lignocaine is a vasodilator and is often used with adrenaline to retard absorption and metabolism and allow a greater maximum safe dose.

Bupivacaine is not a vasodilator. Unwanted effects are unusual and generally relate to overdosage. Occasionally a hypersensitivity reaction may occur, manifesting as profound hypotension and tachycardia after only a small dose.

Local anaesthetic blocks fall into three categories:

i. diagnostic
ii. prognostic
iii. therapeutic

A local anaesthetic nerve block confirms whether a pain is related to compression of a specific nerve and acts as a predictor of the likely outcome of a subsequent neurolytic procedure. Most anaesthetists use a local anaesthetic routinely before a peripheral (as distinct from intrathecal) block.

Neurolytic agents (e.g. alcohol, phenol and chlorocresol) cause demyelination and degeneration of the nerve roots. Following intrathecal administration, patchy damage to fibres of all sizes, extending into the dorsal column of the spinal cord, may occur. Neurolytic procedures are normally carried out only in cancer patients with a short life expectancy, by suitably-trained anaesthetists. If there is a good chance of successful anti-cancer treatment, or the patient is expected to survive for several years, neurolytic blocks are best avoided. Complications include sensory loss, motor weakness, urinary dysfunction and faecal incontinence. The pain eventually recurs, even following a successful block, and the duration of relief varies from two or three weeks to several months.

During the terminal stages of cancer, when most patients have a variety of symptoms, often including several pains, drug therapy generally has more to offer than neurolysis. However, if a patient has a relatively localised unilateral pain caused by neoplastic nerve compression, a nerve block may be the treatment of choice. This is particularly true if the risk of urinary or anal sphincter dysfunction is small, as with blocks in the upper lumbar spine.

Sympathetic block

Many painful states, especially when caused by partial injury to a large mixed peripheral nerve, are accompanied by features of autonomic dysfunction, vasoconstriction, sweating and nail changes. There is also marked allodynia and the patient protects the part against all stimuli. This syndrome, especially in the upper limb, may respond to sympathetic block, notably with regional intravenous guanethidine.

Neurosurgery

Although occasionally used in non-malignant conditions, neurosurgery is generally reserved for cancer pain that has failed to respond to other measures. Cordotomy (anterolateral tractotomy) is the procedure most commonly used. There are two types: surgical and percutaneous.

Percutaneous cordotomy is achieved by inserting a needle in the C2/C3 interspace under x-ray control. A thermal lesion is made in the anterolateral quadrant of the spinal cord using radio frequency waves. Surgical cordotomy requires a general anaesthetic, is usually done in the upper thoracic region, and the anterolateral quadrant of the cord is cut under direct vision. Cordotomy is used mainly for intractable unilateral pain located in segments from the mid-thorax downwards. Bilateral percutaneous high cervical cordotomy is hazardous because of the likelihood of sleep apnoea caused by interruption of the motor fibres to the diaphragm.

Cordotomy of either variety has limitations. The alleviation of the unilateral pain may 'unmask' a severe pain on the contralateral side. Moreover, although seemingly permanent, the versatility of the central nervous system is such that relief does not often last for more than 6–18 months. Although this is sufficient for many patients with terminal cancer, for a substantial minority it is not.

Ablation of the pituitary gland with alcohol is used occasionally to relieve *bone* pain in cancer when other

---

Table 18.5

Neuromuscular Classification of Pain: Implications for Therapy

Type of pain	Treatment
1. Muscle spasm	baclofen diazepam
2. Nociceptive	analgesics
3. Nerve compression	analgesics corticosteroids nerve blocks
4. Nerve destruction (dysaesthetic) peripheral nerve – occasionally useful; cord lesion – of no benefit	psychotropic drugs (especially antidepressants) opioids corticosteroids nerve blocks cordotomy
5. Mixed nerve compression and destruction (partly dysaesthetic)	treated as mixed 3 and 4 (?) stellate ganglion block for upper limb pain

methods have failed. It helps the majority of patients, whether the tumour is hormone-dependent or not. It should be stressed that cordotomy and pituitary ablation are necessary only in a relatively small number of cancer patients.

Immobilisation

Some patients continue to experience pain on movement or weight-bearing, despite analgesics, drugs, radiotherapy and nerve blocks. In these the situation may be improved by explaining the mechanism of pain and suggesting commonsense modifications to daily activity. Individually-designed plastic supports for patients with multiple collapsed vertebrae or Thomas splints for femoral pain are occasionally necessary to overcome intolerable pain on movement in bedfast patients. The humerus can be immobilised in the bedfast patient by an arm sling fastened to a torso jacket by means of interlocking Velcro.

DRUGS

Many drugs influence pain. Some affect it indirectly, such as antibiotics in cystitis and anti-inflammatory drugs in rheumatoid arthritis. These drugs act by modifying the pathological process and fall outside the definition of analgesic. Spasmolytics are another group of pain-modulating drugs. The use of analgesics is best seen as one way of elevating a patient's pain threshold. Analgesics, including narcotics, do not usually relieve pain caused by nerve damage (dysaesthetic and stabbing pains). The site of the neurological lesion and the types of pain determine which pharmacological measures are appropriate (Table 18.5).

Care of the Patient

THE ACUTE NEUROLOGICAL ILLNESS

In many major acute neurological illnesses the essential principles of management are similar. The care and rehabilitation of the patient often requires a team approach utilising several different services (Table 19.1). One of the principal tasks of the doctor is to decide when the help of these services should be enlisted. Early involvement of paramedical staff often helps in identifying the factors likely to cause prolonged disability and hence delay a return to normal life (Table 19.2). The major causes of neurological disability in the UK are shown in Table 19.3.

The patient may often be dependent on the nursing staff for all his immediate needs, due to paralysis or impairment of cerebral function. He will require careful positioning to maximise comfort, to protect pressure areas and prevent contractures: the unconscious patient needs to be positioned with protection of the airway as the primary consideration. Lifting and moving the ill patient, particularly when there is limb weakness,

is a skilled procedure of which medical staff usually have little knowledge. Thus patients should never be dragged to the sitting position by their arms or shoulders as this quickly leads to stretching of the joint capsule with subsequent pain and further loss of function.

Fluids and Nutrition

Great care should be taken initially in the administration of fluids and nutrition by mouth until it is clear that the patient has intact bulbar function: patients particularly at risk in this respect are those with an impaired conscious level, with brainstem disease, and with conditions such as myasthenia gravis and Guillain–Barré syndrome. Aspiration of food, fluids or vomit may not only cause pulmonary problems but also a deterioration in neurological status due to hypoxia, hypercarbia and infection. The use of a nasogastric tube or the intravenous route for fluids and feeding will be determined by several factors, including the ability to

---

Table 19.1

Agencies Involved in Rehabilitation

---

1. Physiotherapy, Remedial gymnast, Orthotist
2. Occupational therapy
3. Speech therapy
4. Clinical psychologist
5. Nursing services especially in management of incontinence
6. Social services (housing welfare, allowances)
7. Disablement Resettlement Officer/Job Centre/Industrial Training

---

Table 19.2

Major Factors Affecting Return to Normal Life in Acquired Neurological Disease

a. Disordered higher function   dementia, confusion, poor concentration
impaired language function
impaired visuospatial perception
loss of motivation
altered mood

b. Loss of mobility   weakness
incoordination of limbs or trunk
akinesia and rigidity
spasticity and loss of fine motor control
sensory loss and impaired postural control
apraxia

c. Incontinence

Table 19.3

Estimated Prevalence of Disabling Neurological Conditions per 10 000 Population

Epilepsy	50
Stroke	25
Multiple sclerosis	8
Severe head injury	1
Blindness	20
Deafness	5
Others requiring rehabilitation:	Spinal injuries
	Polyneuritis (Guillain–Barré syndrome)
	Parkinson's disease

pass a nasogastric tube safely without provoking vomiting, on whether or not bulbar function is intact, and on whether there are craniofacial injuries which make it physically difficult or undesirable to pass a tube.

Careful regulation of intravenous and oral fluids is important in many acute neurological disturbances because of the risk of dehydration or, more commonly, of an excess water-load resulting in hyponatremia with the possibility of seizures and further deterioration. Many acute intracranial disorders have a tendency to cause temporary inappropriate antidiuretic hormone secretion; the regular monitoring of urine and plasma osmolalities is the most effective way of detecting this.

In a patient who is likely to have a protracted illness it is essential to start adequate nutrition, whether oral or intravenous, early. Major paralysing diseases quickly result in severe muscle-wasting and a large negative nitrogen balance, which is compounded by the frequent use of corticosteroids, by infection, and by lack of dietary calories and protein. In the longer term, vitamins, trace elements and minerals also need replacement.

Bladder, Bowels and Sexual Function

Not only is the care of the bladder and bowel function of medical importance but it is frequently a source of concern to patients, who may for the first time find themselves dependent in this respect on others. In the acutely ill or unconscious patient there may be little alternative initially to bladder catheterisation in women and either catheterisation or an external condom drainage system in men. The disadvantage is the inevitable infection of urine with catheterisation but the advantage is a reduced likelihood of macerated skin and pressure areas due to repeated incontinence. In most neurological disorders it is possible to remove the catheter once the patient is well enough to get out of bed.

If higher function is relatively intact, and the bladder has not been damaged by overdistension and repeated infections, patients with spinal cord lesions who cannot pass their urine initially may develop satisfactory reflex emptying when the lower cord and cauda equina is intact. Intermittent self-catheterisation is, in the long run, more satisfactory than chronic indwelling catheter in those with severe urinary retention. The advice of a genito-urinary specialist with access to detailed urodynamic investigations is often of great help when deciding on appropriate long-term management.

Oral medication has a part to play in less severe urinary symptoms, such as urgency and urge incontinence, and frequency and nocturia, where these symptoms are due to loss of inhibition of reflex emptying as in multiple sclerosis. Anticholinergic drugs such as propantheline or amitryptiline in low dose are helpful and the carefully-controlled use of arginine vasopressin has been advocated to reduce nocturia and nocturnal incontinence. These medications should not, however, be used if the major urinary problem is inadequate bladder emptying due either to detrusor inactivity or to failure of relaxation of the bladder sphincter, since they will promote further urinary retention, infection, and chronic damage to the urinary tract. Sphincter overactivity, once accurately diagnosed, may be relieved by alpha-blocking agents such as phenoxybenzamine, or by local injection of phenol. Whatever the symptoms, adequate bladder emptying without residual urine remains the primary aim of medical or surgical treatment.

Avoidance of constipation and faecal impaction is most important in patients with severe weakness. A regime is required for each patient which will enable him to have a regular bowel action at a convenient time. To this end it is necessary to maintain adequate bulk in the diet with the addition of fibre or bran and, if normal bowel control is absent, to use laxatives by mouth or suppository to regulate the bowel action. In the early stages of a long illness, regular rectal examination is important to detect impaction. Occasionally, an enema or manual removal of faeces is necessary on a regular basis.

Many major neurological illnesses impair sexual function completely or in part, and this is a further source of distress to the patient and his or her partner. Discussion of these problems is often helpful and, if necessary, referral for detailed counselling about techniques and appliances can be useful.

Physiotherapy

In the early stages of a major illness the physiotherapist will be particularly concerned with care of the chest and airway, utilising breathing exercises, postural drainage, intermittent positive pressure breathing, percussion and suction, and encouraging coughing. The physiotherapist will also advise about limb positioning to prevent pressure areas, pressure palsies and contractures. As recovery occurs the physiotherapist's guidance regarding mobilisation is essential, and discussion with him about subsequent aspects of mobility and use of limbs is routine. Measures to strengthen weak muscles or to reduce disadvantageous spasticity, and the use of aids such as sticks, crutches and walking frames, as well as advice about splintage of limbs where there is chronic and severe foot drop or wrist drop are all matters to be considered with the physiotherapist.

Apart from their physical roles, the physiotherapist and the nursing staff have a major role, together with the medical staff, in explaining the illness and its consequences to the patient (see p. 278).

Occupational Therapy

As the patient recovers from the acute illness or injury, the rehabilitative process gains momentum. The OT has special skill in assessing disability as it affects activities of daily living. Assessment of the patients' capabilities, bearing in mind the potential for recovery and his previous activities, may be necessary before his ultimate needs at home can be clarified. Specific attention is paid to feeding, dressing, going to the lavatory, bathing, washing and grooming, mobility, writing, cooking, and other activities initially. Most OT departments have facilities for doing these assessments but at a later stage a visit to the patient's home may be necessary.

The OT (or physiotherapist) will give guidance about mobility with respect to appropriate types of wheelchair, car modification, and the possibility of stair lifts and other structural adjustments which may be needed in the home. In addition, an orthotist may be available to advise about particularly difficult problems of mobility, limb appliances, etc.

Speech Therapist

Disorders of language and speech are major handicaps to any patient. It remains a matter of discussion as to how effective speech therapy techniques are in promoting recovery (as is also the case for physiotherapy, OT, and many medical techniques). Nevertheless, there can be little doubt that the dysphasic patient can be helped in many ways to come to terms with his disability, to understand its nature, and to make the best of his residual capabilities by informed guidance and instruction from the speech therapist. The abilities to read and write are also frequently affected, and advice about appropriate measures for overcoming these handicaps is essential.

Patients with severe dysarthria or dysphonia can be equipped with aids to help them communicate, including various electronic devices which can be operated even if there is minimal limb function.

Clinical Psychologist

The role of the clinical psychologist in rehabilitation is perhaps less well-defined than some of those mentioned above. An important aspect is the diagnositc one. The psychologist is trained to analyse the nature of disturbances of higher cerebral function, and formal assessment of the patient will allow this sphere of disability to be broken down into problems of language, memory, visuospatial disorders, dyspraxia, motivation and mood. Overall assessment of intelligence and its change over time are of value in documenting recovery and in planning for suitable occupations for a patient who has had a major brain illness or injury.

In some centres the clinical psychologist takes a more active therapeutic role in re-educating and retraining the brain-injured patient.

EMPLOYMENT AND FINANCIAL MATTERS

Advice about financial entitlement during prolonged sickness and leave of absence is of great importance.

Patients may have considerable anxieties about their dependent relatives, and the social worker may be able to allay these fears considerably by ensuring that the patient is fully informed about relevant allowances. If a patient is not competent to manage his own affairs, a suitable person may need to be appointed to do this, and it is necessary to take legal advice.

The disablement resettlement officer (DRO), employed by the Manpower Services Commission, can help and advise about future employment for those who are too handicapped to return to their previous work but yet are still able to do some work. Advice about suitability for an industrial rehabilitation unit or a sheltered workshop is also available. It is up to the doctor to try and provide relevant information which will enable the DRO to help. Clearly, factors such as motivation, intellectual ability, language function, mobility, and loss of use of limbs, epilepsy, ability to drive, visual and hearing difficulties, are also significant. A major neurological injury or illness often results in a protracted period of inability to work even if a return is ultimately possible. It is quite unrealistic to expect patients to leave hospital after many months and slot quickly back into their original job. Quite apart from their residual physical disability they are susceptible to fatigue, have frequently lost their usual sense of initiative, may lack concentration, and may become depressed. A rehabilitation unit is of value in assisting the transition from hospital life back into the outside world. Resources in such units are directed at helping to overcome or accept overt disability, increasing physical and mental tolerance, and preparing the ground for a return to home and work. Some patients will clearly not be able to return to their previous jobs because of mental or physical handicap, but they may be suitable for some type of industrial retraining.

HOUSING AND SOCIAL SERVICES

A severe hemiplegia or paraplegia may, depending on individual circumstances, make it difficult or impossible for patients to return to their old accommodation because of stairs, the absence of lifts, doors which will not allow a wheelchair through, or numerous other factors. Any degree of mental impairment will have a disproportionately severe effect on the ability to cope independently. Often the spouse or other relatives will be able to help but will require assistance, reassurance, and practical advice in order to do this. A decision has to be made at some stage as to whether the patient will be able to manage in his own home and, if not, what kind of accommodation is suitable: e.g., should he be rehoused in a ground floor flat; does he need warden-assisted accommodation; does he need a nursing environment? The possibilities will depend only in part on the type and severity of the disability; factors such as the availability of home helps, district nursing services, the possibility of modifying the home, the available relatives, and income all play a part. Thought needs to be given to these matters early in the illness and plans laid only after appropriate discussions with the relevant agencies, the patient and family and the family doctor.

DRIVING A MOTOR VEHICLE

Many neurological disorders affect the ability to drive. The question of epilepsy is dealt with on p. 117. A licence holder in the UK has to inform the Drivers Medical Branch at the Driver and Vehicle Licensing Centre if he or she develops any disability (including any physical or mental condition) which is or may become likely to affect fitness as a driver, unless it is not expected to last more than three months. This implies that, although it is the duty of the patient to notify the licensing authority, the doctor must ensure that the patient is adequately informed.

The eyesight must be sufficient to read approximately 6/12 (corrected) on a Snellen chart. Monocular vision does not usually preclude driving if the field is full. Field defects such as bitemporal or homonymous hemianopias are hazardous and usually preclude driv-ing. Diplopia or oscillopsia, or major degrees of impaired night vision as may occur in retinitis pigmentosa, should be notified.

The position of the driver who has sustained a head injury or had a neurosurgical operation (excluding those with epilepsy) is imprecisely defined. He should be advised, depending on the risk of post-traumatic epilepsy (see p. 108), whether he has other disabling symptoms such as attacks of giddiness, poor concentration or other problems. Driving is normally barred for at least a year after a major head injury or supratentorial craniotomy. Most neurological diagnoses do not necessarily lead to a ban on driving unless mental function, balance or vestibular function, consciousness, or vision are seriously affected. Impaired control of limbs, however, may make it necessary to modify car controls, either from manual to automatic or to special hand controls. Standards of fitness for holders of Heavy Goods Vehicle and Public Service Vehicle Licences are considerably more rigorous than for ordinary licence holders and any significant neurological disability is likely to lead to loss of the licence.

Disabled patients are entitled to certain parking privileges (orange badge scheme) which may greatly facilitate their lives, and a severe difficulty with walking entitles them to the Mobility Allowance. The combination of good advice about type of car and wheelchair may allow a very considerable degree of independence to the paraparetic or quadriparetic patient.

INFORMATION (Table 19.4)

Clinical Notes

The patient's history remains one of the most powerful diagnostic tools in clinical neurology, together with the

---

Table 19.4

Information

What?	Who?
a. Diagnosis	a. The patient
b. Prognosis personal statistical	b. The general practitioner
	c. The family
c. Plan of management and its aims and side-effects	Other agencies – social workers, employers
d. Specific advice e.g. work, pregnancy, driving, the home	

full examination, and shows no sign of being supplanted by the development of new investigation techniques. Therefore, for strict clinical diagnostic reasons as well as the more obvious legal reasons, clear and concise notes are of lasting value. In managing a patient through a long illness over many years there may be a loss of perspective as to how symptoms and signs have changed in relation to normality, and exact documentation of the degree of disability is most helpful. Hence, whilst a detailed description of the type of nystagmus may help in diagnosis, a description of whether the patient can walk independently and whether and what aids are required is of value for later comparison.

The General Practitioner

Communication with the family doctor should be prompt and concerned with relevant essentials. Often the diagnostic details of a particular patient are of little relevance to management, whereas details about the basic diagnosis, the expected prognosis, the information given to the patient and family, and the medication given to the patient are of practical importance. There may be a tendency with many chronic neurological problems for patients to become unduly dependent on the hospital although they may (in the UK) regularly see different doctors in the clinic. This is disadvantageous to the patient, whose interests are usually better served by a well-informed local doctor than by a remote and changing hospital situation. There should be clear reasons for follow-up in hospitals, and the family doctor and the patient should know what these are. Great care should be taken by hospital staff to consult with the family doctor about major problems in the home environment, since the Practice may well take considerable interest in and responsibility for the patient.

In deciding how best to manage difficult problems, the family doctor may be a great help in interpreting the intentions and plans of hospital specialists to the patient and in reassuring him. Conversely, bad news about diagnosis or prognosis is sometimes more appropriately conveyed by a doctor who knows the family well than by someone who has only seen the patient in the clinic once or twice. In all these matters close communication between hospital doctor and family doctor is of the essence.

The Patient and Family

What to tell the patient and his family about a serious diagnosis, when to do it, and how to express it is often difficult to decide. In general patients will ask their doctors questions about diagnosis and prognosis as and when they want to, provided that they are given an opportunity. Frequently one needs to invite questions, which should then be answered truthfully. Many patients wish to know if their prognosis is bad either because they regard it as their right or because they need to make practical arrangements to look after their affairs. In many neurological disorders, because the patient may be under follow-up for many years, a frank discussion of the diagnosis and its possible implications should be undertaken at an early stage once the diagnosis is certain. This often helps to form an atmosphere of trust between the patient and doctor and facilitates explanations when, perhaps, the condition worsens or relapses. Full explanation to the patient is of particular importance if the diagnosis has implications for others, especially relatives and children. This is a matter of major concern in the genetically-determined disorders, where not only is detailed genetic counselling often appropriate but practical steps may be available for preventing transmission of the condition. In this type of case the first approach should usually be to the patient and not to enquiring relatives.

When a condition affects an individual's insight, or occurs in a minor, it will frequently be appropriate to discuss diagnosis and prognosis with those who are caring for him or her (usually the spouse or parents). A serious diagnosis *per se* does not, however, imply that the family should be informed before the patient, which may have the effect of creating a rift between the patient and those close to him. Sensitive handling of these issues, and primary consideration for the welfare of the patient, with an awareness of the background family situation helps to resolve the issue.

From a practical point of view there is little to be gained from confronting the patient with a serious diagnosis before a rational plan of management has been decided on. This means that the matter must be discussed by the medical team and a clear plan evolved and then conveyed to others who will have to deal with the patient. Nothing causes a patient to lose confidence so fast as receiving conflicting information from medical advisers.

It is often necessary to write medical reports for non-medical agencies, such as solicitors, compensation boards, employers, insurance companies, etc. Although such reports are usually in the interests of the patient, it is important to obtain written permission to make them. Similarly, social services departments do not have automatic right of access to a patient's medical records and confidentiality should be respected.

Further Reading

Asbury A.K., Gilliatt R.W. (1984). *Peripheral Nerve Disorders – A Practical Approach*. London: Butterworths.

Bannister B.A. (1983). *Infectious Diseases*. London: Baillière Tindall.

Bannister R. (1983). *Autonomic Failure*. Oxford: Oxford University Press.

Brett E.M. (1983). *Paediatric Neurology*. Edinburgh: Churchill Livingstone.

Brodal A. (1981). *Neurological Anatomy (In Relation to Clinical Medicine)*, 3rd Edn. Oxford: Oxford University Press.

Dalessio D.J. (1980). *'Wolff's Headache and Other Head Pain'*, 4th Edn. Oxford: Oxford University Press.

Donaldson J.O. (1978). *Neurology of Pregnancy*. Philadelphia: W.B. Saunders Co.

Dubowitz V. (1978). *Muscle Disorders in Childhood*. Philadelphia: W.B. Saunders Co.

Dyck P.J., Thomas P.K., Lambert E.H., Bunge R. (1984). *Peripheral Neuropathy*, 2nd Edn. Philadelphia: W.B. Saunders Co.

Ellis R. (1980). *Inborn Errors of Metabolism*. London: Croom Helm.

Fowler T. (1982). *Guide for House Physicians in the Neurological Unit*. London: Heinemann.

Glaser J.S. (1978). *Neuroophthalmology*. Maryland: Harper & Row.

Halliday A.M. (1982). *Evoked Potentials in Clinical Testing*. Edinburgh: Churchill Livingstone.

Hallpike J.F., Adams C.W.M., Tourtellotte W.W. (1982). *Multiple Sclerosis*. Chapman and Hall.

Harding A.E. (1984). *The Hereditary Ataxias and Related Disorders*. Edinburgh: Churchill Livingstone.

Henson R.S., Urich H. (1982). *Cancer and the Nervous System (The Neurological Manifestations of Malignant Systemic Disease)*. Oxford: Blackwell.

Jennett B., Galbraith S. (1983). *An Introduction to Neurosurgery*, 4th Edn. London: Heinemann.

Jennett B., Teasdale G., Davis F.A. (1981). *Management of Head Injuries*. Philadelphia.

Kiloh L.G., McComas A., Osselton J.W., Upton E. (1981). *Clinical Electroencephalography*, 4th Edn. London: Butterworths.

Kimura J. (1983). *Electrodiagnosis in Diseases of Nerve and Muscle: Principles and Practice*. F. A. Davis.

Laidlaw J., Richens A. (1982). *A Textbook of Epilepsy*, 2nd Edn. Edinburgh: Churchill Livingstone.

Lambert H. (1983). Management Problems in Meningitis. *British Journal of Hospital Medicine*: **29**: 128.

Lance J.W. (1982). *Mechanism and Management of Headache*, 4th Edn. London: Butterworths.

Lenman J.A.R., Ritchie A.E. (1983). *Clinical Electromyography*, 3rd Edn. London: Pitman Medical.

Marsden C.D., Fahn S. (1982). Movement Disorders. *International Medical Reviews: Neurology 2*. London: Butterworths Scientific.

Matthews W.B. (1975). *Practical Neurology*, 3rd Edn. Oxford: Blackwell.

Mattingley S. (1981). *Rehabilitation Today in Great Britain*. London: Update Books.

McAlpine D., Lumsden C.E., Acheson E.D. (1972). *Multiple Sclerosis: A Reappraisal*, 2nd Edn. Edinburgh.

Medical Research Council Memorandum No. 45 (1976). *Aids to the Examination of the Peripheral Nervous System*. London: HMSO.

Miller N.R. (1984). *Walsh and Hoyt's Clinical Neuro-ophthalmology*, 4th Edn. Baltimore: Williams and Wilkins.

Parsons M. (1979). *Tuberculous Meningitis: A Handbook for Clinicians*. Oxford: Oxford University Press.

Raffle A. (1976). *Medical Aspects of Fitness to Drive*. Pub. by Medical Commission on Accident Prevention.

Ross Russell R.W. (1983). *Vascular Disease of the Central*

Nervous System, 2nd Edn. Edinburgh: Churchill Livingstone.

Rossor M.N. (1982). Dementia. *Lancet*; **ii:** 1200–4.

Rudge P. (1984). *Clinical Neuro-otology*. Edinburgh: Churchill Livingstone.

Silver J.R. (1983). Immediate Management of Spinal Injury. *British Journal of Hospital Medicine*; **29:** 412.

Stålberg E., Young R.R. (1981). *Clinical Neurophysiology*. Butterworths International Medical Reviews: Neurology I. London: Butterworths.

Swash M., Kennard C. (1984). *Scientific Basis of Clinical Neurology*. Edinburgh: Churchill Livingstone.

Thomas D.G.T., Graham D.I. (1980). *Brain Tumours: Scientific Basis, Clinical Investigation and Current Therapy*. London: Butterworths.

Twycross R.G., Lack S.A. (1983). *Symptom Control in Far-advanced Cancer: Pain Relief*. London: Pitman Books.

Tyrer J. (1980). *The Treatment of Epilepsy*. Lancaster: MTD Press.

Valentine A.R., Pullicino P., Bennan E. (1981). *A Practical Introduction to Cranial CT*. London: Heinemann.

Wall P.D., Melzack R. (1984). *Textbook of Pain*. London: Churchill Livingstone.

Walton J.N. (1982). *Disorders of Voluntary Muscle*, 4th Edn. Edinburgh: Churchill Livingstone.

Index

(*Abbreviations:* CSF cerebrospinal fluid; CT computerized tomography.)

283

central pontine myelinolysis 144, 213
cerebellar ataxia 135, 194–7
cerebellar degenerations 194–7
    carcinoma-induced 220
cerebellar syndrome 208, 213
cerebellum 19–20
    hypoplasia radiation-induced 175
    tumours 100–2
cerebral angiography 104
cerebral anomalies 181
cerebral atrophy 75, 213
cerebral blood supply 126–7, 128
cerebral cortex
    motor area 15, 17
    sensory area 25
    vestibular area 42
    visual area 30–2
cerebral embolism 130
    see also stroke
cerebral haemorrhage 130–3 *see also* stroke
cerebral hemisphere specialisation 31
cerebral infarction 130; *see also* stroke
cerebral oedema 130
cerebral palsy 184–5
cerebral thrombosis 129–30; *see also* stroke
cerebral veins 141–2
cerebrospinal fluid (CSF) 76–79
    in meningitis 225–6
cerebrovascular diseases 126–42
    clinical syndromes 133–42
    management 136–9
    pathogenesis 129–33
    pathophysiology 127–30
cervical plexus, malignant infiltration 243
cervical rib 243
cervical root irritation 124
cestodes (tapeworm) 237
Charcot–Marie–Tooth disease 144, 202–3
Charcot's joints 171
Cheyne–Stokes respiration 52–3
Chiari malformation 172, 180
    hydrocephalus due to 81, 180
    vertical nystagmus 44
chlormethiazole 116
chloramphenicol 227
cholinergic projections to cerebral cortex 189, 191
chorea 159–61, 216
choreoathetosis, congenital 184
choroid plexus 77, 80
chronic pain syndrome 268
Chvostek sign 216
ciliary arteritis 30
circle of Willis 69, 126
circulatory arrest, acute 209
cisternal puncture 72
clinical psychologist 276
clobazam 116

clonazepam 114, 116, 163
clonidine 123
Cloward's procedure 168
cluster headache (migrainous neuralgia) 122, 123
cobalamin (vitamin B$_{12}$) deficiency 208, 210, 211, 245
cochlea 44–5
Collier's sign 38
colour vision 31
    tests 33
coma 51–54
combined malformations 181
common peroneal nerve 21, 244
concussion 84–5
confused patient, examination 50–3
congenital ataxias 184
congenital choreoathetosis 184
congenital disease of central nervous system 175–86
congenital herpes simplex 186
congenital neurosyphilis 175, 185
congenital rubella 175, 185
congenital varicella 186
consciousness 51, *see also* coma
conus medullaris damage 56
convulsive syncope 108
coprolalia 162
cordotomy 271
corneal reflex 39
corpus callosum
    agenesis 175, 181
    glioma 98
    lesions 50
    tumours, dementia due to 192
cortical venous infarction 230
cortical venous thrombosis 230
corticobulbar tract 15
corticospinal tract 15
corticosteroid 91, 123, 216, 221, 249, 260–1, 271
counter-irritant cutaneous stimulation 269–70
cramp, occupational 161–2
cranial (temporal) arteritis 30, 142
cranial mononeuropathies 247–9
cranial nerves
    comatose patient 52
    nuclei 15, 34
    1st (olfactory) 26–7
    2nd (optic) 27–33
    3rd (oculomotor) 33, 35–7, 248
    4th (trochlear) 33, 35–7, 248
    5th (trigeminal) 38–40, 52, 123
        see also trigeminal neuralgia
    6th (abducens) 33, 35–7, 248
    7th (facial) 39–41, 52, 248
    8th (auditory) 42, 103, 106, 249
    9th (glossopharyngeal) 45–7, 249
    10th (vagus) 45–7, 249
    11th (accessory) 47
    12th (hypoglossal) 47–8, 249